Image-Guided Percutaneous Spine Biopsy

A. Orlando Ortiz

Image-Guided Percutaneous Spine Biopsy

Springer

A. Orlando Ortiz
Department of Radiology
Winthrop-University Hospital
Mineola
New York
USA

ISBN 978-3-319-43324-0 ISBN 978-3-319-43326-4 (eBook)
DOI 10.1007/978-3-319-43326-4

Library of Congress Control Number: 2017931601

Printed on acid-free paper

This Springer imprint is published by Springer Nature
The registered company is Springer International Publishing AG
The registered company address is: Gewerbestrasse 11, 6330 Cham, Switzerland

Contents

Contributors

Amit Aggarwal, MD Neuroradiology Fellowship, Mount Sinai Hospital, New York, NY, USA

Allan L. Brook, MD, FSIR Albert Einstein College of Medicine, Montefiore Medical Center, Bronx, NY, USA

Michael K. Brooks, MD Section of Musculoskeletal Radiology, Department of Radiology, Winthrop-University Hospital, Mineola, NY, USA

Amish H. Doshi, MD Division of Neuroradiology, Neuroradiology Fellowship, Mount Sinai Hospital, New York, NY, USA

Steven A. Drexler, MD Department of Pathology, Winthrop-University Hospital, Mineola, NY, USA

Man Hon, MD Department of Radiology, Winthrop-University Hospital, Mineola, NY, USA

Joel Marden, LRT-CT Department of Radiology, Winthrop-University Hospital, Mineola, NY, USA

Joseph P. Mazzie, DO Section of Musculoskeletal Radiology, Department of Radiology, Winthrop-University Hospital, Mineola, NY, USA

Todd Miller, MD Department of Radiology Quality/Safety Officer, Montefiore Medical Center, Bronx, NY, USA

A. Orlando Ortiz, MD, MBA, FACR Department of Radiology, Winthrop-University Hospital, Mineola, NY, USA

Yuri Peterkin, MD Department of Radiology, Winthrop-University Hospital, Mineola, NY, USA

Javin Schefflein, MD Department of Radiology, Mount Sinai Medical Center, New York, NY, USA

Richard Silbergleit, MD Oakland University William Beaumont School of Medicine, Royal Oak, Michigan, USA

1 Pre- and Periprocedural Planning and Patient Management for Spine or Rib Biopsies

Richard Silbergleit and A. Orlando Ortiz

Learning Objectives

1. To understand the critical role that proper patient preparation plays in image-guided percutaneous spine or rib biopsy
2. To optimize patient screening practices
3. To improve patient safety by the appropriate application of key patient safety initiatives such as "time-out," hand hygiene, and patient education

1.1 Introduction

Performing a biopsy or biopsies of a spinal, paraspinal, or rib lesion can be a complex procedure. What initially may seem like an innocuous spine or rib biopsy can, without appropriate preparation, quickly become a difficult, if not complicated, procedure. Proper strategic planning before, during, and after the procedure will increase patient safety, patient comfort, and patient satisfaction as well as increase the efficiency and efficacy of the biopsy process. This starts with a thorough review and discussion of the request for the biopsy and a review of the indications for the procedure. Communication between the operator performing the procedure and both the patient and the referring clinician is an important part of the process. The patient and/or the patient's representative should understand the reason for the procedure, the steps necessary for patient preparation, the potential risks of the procedure, and the expected post-procedure care and recovery process. The patient's medications may have to be adjusted or held. Patient-specific information may alter plans for patient positioning or sedation/analgesia. From the perspective of the patient, a spine or rib biopsy is an invasive procedure, and the operator is acting as their physician advocate when not just performing the procedure but also when considering the biopsy request, planning the biopsy procedure, recovering the patient and following up with the patient, and referring and consulting clinical services.

1.2 Before the Procedure

1.2.1 Prescreening and Scheduling

The request for a biopsy may come via the electronic medical record, a written prescription, or verbally either in person or by telephone. A verbal request must be confirmed with an electronic or written request. The request should identify the patient with at least two identifiers which usually include name and either date of birth or a unique medical record number. It is useful to have multiple ways to contact the patient when scheduling an outpatient. Requesting the patient's home, work,

The original version of this chapter was revised. An erratum to this chapter can be found at DOI 10.1007/978-3-319-43326-4_12

A.O. Ortiz, *Image-Guided Percutaneous Spine Biopsy*, DOI 10.1007/978-3-319-43326-4_1

and cell phone numbers improves the ability to contact the patient both before and after the procedure. All staff should be reminded that personal health information should not be left on an answering machine, voice mail, or other unsecured communication. Contacting inpatients is usually more easily accomplished although contact information may be needed for the patient's representative if the patient is not capable of providing the needed clinical information, understanding the procedure, or providing informed consent.

It is extremely useful to have contact information for the requesting physician if questions arise about the appropriateness of the procedure, safety of the procedure, the need to adjust medications, or to suggest another study or procedure if indicated. The request should include the clinical history (signs/symptoms/ICD 10 code) providing the medical indication for the biopsy as well as any other pertinent medical information. Information about the study that prompted the biopsy request including the dates of the prior study and the type of study such as a CT, MRI, ultrasound, radiograph, bone scan, or PET scan should be included. If the study was from outside of the medical practice requested to perform the biopsy, it should be made available for review. The level to be biopsied should be indicated although this may be adjusted after review of the history and imaging studies. Additional information such as if the referring physician thinks the patient will need general anesthesia for the procedure is also acquired.

The operator who is to perform the biopsy should review the study that prompted the request for the biopsy as well as all pertinent clinical information. A careful review of the patient's prior imaging studies is a key prerequisite in the biopsy planning process. It may be determined that the biopsy is not indicated or that there is a safer lesion to biopsy that the referring physician may not be aware of. If it is determined that the lesion should not be biopsied or that a different lesion should be biopsied, communication with the referring physician is essential. Once he/she decides to perform the biopsy, the operator should then determine whether it should be scheduled in CT, fluoroscopy, ultrasound, or MRI (CT and fluoroscopy are most often utilized).

A careful review of the patient's prior imaging studies is a key prerequisite in the biopsy planning process.

Having experienced personnel involved in scheduling, the procedure is useful after it has been determined that the biopsy is indicated. A brief history is obtained to determine if the patient has any medical conditions that may affect the ability to perform the biopsy. Conditions such as respiratory compromise, seizures, inability to stay in the preferred position, anxiety, or heightened sensitivity to pain may require special planning. The presence of an active infectious process may lead to delaying the procedure if the purpose of the biopsy is not to evaluate the infectious process. Information on allergies is collected and placed in the patient's medical record.

Biopsy procedures are often elective, but can also be urgently requested. In the case of the former, there is often sufficient time to acquire the appropriate imaging and clinical information to review as part of the biopsy planning process. Additionally, it can be very helpful, especially if the patient is available, to arrange for a preprocedure consultation with the patient. This is a good opportunity for the operator to review all of the pertinent medical and radiologic information, to examine the patient, to order any necessary laboratory tests, to perform medication reconciliation, and to advise on periprocedural medication adjustments as necessary. Allergies and adverse responses to specific medications should be documented. The latter not only includes oral anticoagulants and antiplatelet medications but also diabetic medications, specific vitamins, and herbal agents. At the time of consultation, the operator may be able to determine which positions the patient can tolerate. Based upon the complexity of the procedure, the patient's comorbidities, and the patient's preference, a determination can be made of the type of anesthesia to be used for the biopsy procedure. This is a tremendous opportunity for the patient and their family to develop a healthy relationship with their doctor and to ease fears or concerns regarding the biopsy procedure and the results. The operator can also provide an overview of what to expect just before, during, and after the biopsy procedure. A brief explanation of the procedure, in layman's terminology, can also help the patient and their family to better understand what will happen. The patient will want to know the risks and benefits of the intended biopsy procedure and will also want to know if there are any other diagnostic alternatives. This information is part of the informed consent process, and depending on the regional regulations, it may be possible to obtain the informed consent at the time of the consultation. This information can be expeditiously reviewed with the patient and their family at the time of the procedure. At the time of the consultation, a patient information guide, if available, can be given to the patient; many patients are often anxious and forget what they were told – these educational guides help to remind them and ease their anxiety levels (RadiologyInfo.org: Biopsies – Overview 2016). Printed patient instructions are also helpful for the very same reason (see sample instructions – *Spine Biopsy: Pre-Procedure Patient Instruction Sheet*).

In an urgent care setting, the patient may present directly for the biopsy procedure, as a direct outpatient referral or as an inpatient. A concise evaluation should be performed with respect to image review, medical evaluation, and acquisition of the pertinent laboratory parameters. As informed consent for the procedure will be required, this can be the operator's opportunity to explain the procedure and answer any questions. The medication history is reviewed with the patient. Anticoagulant and antiplatelet agents are the most common medications to affect scheduling of the procedure (refer to Chap. 2). If the biopsy is being performed for evaluation of a potential infectious process, the patient should preferably not be on antibiotics as these can potentially result in a false-negative or nondiagnostic biopsy result. The procedure is explained to the patient or the patient's representative in sufficient detail to ensure that the nature of the procedure is understood. This conversation is not meant to replace the informed consent that is obtained before the procedure by a member of the team who is credentialed to perform the biopsy. This consultation prevents patients from coming into the radiology department thinking that they are having a radiograph and allows for the patient to schedule time off from work for both the procedure and recovery and to have transportation arranged. Depending on the planned sedation, the patient will be instructed to be NPO for at least 4 h, and if general anesthesia or deep sedation is planned, the patient is NPO for at least 8 h unless there is a contraindication. This may require management of insulin therapy or oral diabetic medications in patients with diabetes. Patients with diabetes will also require glucose monitoring before and after the procedure. If a diabetic patient is using an insulin pump, then this device should be disconnected prior to the procedure. The insulin pump can be reconnected in the recovery area.

Most procedures are performed on an outpatient basis. Complex procedures may require a short stay admission and occasionally an inpatient admission, particularly on medically fragile or complex patients. The admitting service may be the performing operator, radiology if radiologists are privileged for admissions, the referring service, or a hospitalist service. If another service is admitting the patient, the individual who is to perform the procedure should be available for consultation.

1.2.2 Informed Consent

Informed consent should be obtained from the patient or the patient's representative before the procedure. This typically occurs on the day of the procedure for outpatients but may be obtained during a clinic visit before the day of the procedure. Inpatients are often consented the day before the procedure or the day of the procedure. The informed consent includes a discussion of the procedure, indication for the procedure, risks, potential complications, alternatives to the procedure, and expected benefits of the procedure (Table 1.1).

When contemplating an image-guided percutaneous spine or rib biopsy, the operator should be

Table 1.1 Benefits and risks of percutaneous image-guided spine or rib biopsy

Benefits	
Identify and characterize the abnormality that has been previously identified	
Assess for neoplasm	
Assess for infection	
Assess for inflammation	
Assist in pretreatment planning	
Avoid, as much as possible, the possibility of an open biopsy	
Risks	
Bleeding	Neural injury
Infection	Pneumothorax
Pain	Solid organ injury
Nondiagnostic biopsy	
Contrast agent reaction (when intravenous iodinated contrast agent is used)	
Anesthesia (respiratory compromise, cardiovascular collapse, death)	

clearly able to answer in the affirmative to the question: will the results of this procedure significantly impact on the clinical management of the patient? As shown in Table 1.1, this procedure should have a well-defined benefit. Image-guided percutaneous spine or rib biopsy is associated with a very low complication rate. The majority of these complications are related to injury caused by the needle device. Fortunately, with appropriate image guidance and with proper pre-procedure planning and patient selection, these complications can be kept to a minimum (Ortiz et al. 2010). The possibility of a nondiagnostic biopsy, albeit uncommon, should be discussed with the patient. This may necessitate a repeat percutaneous biopsy or an open biopsy by a surgeon. The patient should understand that there are alternatives, though to a certain extent less desirable, to performing image-guided percutaneous spine or rib biopsy. The competing alternative, open biopsy, is more invasive and more labor and equipment intensive and will carry a similar profile of complications with a somewhat higher complication rate and greater post-procedure morbidity and recovery time. Many of these patients are already being sent to you by spine or thoracic surgeons in order to have this procedure – so this portion of the conversation with the patient moves quickly. In terms of the other alternatives, many patients will want an answer to their medical condition and are therefore eager and willing to undergo the biopsy procedure as opposed to waiting months, or what they perceive is an eternity, for continued imaging surveillance and laboratory testing. Lastly, clinicians will be reluctant to subject their patients to empiric treatments, which also carry risks and complications, and will want a definitive diagnosis before commencing with a given treatment plan.

The biopsy alternatives that can be discussed with the patient include:

1. Percutaneous biopsy
2. Open biopsy
3. Continued imaging surveillance of the detected abnormality
4. Empiric therapy (e.g., broad-spectrum antibiotics for suspected infection)

If anesthesiology is providing sedation or anesthesia, a separate consent is obtained by the anesthesiologist. If the person performing the procedure is responsible for sedation, it is included with the procedure consent. The patient should be given an opportunity to have all questions answered. Many institutions have a recorded consent line that is made part of the permanent record if consent cannot be obtained from the patient's representative in person. Emergent procedures can be performed without consent if there is great risk to the patient and consent cannot be obtained. It is important to follow both hospital policies and local laws when making this determination. There should be documentation from both the physician performing the procedure and the physician caring for the patient that the procedure is emergent and that there is significant risk to delaying the procedure. This is a rare occurrence, and only a very small percentage of biopsies will fall into this category. The signed consent form should be witnessed at the time of the consent process, and this can be performed by another staff member.

1.3 At the Time of the Procedure

1.3.1 Patient Sedation

Sedation should be planned based upon the patient's medical condition and comorbidities and the complexity of the procedure (Mueller et al. 2000). Additionally, a patient's preference may factor into this decision. The Joint Commission and the American Society of Anesthesia (ASA) describe sedation as mild, moderate, deep, and general anesthesia (American Society of Anesthesiologists Task Force on Sedation and Analgesia by Non-Anesthesiologists 2002). The patient's cardiovascular function, airway, and ventilation are not impaired when administering minimal sedation. Moderate sedation is greater sedation than minimal, but the airway does not require protection. The patient may require greater verbal or tactile stimulation to respond to questions than with minimal sedation. Physicians must be credentialed by their institution in moderate sedation to administer this level without an anesthesiologist or nurse anesthetist present. A staff member other than the one performing the procedure should be responsible for monitoring the patient while under moderate sedation. The levels of sedation are a continuum, and the intended moderate sedation may unexpectedly become deep sedation. Staff should be trained and equipment available to handle the possibility of deeper sedation. Deep sedation and general anesthesia are best managed by an anesthesiologist because of the greater likelihood of need for airway protection and greater support of cardiovascular function. Moderate or greater sedation requires a patient evaluation that includes documentation of the ASA physical status:

I. Normal healthy patient
II. Mild systemic disease
III. Severe systemic disease
IV. Severe systemic disease that is a constant risk to life
V. Moribund patient
VI. Brain dead/organ donor

Moderate sedation without an anesthesiologist is best suited to patients in ASA class I and II. Consideration can be given to patients in class III and IV. The airway is assessed most commonly by the Mallampati classification which assesses the airway with the mouth open and protrusion of the tongue. Higher classifications correlate with the degree of difficulty in performing intubation.

Moderate sedation most commonly utilizes a combination of a benzodiazepine (sedative) and an opioid (analgesic) (Kohi et al. 2015). The combination allows the use of a lower dose of either drug when used alone. Benzodiazepines are useful in reducing anxiety, inducing a light sleep, and have amnestic properties. Opioids are potent pain relievers. The most frequently used benzodiazepine is midazolam (Versed) because of its short half-life and duration of action. The most frequently used opioid is fentanyl also due to its short half-life and duration of action. There are reversal drugs available for both classes that should be readily available. Naloxone is the reversal agent for opioids, and flumazenil is the reversal agent for benzodiazepines (Martin and Lennox 2003).

By far the most underappreciated, yet critical, step in the patient preparation process is intravenous access. The antecubital fossa should be avoided. The reason for this is that, frequently, the elbows are bent during the procedure. This either impairs intravenous access or compromises intravenous access. We have often seen a frustrated operator and anesthesiologist perplexed by the relative lack of sedation during a procedure in which the intravenous catheter has been dislodged or obstructed by a bent elbow; in the latter scenario, the patient immediately falls asleep once the arm is straightened. It is highly recommended to use either the forearm or hand for efficient intravenous access. Intravenous access should be maintained until the patient fully recovers from the procedure as additional pain medication can be efficiently administered after the procedure.

Try to avoid the antecubital fossa as a site for intravenous access.

The patient should be monitored during the procedure including pulse oximeter, electrocardiogram, blood pressure, and respiratory rate. These devices should be placed in areas that are removed from the intended biopsy site; keep in mind that cables should be removed from the side of the patient at the biopsy level as these may obscure the biopsy site during lateral fluoroscopy. Monitoring is continued after the procedure until the patient returns to their baseline level of consciousness. It is important to realize that sedation may deepen after the procedure if reversal agents are given because they may have a shorter duration of action than the sedation agents.

A "time-out" protocol is required before an invasive procedure such as a spine or rib biopsy (The Joint Commission 2016). This should be a focused process involving everyone participating in the procedure with patient involvement when possible. Involving the patient in the time-out reduces medical error, increases patient confidence in the professionalism of their healthcare team, and reduces patient anxiety. All other activities should temporarily cease during the time-out. The patient is identified with two identifiers. Valid medical identifiers usually include the patient's name and another identifier such as medical record number or date of birth. The procedure is confirmed with a source document, either a paper request or a request in the electronic medical record. The name and other identifiers on the specimen containers are compared to the patient's wristband. Anatomic counting and marking is performed and confirmed to avoid wrong side or wrong level procedures. Available imaging is reviewed prior to the procedure and displayed on a monitor in the procedure suite if possible. Correct patient positioning and the availability of all needed equipment is confirmed.

1.3.2 Imaging Guidance and Contrast Agents

Most spine biopsies are performed with fluoroscopy or CT guidance without intravenous iodinated contrast agent injection. Most percutaneous rib biopsies are performed with un-enhanced CT guidance. Occasionally, intravenous iodinated contrast agent injection is useful for identification of a paraspinal soft tissue mass or to define a critical vascular structure that should be avoided. If there is a history of or a suspicion of renal impairment, renal function studies should be obtained prior to injecting intravascular iodinated contrast material. Diabetic patients taking metformin (Glucophage) should stop taking the drug at the time of the procedure and wait 48 h prior to resuming this medication (Beckett et al. 2015). In some cases, depending on the patient's clinical condition, metformin may be held until renal function is confirmed to be normal. This protocol is necessary in order to avoid the potential for lactic acidosis.

1.3.3 The Biopsy Procedure

The patient is positioned on the table, placed on the appropriate monitoring devices, shaved with clippers (when necessary), prepped, and draped in sterile fashion (Kohi et al. 2015). Strict adherence to aseptic technique by all members of the biopsy team is a prerequisite to a safer procedure (The Joint Commission 2013) (Table 1.2).

The application of local anesthetic (such as 1% or 2% lidocaine) at the skin puncture site and along the intended biopsy tract up to the periosteum of the vertebral or rib cortex can reduce patient discomfort, thereby reducing patient motion as well as potentially reducing the required dose of intravenous sedative and/or pain

Table 1.2 Infection prevention

Pre-procedure aspects
Remove hair with clippers (avoid shaving with razor)
Pre-procedure antibiotic prophylaxis – not required unless patient is immune compromised and biopsy is being performed to assess for neoplastic process; antibiotics for biopsies intended to assess for infection are discouraged
Intra-procedure care
Aseptic technique is paramount
Strict hand hygiene
Post-biopsy care
Wound care (educate patient and family)

medication. As a result of being properly prepared, the operator will have the appropriate instrumentation to perform the biopsy procedure. The operator will utilize the advantages of imaging guidance in order to safely and efficiently place the biopsy devices. Coaxial technique can be helpful as it provides a onetime access to the margin of the lesion and allows for multiple passes with biopsy instruments. Imaging guidance should be utilized to monitor all needle insertions and advancements and to monitor the position of the biopsy needle tip relative to the lesion and critical structures.

Once the biopsy procedure is initiated and performed, all of the specimens are placed within the appropriate containers as they are obtained. If pathology support is available and fine needle aspirations are being performed, these specimens can be assessed for adequacy at the time of the biopsy. All specimen containers should be properly labeled, with at least two patient identifiers, and immediately transported to their appropriate destinations by trained personnel (Kohi et al. 2015). Unfortunately, biopsy specimens are at risk for getting lost – yes, this can happen, has happened, and will happen again unless skilled personnel, great care, and accurate processes are in place for specimen transport and tracking. Therefore, post-procedure completion should be emphasized as much as the biopsy procedure itself (Siewert and Hochman 2015)!

Once the operator is satisfied that sufficient specimens have been obtained and removes the biopsy needle system, hemostasis is obtained by hand compression at the biopsy site. The operator should hold moderate pressure at the biopsy site for 3–5 min. A sterile dressing, such as a Steri-Strip or bandage, can be placed at the puncture site. The operator and/or a designee should monitor the biopsy site for at least 5 more minutes to assess for bleeding or swelling at the biopsy site. In specific situations, such as when performing a biopsy on a suspected vascular lesion, or in patients who have been receiving antiplatelet agents or anticoagulants, or when the operator has encountered bleeding via the biopsy tract, it may be necessary to seal the biopsy tract with a small volume of Surgifoam (refer to Chap. 2). This can be injected directly through the guiding cannula of a coaxial system or using a 20 gauge spinal needle through the area of the biopsy tract. Surgifoam powder is mixed with 8 mL of normal sterile saline just prior to use – this should form the consistency of mashed potatoes and can be back loaded into a 10 mL syringe prior to injection.

1.4 After the Procedure

1.4.1 Patient Recovery

Following a biopsy procedure, the patient is transferred to a recovery area. Patients are usually observed and monitored for at least 2 h after their procedure. The biopsy site is monitored for signs of active bleeding or increasing swelling. The patient may be given additional pain medication. Patients are allowed to drink and eat after they are recovered from their anesthesia and have returned to their baseline mental status. Intravenous access may be discontinued when the patient is fully recovered, demonstrating satisfactory oral intake, and is no longer in need of intravenous medication. Post-procedure care instructions are given to, and reviewed with the patient and/or family member, just prior to discharge. If the biopsy specimens include osseous material, then the patient is reminded that it will take 2 days to process (decalcify) the specimen prior to analyzing it in the pathology department. The patient is instructed to follow up with the referring physician in order to review the biopsy results. It is often helpful to communicate with the referring physician in order to let them know that the biopsy was performed and that the patient is doing well and to expect the biopsy results.

If a biopsy complication occurs, then it is imperative that the operator immediately evaluates the patient. The complication, whether local or systemic, must be promptly addressed by the operator, and the patient should be stabilized. A complication should be documented in a factual manner within the medical record. Most complications are related to hemorrhage, and the management of these types of complications is discussed in the *chapter dealing with anticoagulation management*. Vascular injury may require an endovascular procedure or an open vascular procedure by a vascular surgeon. Neural injury may require supportive care, steroids, or, rarely, an attempt at surgical decompression. If infection occurs, then an imaging study, such as a contrast enhanced MRI or a nuclear medicine study such as a gallium scan, can be performed to confirm the diagnosis and to assess for the presence of abscess formation which may require drainage depending on its size and location. The likely organism is usually *Staphylococcus*, and appropriate antibiotic therapy can be promptly initiated. Once it is established that a biopsy-related complication has occurred, then the operator should discuss and document the clinical situation and its management with the patient and their family. The operator should follow up with the patient on a regular basis, even when other consultants are directly caring for the patient.

When a spine or rib biopsy complication occurs:

1. Promptly evaluate and assist the patient.
2. Obtain the appropriate studies and consultations.
3. Discuss the situation with the patient and their family.
4. Treat the patient.
5. Follow up with the patient.
6. Remain available to the patient and their family.

1.4.2 Patient Follow-Up

While the patient discharge instructions include specific detailed instructions about the type of procedure that was performed, signs and symptoms to watch out for in terms of delayed complications (bleeding, swelling, increasing pain, fever), and a phone number with whom to contact if there are any questions or problems, a follow-up telephone call to the patient on the day after the procedure can be performed in order to ascertain the patient's condition and to address any of the patient's concerns. The operator should have a process in place for obtaining the biopsy results, documenting this, and making sure that the referring physician has also received a copy of the test results. With respect to microbiology results, the operator may have to check results for several weeks; for example, *Mycobacteria* requires 4–6 weeks of follow-up. Patient and biopsy result follow-up close the loop on the spine or rib biopsy procedure.

The operator should have a process in place for obtaining the biopsy results, documenting the results, and making sure that the referring physician has also received a copy of the test results.

Key Review Points

1. Communication between the patient, the referring physician, and the operator improves quality of care and patient satisfaction.
2. The request for the biopsy should include patient identification, patient contact information, and clinical history providing the medical necessity information for the procedure.
3. Review of the imaging study or studies that prompted the request for the biopsy should occur before scheduling the patient for the procedure.

4. The choice of the imaging modality for performing the biopsy should be based on the particular anatomic characteristics of the lesion and operator preference.
5. Biopsies for infectious processes have a higher diagnostic yield if the patient is not taking antibiotics at the time of the procedure.
6. The informed consent discussion should include the possibility of a "nondiagnostic biopsy" as an outcome of the procedure.
7. The "time-out" procedure enhances patient safety and contributes to better patient care.
8. Follow-up is important with respect to patient, referring physician, and biopsy results.

Spine or Rib Biopsy: Pre-procedure Patient Instruction Sheet

Patient Name: __________________

Date of Birth:________________

1. You are scheduled for a spine biopsy procedure on: (date and time)

   At: location (specific address as to where the patient should first arrive)

2. Please do not eat or drink anything

   __After the midnight before your procedure

   __After ___:___(time) on the day of your procedure
3. *On the day of your procedure please bring with you:

   ___Your prescription for the procedure

   ___Your radiology studies (CDs or Films)

   **FAILURE TO FOLLOW THIS IMPORTANT STEP COULD POSTPONE YOUR PROCEDURE*
4. If you are a diabetic patient, please check your morning blood sugar and notify the nursing staff of the result when you arrive in our department. If your blood sugar is not within the normal range, then we will treat you appropriately. We recommend that you do not take your diabetes medication in the morning of your procedure, but please consult with your physician prior to changing any medicine. Please alert us if you are using an insulin pump.
5. We recommend that you STOP only your blood thinner and any medicines or supplements that may interfere with the clotting of your blood _____ days before your procedure, unless otherwise instructed by your physician(s):

   __Aspirin, Ecotrin __Plavix (clopidogrel) __Persantine (dipyridamole)

   __Pletal (cilostazol) __Coumadin (warfarin) __Other (Pradaxa, Eliquis)

   __Ibuprofen (Advil, Motrin) __Naproxen (Aleve) __Vitamin E, fish oil

6. Please take your other usual medications in the morning of your procedure as you normally would with small sips of water.
7. If you have been given a prescription for specific blood work:

   Please have it drawn at: (location and phone number)

   Please have it drawn _______day(s) before your procedure

   If this is an independent laboratory, then please have results immediately sent to our facility: (address and facsimile telephone number)
8. Please call us at (telephone number), if there is a significant change in your physical health prior to your procedure or if you have any additional questions or concerns.
9. Please leave your jewelry at home and wear loose, comfortable clothing.

Patient Information Guide: Spine Biopsy

What is a spine biopsy?

A spine biopsy is the removal of a small sample of tissue from the spinal column or adjacent structures in order to examine it for possible disease (cancer, infection, inflammation).

How is a spine biopsy performed?

A spine biopsy is performed using special needles that can acquire small samples of tissue. A needle is placed through the skin, near the area to be sampled, under imaging guidance such as x-ray (fluoroscopy) or computed tomography (CT). The procedure is performed by a qualified operator as part of a team that will help to monitor you and keep you safe and comfortable before, during, and after the procedure.

Is the spine biopsy procedure safe?

Image-guided percutaneous spine biopsy has been shown to be a safe and effective procedure. The benefit of the procedure is to obtain sufficient tissue from a specific area of the spine and analyze this tissue in order to establish a diagnosis. This diagnosis will help to determine your treatment plan. The risks of the procedure are uncommon (well under 1%) and include bleeding, infection, and injury to small nerves, blood vessels, or other structures near or in the path of the biopsy needle. Alternatives to percutaneous spine biopsy include continued observation and monitoring of your condition or open surgical spine biopsy in an operating room performed by a spine surgeon. Your doctor will discuss these benefits, risks, and alternative treatments when obtaining your informed consent for the procedure.

Will it hurt?

Most patients receive intravenous medications to help them remain relaxed, comfortable, and hold still during the procedure. Spine biopsy can be performed using different types of anesthesia. First, local anesthetic such as lidocaine will be applied at and beneath the skin at the biopsy site in order to minimize any pain. For additional anesthesia, an intravenous (IV) line will be inserted into your arm or hand so that medication can be given to relax you (sedation) and to provide pain relief (analgesia) during the procedure. Alternatively, an anesthesiologist may assist in your care and administer a medication (such as propofol) in order to have you more deeply sedated during the procedure.

What will I experience during the procedure?

Before your procedure is started, you will be asked your name, date of birth, and what type of procedure you are having. Your healthcare team members will introduce themselves and let you know why they are in the room with you. Nurses, technologists, and other staff will help position you safely and comfortably on the procedure table. The procedure is performed using sterile technique, so everyone within the procedure suite will be wearing surgical caps and masks.

Depending upon what type of spine biopsy procedure you are having, you will be placed on your stomach or on your back or on your side. Once you are positioned properly, you will need to remain still throughout the procedure. You may have the area of the biopsy shaved by one of the staff members. The spine level of your biopsy will be marked once you are properly and comfortably positioned. Monitoring equipment will be used during your procedure so you will have a pulse oximeter placed on one of your fingers, electrocardiogram leads placed on your skin, a blood pressure cuff placed around your arm, and possibly a nasal cannula placed under your nose. You will hear the beeping sounds of these devices and feel the pressure of the blood pressure cuff on your arm from time to time. Your skin will be cleansed with sterilizing solutions, this may feel cold, and the biopsy area will be covered with sterile sheets. The intravenous medication that is initially administered may cause some temporary irritation or burning at the time it is first given. You will feel a pinch and then pressure or temporary discomfort at the site where the local anesthetic (numbing medicine) is applied.

What will I experience after the procedure?

You may feel sore at the biopsy site for a day or so. You can apply a cold compress to the biopsy site as well as take your usual pain medication. Keep the biopsy area dry with the bandage on for 24 h after the procedure. After this time you may bathe and the bandage can be removed. Please refer to your discharge instructions for any care instructions that are specific to your procedure and for a telephone contact number to call if you have any urgent concerns or questions after your procedure.

When will I get my biopsy results?

Please follow up with your referring doctor in order to obtain the biopsy results. This may take several days as spine biopsy specimens often have to be processed prior to being analyzed. The biopsy specimens may be studied by a pathologist and/or a microbiologist, depending on the reason for your procedure – they will send the result to your doctor.

Please be aware that sometimes, despite obtaining the appropriate amount of tissue samples, the diagnosis may still not be made and you may require additional evaluation, including another biopsy.

What should I do before the procedure?

1. Arrange for transportation to your home after the procedure as you are advised not to drive.
2. The night before your spine biopsy procedure, do not have anything to eat or drink after midnight. If you take daily medications, take them with a small sip of water.
3. Shower or bathe before you come to the hospital and wear loose, comfortable clothing.
4. Please leave your jewelry at home.
5. Bring your spine x-rays and other imaging studies including CTs and MRIs and your prescription for the procedure with you to your appointment.
6. Notify the doctor who is performing your procedure if you have been taking medications, such as blood thinners, that affect your blood's ability to clot.
7. Tell your doctor if you are allergic to any medications.
8. If you are a diabetic, you should discuss this ahead of time with the doctor and follow the specific instructions that are unique to your care.
9. Plan to invest about 4 or more hours of your time in the medical center that is performing your procedure.

Safe Biopsy Checklist

Before starting the procedure

Patient verification (double identifier)
Correct patient, correct procedure, correct level, and correct side.
Verify the correct patient information on the sample tubes and containers.
Are the prior imaging studies available and have they been reviewed?
Review all pertinent laboratory tests (coagulation profile, renal profile, infection/inflammation panel, pregnancy test result (in all females with reproductive capacity)).
Does pathology department need to be contacted?
Are there any special transport media?
Does a pathologist need to be available at the time of the procedure?
Review any anticipated critical events.
Confirm any patient allergies and type of reaction.
Confirm NPO status.
Confirm airway status and aspiration risk.
Is there a risk of significant blood loss?
Is the lesion being sampled suspected to be hypervascular?
Has the patient been recently receiving anticoagulant or antiplatelet therapy?
Check that patient monitoring equipment is operational.
Confirm that radiology equipment is functional and that dose reduction protocols are in effect.
Have procedure table prepared using sterile technique and cover table with a sterile drape.

Before prepping the patient

All staff must introduce themselves to the patient (staff member name and role in procedure).
Optimize patient position.
Remove hair at biopsy site with clippers.
Check that intravenous access is functional.
Place monitoring devices away from area of interest.
Perform the "time-out" with all of the staff present in the procedure suite.
Use imaging guidance in order to mark the level and side of interest on the skin surface.
Verify the correct patient information on the imaging modality monitor screen.
All staff must utilize appropriate hand hygiene protocol.

During the procedure

All staff in room must adhere to strict aseptic technique.
Expose the covered procedure table.
Prep the skin with appropriate antiseptic and cleansing agents.
Drape the patient.
Assure that patient is adequately sedated.
Use appropriate amount of local anesthetic agent for subcutaneous and periosteal application.
Make small crosshair incision on skin surface and monitor not only for bleeding but for ability to obtain hemostasis by hand compression.
Use coaxial techniques whenever possible.
Monitor placement, advancement, and location of instruments and needle tips with imaging guidance.
Place all specimens in their properly labeled containers.
After removing all instruments, obtain hemostasis by hand compression for 3–5 min.
Monitor skin surface and biopsy site for signs of active bleeding or swelling for at least 5 min after hand compression.
Apply sterile dressing to biopsy site.

After the procedure

Nurse or assistant confirms specimen labeling and use of appropriate containers and transport media.
Carefully move the semi-sedated patient onto a recovery stretcher.
Continue to actively monitor patient and vital signs.
Monitor for signs of bleeding or swelling at biopsy site.
Any concerns for patient recovery or management are discussed by the team.
Recovery periods vary, but consider recovering patient for at least 2 h.
A paper or electronic requisition is completed and matched with the labeled specimens.
The correctly labeled specimen container(s) are transported by accountable and responsible personnel to the appropriate laboratories.

References

American Society of Anesthesiologists Task Force on Sedation and Analgesia by Non-Anesthesiologists. Practice guidelines for sedation and analgesia by non-anesthesiologists. Anesthesiology. 2002;96:1004–17.

Beckett KR, Moriarity AK, Langer JM. Safe use of contrast media: what the radiologist needs to know. RadioGraphics. 2015;35:1738–50.

Kohi MP, Fidelman N, Behr S, Taylor AG, Kolli K, Conrad M, Hwang G, Weinstein S. Periprocedural patient care. Radiographics. 2015;35:1766–78.

Martin ML, Lennox PH. Sedation and analgesia in the interventional radiology department. J Vasc Interv Radiol. 2003;14:1119–28.

Mueller PR, Biswal S, Halpern EF, Kaufman JA, Lee MJ. Interventional radiologic procedures: patient anxiety, perception of pain, understanding of procedure, and satisfaction with medication – a prospective study. Radiology. 2000;215:684–8.

Ortiz AO, Zoarski GH, Brook AL. Image-guided percutaneous spine biopsy. In: Mathis JM, Golovac S, editors. Image-guided spine interventions. New York: Springer; 2010. p. 75–106.

RadiologyInfo.org. For patients. Biopsies- overview. Accessed 16 Sep 2016. http://www.radiologyinfo.org.

Siewert B, Hochman MG. Improving safety through human factors engineering. RadioGraphics. 2015; 35:1694–705.

The Joint Commission. The Joint Commission's implementation guide for NPSG.07.05.01 on surgical site infections: The SSI change project. 2013.

Universal protocol for preventing wrong site, wrong procedure, wrong person surgery. The Joint Commission Web site. Accessed 16 Sep 2016. http://www.jointcommission.org/PatientSafety/UniversalProtocol/2016.

2 Anticoagulation Management

Man Hon, Richard Silbergleit,
and A. Orlando Ortiz

Learning Objectives

1. To learn how to evaluate and manage patients on anticoagulant and/or antiplatelet therapy prior to performing a spine or rib biopsy
2. To review and update our understanding of current anticoagulant and antiplatelet medications
3. To learn how to promptly address bleeding complications when they occur during or after a spine or rib biopsy

2.1 Introduction

A significant percentage of the general population is affected by medical conditions such as stroke or venothromboembolic disease or prior medical interventions such as cardiac stent placement. Another group of patients has risk factors, such as atrial fibrillation, that may predispose these patients to these medical conditions. Patients with preexisting neoplastic conditions may have hypercoagulable states that require anticoagulation therapy. Therefore, it is no surprise that many patients that are referred for a spine or rib biopsy are on antiplatelet or anticoagulant medications. Additionally, they may also be taking other medications, vitamins, or herbal supplements that alter their coagulation status. Since image-guided percutaneous spine or rib biopsy requires the use of needles and devices that may range in size from 25 gauge up to 8 gauge diameter, bleeding and hematoma formation are possible local complications that can be caused by the percutaneous insertion of these devices. When considering and planning an image-guided percutaneous biopsy procedure, it is important to not only to identify which medications that a patient is using but to determine if they have any anticoagulant properties and, if so, to decide on how to manage the administration of these latter types of medications. Managing the hemostasis risk in these patients is becoming increasingly complicated as more patients are receiving these medications and new agents are continuously being introduced into clinical practice.

The first challenge with respect to anticoagulant or antiplatelet agent management is that guidelines for holding medications vary widely and are dependent on the perceived risk of the procedure. Procedures are usually categorized as low risk, moderate (intermediate) risk, and high (significant) risk for a bleeding complication (Kohi et al. 2015). The second challenge is that different authors and professional medical societies categorize some of these procedures differently. The recommendations on holding anticoagulants and antiplatelet medications differ for the various risk categories. The third challenge is that these guidelines do not include image-guided percutaneous spine or rib biopsies in their listed procedures. Procedures that can result in intraspinal hemorrhage are considered

A.O. Ortiz, *Image-Guided Percutaneous Spine Biopsy*, DOI 10.1007/978-3-319-43326-4_2

by some experts to be high risk (Baron et al. 2013). The Society of Interventional Radiology (SIR) 2012 Consensus Guidelines for Periprocedural Management of Coagulation Status and Hemostasis Risk in Percutaneous Image-guided Interventions does not list spine biopsy but lists spine procedures including vertebroplasty and kyphoplasty as having moderate risk of bleeding (Patel et al. 2013). The American Society of Regional Anesthesia and Pain Medicine (ASRA) Guidelines on Interventional Spine and Pain Procedures in Patients on Antiplatelet and Anticoagulation Medications also does not include spine biopsies but lists vertebral augmentation (vertebroplasty and kyphoplasty) as high-risk procedures (Narouze et al. 2015). Lastly, the grades of bleeding severity are not specified or standardized across the specialties that perform image-guided percutaneous spine interventions (Baron et al. 2013).

In the setting of guidelines that are helpful but different and in risk stratification categories that are also helpful but different, what is the best way to approach the patient who is on anticoagulant and/or antiplatelet therapy and requires a spine or rib biopsy? Vertebroplasty and kyphoplasty might be considered reasonable surrogates for spine biopsy much of the time because the instruments used are similar and occasionally identical. Large needles ranging from 13 to 8 gauge in diameter are typically used for vertebral augmentation and many bone biopsies. But there is a difference between the two procedures. Vertebral augmentation procedures usually involve a single transpedicular pass and entry, either through one or both pedicles, and entail injection of acrylic bone cement within the vertebral body. Spine biopsies may entail multiple passes, with multiple tracts and entry sites, with variable access routes in addition to the transpedicular approach, with different targets in addition to the vertebral body (such as the intervertebral disk or the paraspinal soft tissues), and with no material being deposited within the biopsy site. The use of large needles in a deep location, with a variable number of passes and needle tracts, next to vital structures such as the spinal canal where bleeding cannot be easily controlled by manual compression suggests categorization as a high-risk procedure. Nevertheless, extensive experience with biopsy procedures has led many to suggest that they are of moderate risk. In practice, each biopsy is different. A biopsy of a lytic lesion in a lumbar spinous process that is not deep and that can be sampled with a smaller needle may be considered a low-risk procedure. The biopsy of suspected vascular lesion such as a metastasis from renal cell carcinoma in the cervical or upper thoracic spine would likely be considered a high-risk procedure. Image-guided percutaneous spine biopsy is a closed procedure, and since potentially uncontrollable hemorrhage can develop around and inside the spinal axis, with catastrophic consequences if not addressed emergently, it is recommended that all operators be aware of this risk and manage each case wisely: careful pre-procedure patient management, familiarity with anticoagulant and antiplatelet medications and supplements, active communication with the referring clinician and patient, and consistent post-procedure patient care (Layton et al. 2006).

Image-guided percutaneous spine biopsy is a closed procedure, and since potentially uncontrollable hemorrhage can develop around and inside the spinal axis, with catastrophic consequences if not addressed emergently, it is recommended that all operators be aware of this risk and manage each case wisely: careful pre-procedure patient management, familiarity with anticoagulant and antiplatelet medications and supplements, active communication with the referring clinician and patient, and consistent post-procedure patient care.

2.2 How to Prevent a Bleeding Complication

The best way to avoid a bleeding complication during an image-guided percutaneous spine or rib biopsy procedure is to prevent it (Hunt 2014). It is extremely important for the operator to meet the patient, review the patient's medical history, and examine the patient. This will provide information as to the necessity for the anticoagulation and/or antiplatelet regimen. The patient may inform the operator that they have withheld these types of medications in the past for other invasive procedures. The patient can also inform the operator as to the clinician who placed them on the specific anticoagulant or antiplatelet agent. This will enable the operator to quickly contact this clinician and develop the biopsy treatment plan. Documentation of the anticoagulant/antiplatelet agent management strategy is advised. The two risks that are being balanced during this communication are the risk of procedure-related hemorrhage versus the risk of a thromboembolic event. The operator or an assistant should ask the patient if they experience easy bruising (you should also examine the arms and legs) and if they have had any bleeding problems with any other types of medical or dental procedures. Not only should the operator inquire about anticoagulant or antiplatelet medications but also about vitamins (vitamin E), fish oils, and other herbal compounds (garlic, *Ginkgo biloba*, ginseng, danshen, dong quai) that may affect the blood's normal ability to form clots. At the time of the patient's clinical evaluation, the operator can determine the type of anesthesia that may be required for the procedure. Preventing unnecessary patient movement and maximizing patient comfort during the procedure increase the likelihood of a safer procedure. Hence, the importance of identifying an uncooperative patient cannot be emphasized enough. Reviewing the prior imaging studies helps in identifying vascular structures that should be avoided and in determining optimal biopsy trajectories.

The operator should conduct a thorough investigation of the patient's medication, vitamin, and herbal supplement use; this information should be documented in the patient's medical record.

The operator should obtain baseline hematologic studies. This includes a coagulation profile: hematocrit and hemoglobin, platelets, prothrombin time (PT), partial thromboplastin time (PTT), and international normalized ratio (INR). A renal profile should also be obtained as many of dosing and holding recommendations for the newer anticoagulants are based on renal function: BUN, creatinine, and glomerular filtration rate. These baseline values are a useful reference in case the patient experiences a hemorrhagic event, and the new serum hematologic profile can be compared to the original values.

It is important for the operator to know the most commonly used anticoagulant and antiplatelet medications and to be aware of the newly introduced agents. Similarly, the operator should be up to date with the guidelines for the use of these agents – not only do the medications change, but the guidelines can be revised. The operator should be familiar with the use and application of bridging strategies (Tables 2.1 and 2.2). If there is any uncertainty as to whether or not an anticoagulant and/or antiplatelet agent can be held prior to arranging a biopsy procedure, then the operator should wait until the pertinent clinical issues are discussed and a biopsy management strategy is agreed to by the operator, the referring clinician, and the patient.

Table 2.1 Example of a bridging strategy using intravenous heparin

Patient admitted into hospital	
Patient's usual anticoagulant medication	Stopped
Intravenous heparin therapy	Started immediately
Intravenous heparin therapy	Temporarily held ~4 h prior to procedure
Procedure performed	Hemostasis at puncture site confirmed
	Biopsy site monitored (at least 2 h)
Intravenous heparin therapy	Resumed ~4 h after the procedure
Patient's usual anticoagulation medication	Started
Intravenous heparin therapy	Stopped
Patient discharged from hospital	

Table 2.2 Example of a bridging strategy using Lovenox

Subcutaneous therapeutic dose of Lovenox	Started
Patient's usual anticoagulation medication	Stopped
Perform procedure just prior to the next scheduled Lovenox dose	Hold
Lovenox can be resumed as early as 4 h after procedure or can wait until next scheduled administration (12 or 24 h depending on dosing schedule)	Resume
Resume patient's usual anticoagulation	Resume
Warfarin – resume usual evening dose on same day as procedure	
New anticoagulant: can start dosing after 4 h and STOP Lovenox based on effective onset of new anticoagulant (refer to Table 2.4)	

If there is any uncertainty as to whether or not an anticoagulant and/or antiplatelet agent can be held prior to arranging a biopsy procedure, then the operator should wait until the pertinent clinical issues are discussed and a biopsy management strategy is agreed to by the operator, the referring clinician, and the patient.

In the next sections, suggestions on holding medications are made based on times necessary to reverse enough of the antiplatelet or anticoagulant effect to decrease the risk of procedurally induced bleeding to a level similar to a patient who is not on these medications. It must be recognized that this is often a challenging clinical situation for both the clinician and the patient. Patients are usually placed on these agents for a medically indicated reason. Minimizing the risk of a biopsy-related hemorrhage by holding antithrombotic medications may result in a variety of complications such as stroke, myocardial infarction, deep venous thrombosis, or pulmonary embolism. The decision to hold these medications should be made in conjunction with the service that prescribed the antithrombotic to determine if holding the medication is feasible. A spectrum of decisions may be made such as that the biopsy cannot be safely performed, the biopsy can be performed but with less than the typically recommended holding time for that agent, the biopsy can be performed after holding the specific anticoagulant or antiplatelet agent for a standard period of time, or that bridging therapy, to minimize the amount of time off antithrombotic medication, is indicated in order to perform the biopsy (Tables 2.1 and 2.2). Bridging anticoagulation therapy is used to reduce the risk of thromboembolism in patients at high risk for recurrent thromboembolic events when their anticoagulation therapy is suspended (Baron et al. 2013).

Bridging therapy may be required in patients on anticoagulation with the following conditions (Baron et al. 2013):

Mechanical heart valve	Mitral valve replacement, two or more mechanical valves, aortic valve replacement of the non-bileaflet type or with other risk factors
Atrial fibrillation	With prior stroke or embolic event, cardiac thrombus, or CHADS score of 4 or more (1 point for congestive heart failure, hypertension, diabetes mellitus, and age 75 or older; 2 points for prior stroke or transient ischemic attack)
Venous thromboembolism	Within prior 3 months; severe thrombophilia (protein C or S or antithrombin deficiency; antiphospholipid syndrome; homozygous for factor V Leiden or mutation in prothrombin gene G20210A or compound heterozygous mutation of these two genes)

2.3 Antiplatelet Agents

2.3.1 Aspirin (Acetylsalicylic Acid, ASA)

Aspirin has a potent effect on platelet function that is irreversible. Its major action is through the acetylation of serine which inhibits platelet cyclooxygenase enzyme 1 (COX-1). Humans replace approximately 10% of their platelets each day. After 5 days, most patients will have 50% of their platelets functioning. Platelet transfusion can be used to restore clotting function more rapidly when necessary. There is no universally accepted test to evaluate aspirin's effect on hemostasis. Many patients take aspirin for primary prophylaxis without a history of a cardiovascular event such as stroke or myocardial infarct. Aspirin is frequently held in these patients. When a patient with known cardiovascular disease or an implanted intravascular device is taking aspirin, this is considered secondary prophylaxis (Diener et al. 1996). Holding aspirin in a patient on secondary prophylaxis requires a careful balance of the risks of a hemorrhagic complication from the procedure with the risks of a thrombotic event related to the underlying cardiovascular condition. The latter situation is particularly concerning in patients who have undergone recent intravascular stent placement. For example, patients with coronary artery stents are usually placed on dual antiplatelet therapy for 1 year. If an elective procedure that is associated with a high risk of bleeding is being considered, then it should be delayed for at least 6 weeks in patients receiving bare metal stents or for 6 months in patients with drug-eluting coronary stents (Jneid et al. 2012). Obviously, a patient who is being considered for a biopsy will likely not be able to wait 6 months for an elective, but necessary, biopsy. Therefore, consultation with the service that prescribed the aspirin to determine the relative risks is important. It is important to realize that numerous prescription and over-the-counter medications include aspirin.

Recommendations on holding aspirin vary widely, from not holding aspirin for spine procedures to suspending aspirin use for at least 7 days (Layton et al. 2006; Baron et al. 2013). The SIR guidelines recommend not holding aspirin for low and moderate risk procedures but holding it for 5 days for procedures with a significant bleeding risk (Patel et al. 2012). ASRA guidelines recommend holding aspirin for high-risk procedures and some intermediate risk procedures, but this should be tailored to both the patient and the type of procedure (Narouze et al. 2015). The recommended holding period is 4 days when the risk is lower and 6 days when the risk is higher. Many of the guidelines do not include a recommendation for the amount of time to wait before restarting antithrombotics. ASRA recommends waiting 24 h before restarting aspirin. As can be seen by these recommendations, there is not one specific approach to this situation, but based upon our experience, we tend to hold aspirin for 5 days before performing an image-guided percutaneous spine biopsy and resume this medication the day after the procedure (Table 2.3).

2.3.2 Dipyridamole

Dipyridamole (Persantine) inhibits adenosine uptake into platelets and potentiates the antiplatelet effects of prostacyclin (26). It has a half-life of 10–12 h. Its duration of action lasts approximately 2 days after its discontinuation (Baron et al. 2013). Aggrenox is a combination antiplatelet containing 200 mg extended release dipyridamole and 25 mg aspirin. This combination should be considered a bleeding risk. The combination should be held for 5 days before a high-risk procedure and can be resumed within 24 h. Rapid reversal of the antiplatelet effects can be achieved with DDAVP and/or platelet transfusions.

2.3.3 Cilostazol

Cilostazol (Pletal) is used to treat claudication in a patient with peripheral vascular disease. It is a phosphodiesterase III inhibitor which effects reversible inhibition of platelet aggregation. It has a clinical onset of action of 2–4 weeks with a half-life of approximately 11–13 h. Cilostazol should be held for 24 h before a high-risk procedure and can be resumed immediately after the procedure (Jaffe et al. 2015). Rapid reversal of its antiplatelet effects can be done with DDAVP and/or platelet transfusions.

Table 2.3 Some common antiplatelet medications and reversal treatment strategies

Medication	Class of drug	Half-life	Hold time	Resume time	Treatment
Aspirin	COX-1 inhibitor	20 min	5 d	24 h	DDAVP (0.3–0.4 mcg/kg) Platelet transfusion
NSAIDS	COX-1 inhibitor	Variable	24 h–10 d 5 half-lives	24 h	DDAVP (0.3–0.4 mcg/kg) Platelet transfusion
NSAIDS (Celecoxib)	COX-2 inhibitor	–	none	–	Does not affect platelet function
Abciximab (ReoPro)	GP IIb/IIIA inhibitor	10–30 min	5 d	8–12 h	Platelet transfusion
Cilostazol (Pletal)	Phosphodiesterase inhibitor	11–13 h	24 h	0 h Immediate	Platelet transfusion DDAVP (0.3–0.4 mcg/kg)
Clopidogrel (Plavix)	ADP receptor antagonist	6 h	7 d	0 h Immediate	Platelet transfusion DDAVP (0.3–0.4 mcg/kg)
Eptifibatide (Integrilin)	GP IIb/IIIA inhibitor	2.5 h	24 h	8–12 h	Platelet transfusion DDAVP (0.3–0.4 mcg/kg)
Prasugrel (Effient)	ADP receptor antagonist	7–9 h	7 d	24 h	Platelet transfusion DDAVP (0.3–0.4 mcg/kg)
Ticagrelor (Brilinta)	ADP receptor Antagonist	7–9 h	7 d	24 h	Platelet transfusion DDAVP (0.3–0.4 mcg/kg)
Tirofiban (Aggrastat)	GP IIb/IIIA inhibitor	2 h	24 h	8–12 h	Platelet transfusion DDAVP (0.3–0.4 mcg/kg)

2.3.4 P2Y12 Inhibitors

The P2Y12 inhibitors include ticagrelor (Brilinta) and the thienopyridine derivatives clopidogrel (Plavix), ticlopidine (Ticlid), and prasugrel (Effient). These drugs bind to the P2Y12 receptor on platelets, preventing adenosine diphosphate (ADP) from activating the glycoprotein IIb/IIIa receptor complex, thereby inhibiting platelet aggregation. P2Y12 inhibitors are often used with aspirin to provide dual antiplatelet therapy. Clopidogrel has a dose-dependent onset of action. A loading dose of 300–600 mg will result in onset of maximum antiplatelet effect in 2–5 h, while a daily dose without the loading dose will take 4–5 days. Its binding is irreversible with 40% of normal platelet function after discontinuation (Cattaneo 2008). Prasugrel with a loading dose has a faster onset of action compared to clopidogrel. Its antiplatelet effect is inversely related to the patient's weight (Hall and Mazer 2011). Its active metabolite irreversibly binds to platelets (Cattaneo 2008). Ticagrelor also has a faster onset of action than clopidogrel but is a reversible antagonist. Platelet function (60%) is restored within 24 h after discontinuation of the medication. These drugs are held 7 days prior to a high-risk procedure. Clopidogrel can be resumed immediately after the procedure, while prasugrel and ticagrelor are held for 24 h (Jaffe et al. 2015). DDAVP and/or platelet transfusions may overcome some of the antiplatelet effects of these medications (Yorkgitis et al. 2014; McCoy et al. 2014).

2.3.5 Nonsteroidal Anti-inflammatory Drugs (NSAIDs)

NSAIDs have a reversible effect on platelet aggregation. These drugs are not typically used for their antithrombotic properties, so it is usually safe to hold NSAIDs before an elective procedure. They have widely varying half-lives leading to different recommended hold times for high-risk procedures. Diclofenac (Zorvolex), ibuprofen (Motrin, Advil), and ketorolac (Toradol) are held for 1 day. Etodolac (Lodine) and indomethacin (Indocin) are held for 2 days. Meloxicam (Mobic) and naproxen (Naprosyn, Aleve, Anaprox, Naprelan) are held for 4 days. Nabumetone (Relafen) is held for 6 days. Oxaprozin (Daypro) and piroxicam (Feldene) are held for 10 days. All are restarted 24 h after a high-risk procedure (Narouze et al. 2015).

2.3.6 Glycoprotein IIb/IIIa Inhibitors

Glycoprotein IIb/IIIa inhibitors tirofiban (Aggrastat), eptifibatide (Integrilin), and abciximab (ReoPro) are potent intravenously administered platelet inhibitors that have a very rapid onset of action (10 min for tirofiban and abciximab and 15 min for eptifibatide). The plasma half-lives range between 30 and 150 min. They are used to treat unstable angina and acute coronary syndromes and are frequently used during coronary artery interventions. Abciximab (ReoPro) should be held 5 days for medium- and high-risk procedures and resumed after 8–12 h (Narouze et al. 2015). Eptifibatide (Integrilin) and tirofiban (Aggrastat) should be held 24 h for medium- and high-risk procedures and can be resumed after 8–12 h. This is a rarely encountered scenario in the potential spine biopsy population given the primary indications for these medications. Platelet transfusions can be used to overcome the antiplatelet effects of these medications.

2.4 Anticoagulants

2.4.1 Warfarin (Coumadin)

Warfarin is an oral anticoagulant that functions primarily by inhibition of factors II, VII, IX, and X which are the vitamin K-dependent coagulation factors. There is also an effect on protein C and S. The peak anticoagulation effect does not occur for 96 h after administration. Patients are often started on heparin while waiting for warfarin to become effective when there is a need for rapid anticoagulation. The effect of warfarin can be evaluated by the international normalized ratio (INR) which is a standardized method of reporting the prothrombin time (PT). INR and PT evaluate the extrinsic and common coagulation pathways. However, the INR is unreliable early in the therapeutic range, so heparin should be continued until there is the full anticoagulant effect of the Coumadin.

Warfarin is usually stopped 5 days before a planned moderate- or high-risk procedure to allow the INR to normalize (Douketis et al. 2012). Because of the delayed onset of action, most procedures can be performed within 12–24 h of initiation of warfarin anticoagulation without checking the INR. After this period, confirmation with measurement of the INR should be performed as there is variability in the duration of action of warfarin. An INR of 1.5 or less is usually not associated with an increased risk of hemorrhage. An INR of between 1.5 and 2.0 is indeterminate. An INR of greater than 2.0 is associated with an increased risk of bleeding, and the risk increases as the INR increases. Vitamin K can be administered to speed the reversal of the action of warfarin. Parenteral administration of vitamin K has a more rapid action but is also associated with severe reactions. Four-factor prothrombin complex concentrate (PCC) (Kcentra) is now used for the urgent or emergent reversal of the anticoagulation effects of warfarin, either for acute major bleeding or preoperatively before an urgent surgery or invasive procedure (Lexicomp Online 2014a, b, c, d). Transfusion of fresh frozen plasma may also be considered for reversing the effects of warfarin. Fresh frozen plasma takes much more time to administer, has a longer onset of action, requires much more fluid to be administered in, and has other potential complications compared to PCC (Patel et al. 2012). Warfarin is usually restarted 24 h after the procedure (Table 2.4).

Table 2.4 Some common anticoagulant medications and reversal treatment strategies

Medication	Class of drug	Half-life	Hold time	Resume time	Treatment
Warfarin (Coumadin)	Vitamin K inhibitor	Effective half-life: 20–60 h (mean 40 h)	5 d	1 d	Monitor INR Vitamin K Four-factor PCC (Kcentra) Fresh frozen plasma
Heparin unfractionated	Antithrombin III activation	30–90 min	4 h	4 h	Monitor aPTT or anti-factor Xa assay Protamine
Low molecular weight heparin enoxaparin (Lovenox/Fragmin)	Antithrombin III activation	Lovenox: 4.5 h Fragmin: 3–5 h (SQ)	24 h	24 h	Protamine (incomplete reversal – 60%) Anti-factor Xa assay Consider activated factor VII for critical bleeding
Apixaban (Eliquis)	Direct factor Xa inhibitor	9–12 h	48–72 h	24–48 h	No antidote If ingested <2 h, give activated charcoal Consider four-factor PCC (Kcentra)
Argatroban	Direct thrombin inhibitor	50 min	4 h	1 h	No antidote Monitor plasma-diluted thrombin time
Bivalirudin (Angiomax)	Direct thrombin inhibitor	20–25 min; 60 min renal failure pts	4 h	1 h	No antidote Monitor aPTT or plasma-diluted thrombin time Consider hemodialysis, hemofiltration, or plasmapheresis for critical bleeding
Dabigatran (Pradaxa)	Direct thrombin inhibitor	12–17 h	72 h	48 h	Idarucizumab (Praxbind) for emergent reversal Monitor plasma-diluted thrombin time If ingested <2 h, give activated charcoal
Desirudin (Iprivask)	Direct thrombin inhibitor	2 h	4 h	1 h	No antidote Monitor aPTT or plasma-diluted thrombin time
Fondaparinux (Arixtra)	Select factor Xa inhibitor	17–21 h	3–4 d	24 h	No antidote Consider factor VII for critical bleeding
Rivaroxaban (Xarelto)	Direct thrombin inhibitor	5–9 h (healthy) 11–13 h (elderly)	48–72 h	24–48 h	No antidote If ingested <2 h, give activated charcoal Consider four-factor PCC (Kcentra)

Warfarin is a common oral anticoagulant with the following advantages: (1) the effects can be monitored with a blood test, (2) a bridging strategy is possible with heparin or Lovenox, and (3) the effects can be reversed on an urgent or emergent basis.

2.4.2 Heparin

Heparin is an anticoagulant that may be administered intravenously or subcutaneously. There are two major classes of heparin, unfractionated heparin and low molecular weight heparin (LMWH). Unfractionated heparin is frequently administered intravenously or subcutaneously. Low molecular weight heparin (LMWH) is infrequently administered intravenously and is typically administered subcutaneously, particularly in outpatients. The use of LMWHs is increasing because of easier dosing and less severe side effects. The effect of unfractionated heparin can be monitored by the activated partial thromboplastin time (aPTT). The anticoagulant effect of unfractionated heparin can be reversed with intravenous protamine. Low molecular weight heparin cannot be monitored with the aPTT and is not fully reversible with protamine.

Intravenous unfractionated heparin is usually stopped 4 h before procedures to normalize the APTT (<35 s) and is not restarted for at least 2–4 h. If a procedure is associated with significant blood loss, then intravenous heparin is not restarted for 24 h (Narouze et al. 2015). Low-dose subcutaneous unfractionated heparin (<10,000 U) is typically held for 8 h and restarted 2 h after the procedure (Narouze et al. 2015). Enoxaparin (Lovenox) is the most commonly used LMWH in the United States. When enoxaparin is used in low doses for venous thromboembolism prophylaxis, it is held for 12 h before procedures (24 h in renal failure). Systemic full anticoagulation doses of enoxaparin are held for 24 h. Either dose of enoxaparin may be restarted 4 h after low-risk procedures, 12 h after medium-risk procedures, and 24 h after high-risk procedures (Table 2.4) (Narouze et al. 2015).

2.4.3 Newer Oral Anticoagulants

Several newer anticoagulants are available that do not have the dietary restrictions that accompany warfarin use. These cannot be followed with serum INR or aPTT testing.

Dabigatran (Pradaxa) directly inhibits both free- and clot-bound thrombin, which impedes the conversion of fibrinogen to fibrin, thus preventing thrombus development (Stangier et al. 2007). It has a rapid onset of action with a peak effect in 1–2 h. It has a half-life of 12–17 h with normal renal function. It is 80% cleared by the kidneys and is dialyzable (Douketis et al. 2012). There is also a reversal agent for dabigatran, idarucizumab (Praxbind) that can be used. Thrombin time is the most sensitive assay, but it is not routinely monitored (Lexicomp Online 2014a, b, c, d). Dabigatran should be held for 72 h for a high-risk procedure with adjustments for patients with impaired renal function. It can be resumed 48 h after the high-risk procedure (Jaffe et al. 2015).

Rivaroxaban (Xarelto), apixaban (Eliquis), and edoxaban (Savaysa) are oral anticoagulation agents that inhibit platelet activation and fibrin clot formation by direct, selective, and reversible inhibition of factor Xa. This decreases the generation of thrombin. These medications have a rapid onset of action with peak effects in 1–3 h. Their half-lives range between 7 and 12 h with a renal clearance of 25–35%. They are not dialyzable and there is no reversal agent (Douketis et al. 2012). There is no consistent assay for monitoring of blood levels. The general recommendation with these agents is to wait five half-lives after the last dose before performing a high-risk procedure. These medications should be stopped 48–72 h prior to the high-risk procedure and can be resumed 24–48 h after the procedure (Douketis et al. 2012; Jaffe et al. 2015; Crockett et al. 2012; Narouze et al. 2015). Options for reversal are limited if a patient requires immediate reversal. Studies that have evaluated the reversal of the new oral anticoagulants have been limited to reversal of drug effect with the use of recombinant activated factor VII and prothrombin complex concentrate (PCC). Current evidence suggests that prothrombin complex concentrate may be the best option and that it reverses the effects of rivaroxaban better than the effects of dabigatran (Lazo-Langner et al. 2013). Prothrombin complex concentrates (PCCs) containing coagulation factors II, VII, IX, and X have shown promise in the laboratory setting for all of the new anticoagulants and in selected case reports, but there is a deficiency of clinical studies (Crockett et al. 2012).

2.4.4 Injectable Anticoagulants

Fondaparinux (Arixtra) is a subcutaneously administered anticoagulant indicated for prophylaxis or treatment of deep vein thrombosis or acute pulmonary embolism. It works by inhibiting factor Xa. The onset of action is 2–3 h with a half-life of 17–21 h. Fondaparinux is held 3–4 days for medium- and high-risk procedures (Narouze et al. 2015). An additional recommendation includes adding a day or two if the creatinine clearance is 50 mL/min or less (Patel et al. 2013). Fondaparinux can be resumed after 24 h. Fondaparinux has no effect on PT and a minimal effect on aPTT. There is no reversal agent. Recombinant factor VIIa and PCC have been evaluated for reversal (Bijsterveld et al. 2002; Desmurs-Clavel et al. 2009).

Argatroban, desirudin (Iprivask), and bivalirudin (Angiomax) are all reversible direct thrombin inhibitors, preventing the formation of fibrin from fibrinogen. They are monitored by aPTT. Argatroban is used to prevent or treat blood clots in patients with heparin-induced thrombocytopenia; it is also used during certain percutaneous coronary artery interventions. Argatroban is given intravenously and drug plasma concentrations reach steady state in 1–3 h. Argatroban is metabolized in the liver and has a half-life of about 50 min. Because of its hepatic metabolism, it may be used in patients with renal dysfunction. If warfarin is chosen as the long-term anticoagulant, this poses particular challenges due to the falsely elevated prothrombin time and INR caused by argatroban. The combination of argatroban and warfarin may raise the INR to greater than 5.0 without a significant increased risk of bleeding complications (Hursting et al. 2005). Desirudin and bivalirudin may, to a lesser degree, also give a falsely elevated INR. Desirudin is given subcutaneously or intravenously. The maximal plasma concentrations are reached in 1–3 h. Approximately 90% of the dose is cleared by the kidneys within 2 h. Bivalirudin is given intravenously. It has a half-life of 20–25 min, but this half-life can be markedly prolonged in patients with renal impairment. It has the advantage of a short half-life and the ability to be partially removed with hemodialysis, hemofiltration, or plasmapheresis. There are no reversal agents for these medications. These medications are held for 4 h before a high-risk procedure. They can be restarted beginning at 1 h after the procedure (Jaffe et al. 2015).

2.5 Thrombolytics

Thrombolytic drugs are used to lyse existing clots. The thrombolytic drugs include tissue plasminogen activator tPA drugs (alteplase (Activase), reteplase (Retavase), tenecteplase (TNKase)), streptokinase (Kabikinase, Streptase), anistreplase (Eminase), and urokinase (Abbokinase). The tPA drugs bind to the fibrin that serves as the matrix for blood clot formation. It catalyzes the conversion of plasminogen molecules that are within the blood clot into plasmin. The plasmin cleaves fibrin thus breaking down the meshwork of the clot. The tPA drugs are fibrin specific and have short plasma half-lives (alteplase (5 min), reteplase (13–16 min), and tenecteplase (20–24 min)) giving an advantage over streptokinase which has a biphasic half-life (initially 18 min and then 83 min). Urokinase has a half-life of 10–20 min. Although the half-lives of the tPA agents are short, there may be a prolonged effect. Thrombolysis may continue for approximately 4 h following administration of alteplase, streptokinase, or urokinase; this hyper-fibrinolytic effect disappears within a few hours following discontinuation of tPA medication. Following administration of anistreplase, thrombolysis may continue for approximately 6 h, and a systemic hyper-fibrinolytic state may persist for more than

2 days. Procedures should be avoided for at least 48 h after administration of thrombolytics. Using thrombolytic agents after a high-risk procedure needs careful input from all involved medical staff due to the risk that the blood clot formed from the needle passage may be lysed, resulting in hemorrhage. Because clots become stable after 10 days, waiting more than 48 h should add an additional margin of safety. Measuring fibrinogen levels can assist in monitoring a patient who may need to undergo a spine biopsy procedure (Layton et al. 2006).

2.6 Other Coagulation Issues

A variety of coagulation issues unrelated to antithrombotic medications may also be encountered in patients scheduled for a spine or rib biopsy. Thrombocytopenia is a low platelet count and may result from many etiologies. Platelet transfusion is used to raise the platelet count to at least 50,000 platelets per microliter for minor procedures and 100,000 for medium- and high-risk procedures.

Classic hemophilia is a genetic disorder resulting in a low level or low function of factor VIII. Factor VIII replacement and desmopressin are both used in treatment of classic hemophilia and in preparation for invasive procedures. Treatment and pre-procedural preparation of patients with hemophilia and rarer disorders of coagulation are best left to hematologists with expertise in these conditions.

2.6.1 Reversal Medications

2.6.1.1 Protamine

Protamine sulfate is used for the neutralization of anticoagulant effect of heparin. The dose of protamine sulfate is determined by the dose of heparin received, route of administration, time elapsed since heparin was given, and blood coagulation studies. For reversal of low molecular weight heparin, a maximum of about 60% of anti-factor X_a activity is neutralized with protamine sulfate administration for overdosage of enoxaparin. Severe hypotension and severe anaphylactic reactions have been reported, particularly with large doses or rapid administration of protamine sulfate, especially in patients with prior exposure to protamine-containing insulin or previous protamine sulfate therapy (Makris and Watson 2001).

2.6.1.2 Vitamin K

Administration of vitamin K overpowers the anticoagulation system and turns on the endogenous activation of the coagulation factors. Vitamin K can be orally or intravenously administered. Both routes of administration are effective at correcting supratherapeutic INRs at 24-h posttreatment; however, intravenous vitamin K can correct the INR much sooner, in as few as 4–6 h (Ansell et al. 2008; Makris and Watson 2001). While intravenous vitamin K has been proven effective, it is not without risks and has been associated with severe anaphylactic reactions (Ansell et al. 2008).

2.6.1.3 Four-Factor Prothrombin Complex Concentrate

Four-factor prothrombin complex concentrate (Kcentra, 4F-PCC) is a purified, heat-treated, nanofiltered, lyophilized, nonactivated plasma protein concentrate made from pooled human plasma (Zareh et al. 2011). Kcentra contains all four vitamin K-dependent coagulation factors (II, VII, IX, and X) and the antithrombotic proteins C and S. PCCs are stored as a lyophilized powder at room temperature and are reconstituted in sterile water immediately prior to use, which means they can be administered much more quickly than FFP. The mean infusion time for PCCs is 21–24 min. In a prospective study of 41 patients requiring rapid reversal of VKA-associated over-anticoagulation, 28 of 29 patients treated with 4F-PCC showed a complete correction of the INR within 15 min (mean INR of 1.3) (Makris et al. 1997).There is no need for ABO matching, so there is no delay for the blood type and cross. 4F-PCC contains known quantities of the vitamin K-dependent coagulation factors in small volumes, which substantially reduces the risks associated with large-volume infusions of FFP (4F-PCC requires 85% less infusion volume compared with plasma). The main concern associated with PCCs is the risk of thromboembolism.

2.6.1.4 Fresh Frozen Plasma

FFP or thawed plasma is the plasma taken from a unit of whole blood. FFP is frozen within 8 h of collection. FFP contains all coagulation factors in normal concentrations. The plasma is free of red blood cells, leukocytes, and platelets. One unit is approximately 250 mL and must be ABO compatible. Prior to use, the blood must be typed and crossed and the FFP thawed (since it is stored at 4 °C). This contributes to a time delay before it can be given to the patient. A retrospective study found that a median time of 6.5 h was needed to infuse 5 U of FFP to patients who suffered from warfarin-induced intracranial hemorrhage (Lee et al. 2006). A major problem with the use of FFP in over-anticoagulated patients is the large volume that is often required to reverse the coagulation defect: it is not uncommon to rapidly transfuse 2–4 L (approximately 8–16 U) in patients with greatly elevated INRs (Aguilar et al. 2007). Rapid transfusion of large volumes can lead to cardiogenic lung edema, and transfusion of FFP specifically has been associated with a noncardiogenic lung edema known as transfusion-related acute lung injury (Bux 2005; Khan et al. 2007).

2.6.1.5 Desmopressin (DDAVP)

Desmopressin (DDAVP) 1-deamino-8-d-arginine vasopressin is a synthetic analogue of the antidiuretic hormone vasopressin that exerts a substantial hemostatic effect by inducing the release of von Willebrand factor from its storage sites in endothelial cells, increasing exposure at damage sites (Levi et al. 2003). It increases the density of platelet surface glycoprotein receptors (improving adhesiveness) and increases plasma activity of factor VIII and levels of plasminogen activator antigen. (Wun et al. 1995; Mannucci et al. 1975). It has proved useful in treating or preventing bleeding episodes in patients with von Willebrand disease, hemophilia A, and platelet function defects (Bulent et al. 2007). DDAVP selectively and markedly enhances the ability to form procoagulant platelets and increases platelet-dependent thrombin generation by enhancing Na^+/Ca^{++} mobilization (Colucci et al. 2014).

2.6.1.6 Idarucizumab

Idarucizumab (Praxbind) is a monoclonal antibody fragment that binds avidly to dabigatran and reverses the anticoagulant effects. The US Food and Drug Administration granted accelerated approval to Praxbind (idarucizumab) in October 2015 for use in patients who are taking the anticoagulant Pradaxa (dabigatran) during emergency situations when there is a need to reverse dabigatran's (Pradaxa) anticoagulant effect. In one study, 89% of 123 patients taking Pradaxa who received Praxbind due to uncontrolled bleeding or because they required emergency surgery experienced full reversal of anticoagulation within 4 h of receiving Praxbind (FDA release, 10/16/2015).

> It is extremely important for the operator to be aware of and understand the antiplatelet, anticoagulant, and thrombolytic medications, their names and mechanisms of action, their half-lives and mode of clearance, their recommended hold and resumption time periods as applies to spine or rib biopsy procedures, and their specific reversal agents, if any, for emergent clinical care.

2.7 During the Procedure

Meticulous planning with review of recent imaging is required prior to any intervention. Any vascular or other vital structure should be avoided. For biopsies, the use of a thinner needle that will obtain reliable diagnostic material will decrease the likelihood of bleeding during and after the procedure. It is not necessary to use a 12 gauge bone biopsy needle if there is a lytic bone lesion with soft tissue extension. An 18 or 20 gauge biopsy cutting needle usually obtains enough tissue for diagnosis. Fine needle aspirates with 21 or 22 gauge needles may be sufficient if only a small amount of material is needed to document malignancy or infection. The use of a guiding needle will limit the number of needle tracts and bleeding through the tract.

Upon completion of the procedure, the needle should never be removed if there is arterial back bleeding thru the hub of the needle. This should prompt an immediate investigation for the source of the arterial bleeding and may require immediate endovascular and/or surgical consultation. Venous bleeding is relatively common with biopsy of the vertebral body as this is a highly vascularized structure. In this latter situation, the needle should be used to obtain hemostasis; placing a stylet or introducer to obstruct the needle lumen for a minute or so will usually stop the majority of venous oozing from the needle hub. Various materials can be injected into the needle to stop bleeding from the needle tract between the periosteal surface of the bone and/or biopsy site and the skin surface. Autologous clot, gelfoam, surgifoam, fibrin glue, thrombin, or collagen mixtures can all be used to stop the bleeding. Platelets can be injected into the needle to saturate the area with platelets in patients who are having platelet transfusions for the procedure, either because of low platelet counts or dysfunctional platelets. The use of combination agents such as gelfoam or surgifoam imbedded with thrombin or platelets may give more control to achieve immediate thrombosis. We typically will use a coaxial system so that there is one guiding needle at the margin of the vertebral cortex or the paraspinal soft tissue mass. This enables multiple biopsy passes to be performed through the guiding needle with a biopsy device. We can then perform tract embolization as we remove the guide needle if the patient is at high risk of bleeding. This is especially important with known or suspected hypervascular lesions. Once the needle has been removed, local direct pressure at the puncture site can control bleeding if it is a superficial procedure or if the bleeding is originating from the tract. This is especially useful when large bore biopsy needles are used.

Surgifoam powder is an excellent material to assist in obtaining local hemostasis. Since it is a powder, it must be mixed, using sterile technique, with a liquid agent (either normal saline or thrombin solution), prior to its use. We keep the surgifoam powder and sterile normal saline available on a standby basis in our procedure suites. The mixture is easy and quick (less than 1 min preparation time) to prepare and can be injected using a 10 mL Luer-Lok syringe and a 20 gauge or larger needle (Fig. 2.1). The latter can be inserted coaxially through the initially placed guide cannula or can be inserted into the previously created needle tract. The surgifoam suspension is slowly injected as the needle is withdrawn from the tract. The volume of surgifoam that is required depends on the length and width of the needle tract, which is also related to the size and length of the biopsy needle system. On average it takes about 1–3 mL of surgifoam suspension to "seal" the tract and, with gentle hand compression for 1–2 min, to obtain hemostasis at the puncture site.

Preparing surgifoam for syringe injection (Fig. 2.1):

1. Add 7–10 mL sterile normal saline or thrombin solution to surgifoam container.
2. Recap the container and shake vigorously for 20–30 s.
3. The surgifoam suspension will resemble a pasty mash potato-like consistency.
4. Remove plunger from sterile 10 mL Luer-Lok syringe, and backfill the surgifoam into the syringe.
5. Replace the syringe plunger.
6. The surgifoam suspension is now ready to be used when needed.

2.8 After the Procedure

Bleeding can occur acutely after the procedure, delayed bleeding after the patient is moved from the procedure table to a stretcher, or when the patient has been placed back on their anticoagulation or antiplatelet medications. Treatment is determined by the severity of the bleeding and its

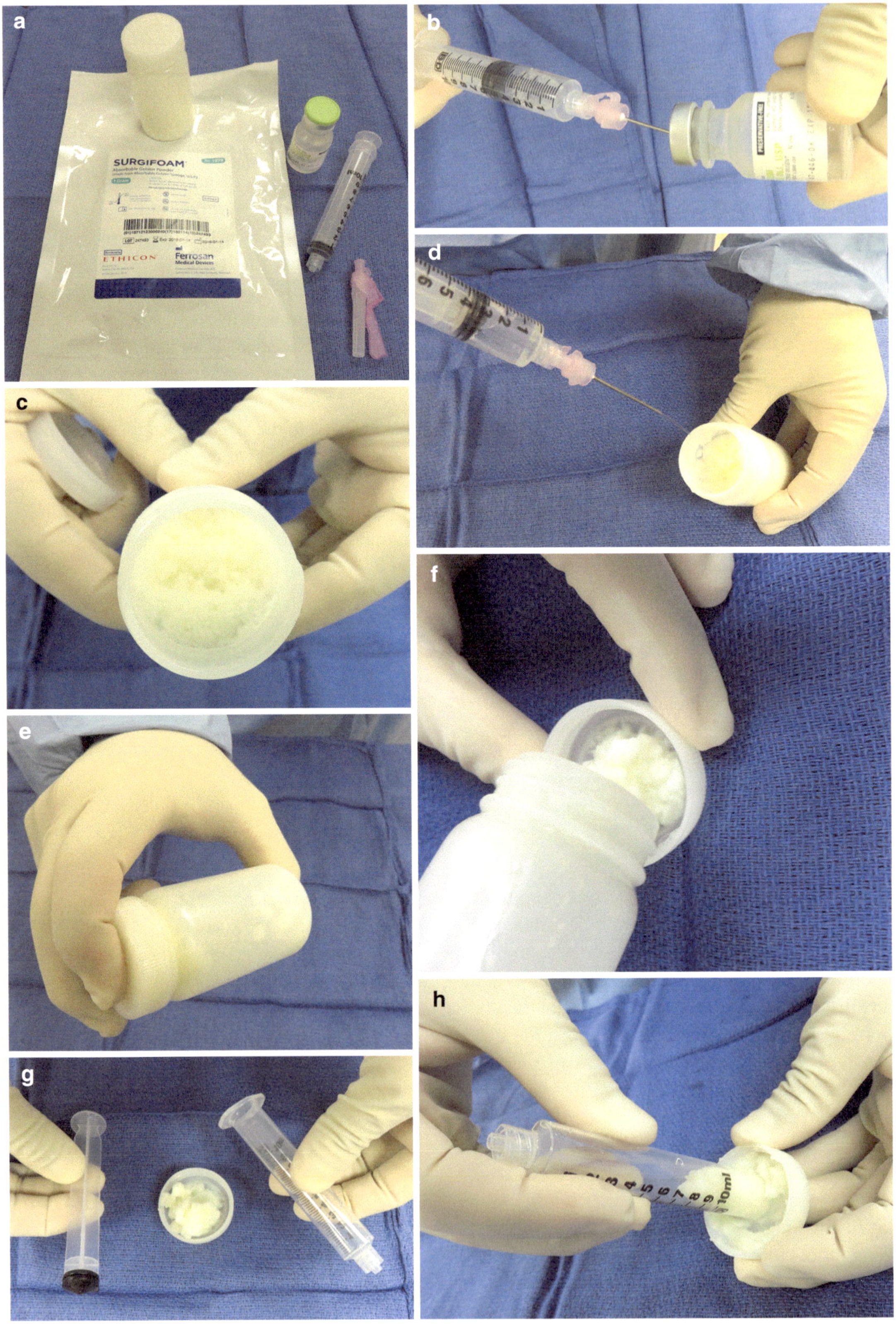
a
b
c
d
e
f
g
h
SURGIFOAM
ETHICON
Ferrosan
Medical Devices

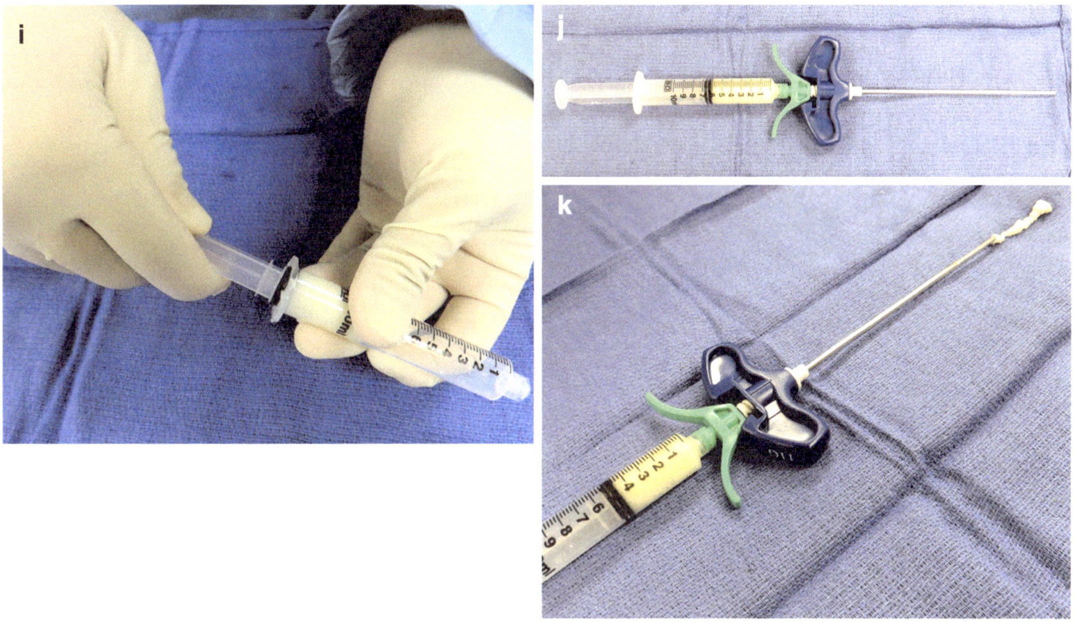

Fig. 2.1 (continued)

presumed cause. The practice of sound post-procedure care will help to promptly identify a bleeding complication. This includes frequent monitoring of the puncture site and monitoring of the patient and the patient's vital signs. Critical time points for examining the puncture site include the first 10 min after the procedure, immediately after the patient is moved onto their stretcher, anytime the patient's position is adjusted during their recovery period, or if the patient complains of severe pain at the puncture site.

With acute hemorrhage with normal coagulation factors and no active anticoagulation or antiplatelet medications in effect, treatment is determined by the severity of the bleed. Patients may have pain and a small hematoma at the biopsy site; this is somewhat common, but can be minimized by using moderate hand compression at the puncture site for a few minutes. In rare cases, urgent imaging with CT may be required to identify an expanding hematoma deep to the skin surface (Fig. 2.2). This is fairly common but can be minimized by using moderate hand compression at the puncture site for a few minutes. However, if pain out of proportion to the procedure or the pain is increasing in severity, then this needs to be immediately investigated. Most post-procedure bleeding is venous and is self-limited. Serial blood work including CBC, platelets, PT/PTT, and INR are

Fig. 2.1 Basic equipment required to prepare surgifoam suspension. (**a**) 1 gram of surgifoam powder comes in a prepackaged sterile container, 10 mL vial of sterile normal saline solution, 10 mL Luer-Lok syringe, and 18 gauge needle. (**b**) Sterile technique is used to draw up 10 mL of the normal sterile saline into the syringe. (**c**) The surgifoam container is opened; the surgifoam is a flaky powder. (**d**) 7 mL sterile saline is injected into the surgifoam container. (**e**) Place the container cap back on and shake vigorously for about 20–30 s. (**f**) The pasty -surgifoam suspension is extruded into the container cap. (**g**) The syringe plunger is removed. (h) The surgifoam suspension has a "mashed potato" consistency and appearance and can readily be back-loaded into the syringe. (**i**) The syringe plunger is carefully reinserted. (**j**) The syringe can be attached to an insert needle which can then be inserted coaxially into the larger needle as shown in this example. (**k**) The surgifoam suspension can be easily injected; an example of a tract created by injecting 1.5 mL of the suspension

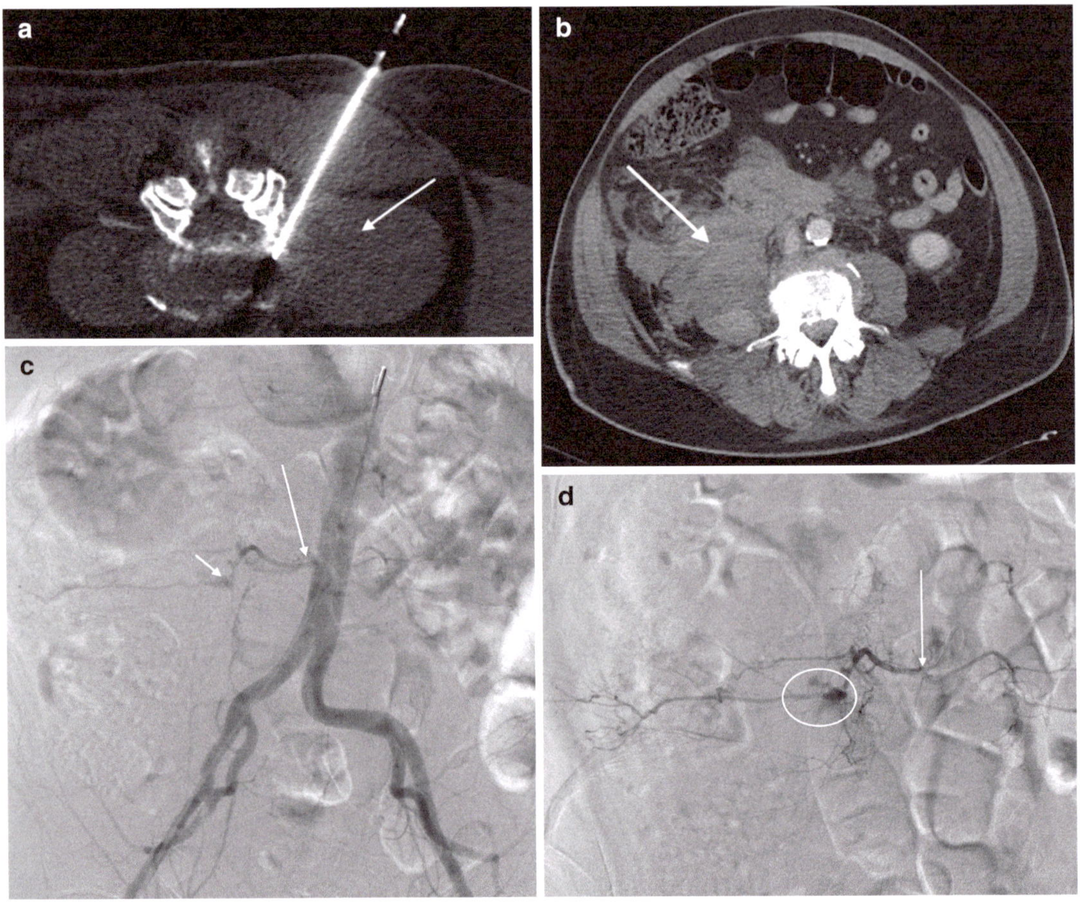

Fig. 2.2 Expanding psoas hematoma following a lumbar disk biopsy in a patient with marginally corrected coagulation status (**a**). Axial CT image during the biopsy shows swelling of the right psoas muscle (*arrow*). (**b**). Follow-up CT of the abdomen shows expanding retroperitoneal hematoma (*arrow*). (**c**). Single frontal projection from aortic angiogram shows prominent right lumbar artery (large arrow) with focus of contrast staining (*small arrow*). (**d**). Frontal projection from selective catheterization of right lumbar artery (*arrow*) shows active contrast extravasation from a distal branch (*oval*). This was immediately embolized with polyvinyl alcohol microparticles and microcoils

used to determine the amount of bleeding. Samples should be sent for type and screen in the event that blood transfusions are needed. Serial imaging may be performed to evaluate if the hematoma is expanding. Emergent computed tomography angiography (CTA) is especially useful when imaging is performed as an arterial source for the bleeding requires immediate intervention with angiography with embolization. The CTA can also be used as a map since the source of the bleeding is identified and traced back to the feeding artery. Catheter angiography with selective catheterization of the identified bleeding artery can then be performed quickly (Fig. 2.2). Once the feeding artery is entered and the optimal positioning of the catheter or coaxial micro catheter obtained, embolization can be performed using various agents such as coils, microcoils, glue, Onyx, gelfoam, Avitene, particles, etc., depending on the preference of the interventional radiologist. In patients who develop neurologic symptoms of spinal cord compression due to possible epidural hematoma, an emergent MRI of the spine is performed in addition to an emergent evaluation by a spine surgeon. Emergency spinal decompression may be required with symptomatic improvement seen in patients who undergo laminectomy within 8 h of onset of neurologic dysfunction (Vanermeulen et al. 1994).

In patients who have resumed their anticoagulation or had incomplete reversal of their anticoagulation prior to the procedure, the cause of the bleeding is likely secondary to the anticoagulation and/or antiplatelet therapy. The immediate treatment is to stop and fully reverse the anticoagulation or antiplatelet therapy (the reversal agents are listed in Tables 2.3 and 2.4). If the effects of the anticoagulation or antiplatelet medications are reversed and there is persistent bleeding, then the steps for treatment of acute hemorrhage should be followed. Generally, once a patient starts bleeding from anticoagulation or antiplatelet effect, it's presumed that they will not stop unless the anticoagulation effects are reversed. The rapidity of the reversal is a clinical judgment determined by the patient's need to be on the medication. Often there is a difficult choice between stopping the bleeding and stopping the medication if the bleeding is not significant. However, moderate to severe bleeding must be stopped, and this overrides the need for the medication in the immediate short term. The use of CTA may be helpful in this situation as the absence of an arterial source of bleeding, a rare cause of delayed hemorrhage, may not require cessation of the medication. Most bleeding will stop with reversal of the anticoagulant or antiplatelet medication and supportive medical treatment including blood pressure control.

2.8.1 Clinical Management of the Patient with Acute Hemorrhage After a Spine or Rib Biopsy

Management of the acutely bleeding patient requires close observation and immediate treatment by the medical staff. Good large bore intravenous access or central venous access is a requirement. The patient is given intravenous fluids to maintain their vascular volume with transfusions of blood products as appropriate. Frequent blood tests are taken to evaluate the amount of blood and coagulation factors. Admission to the intensive care unit is advisable if the bleeding is severe and the patient requires constant vital sign monitoring.

Initially, STAT blood work is drawn, including PT/PTT, INR, complete blood count (CBC) with platelets, basic metabolic profile including BUN and creatinine, and a STAT type and screen. Group O uncrossed-matched blood can be used if there is not enough time to type and screen the patient for packed red blood cell replacement.

2.8.2 Clinical Management of the Patient with an Acute Thromboembolic Event After a Spine or Rib Biopsy

The key to managing acute thromboembolic events is to prevent them. The use of bridging strategies should be considered and employed in high-risk patients. Delaying procedures when possible can also be helpful. Ensuring adequate hydration of the patient after the procedure is important; these patients are often slightly dehydrated due to the NPO status, and a dehydrated state is a procoagulant state. Resuming the patient's antiplatelet or anticoagulant medication therapy should also be clearly explained to the patient, so that the dose is properly timed and not missed or skipped. Patients should be made aware of the possibility of these types of complications at the time of consultation and informed consent. The patient and their family will then at least be aware of the possibility of these types of adverse events after the procedure and can act quickly in terms of seeking immediate medical attention.

The clinical management for an acute thromboembolic event will depend on the type of event: cardiac, stroke, or deep venous thrombosis. Cardiac and neurologic events are managed emergently with a goal of revascularization. Deep venous thrombosis, often seen in the lower extremities, requires emergent evaluation and management as well.

Key Review Points

1. The patient's coagulation status should be reviewed before the procedure.
2. Spine and rib biopsies are infrequently emergent procedures allowing coagula-

tion status and antithrombotic medications to be adjusted or held.

3. There are recommended hold times for antithrombotic medications before and after procedures; however, the risks of hemorrhage must be carefully balanced on an individual basis. There are cases where a biopsy is indicated and the risks of holding the antithrombotic for the recommended time or at all are greater than the risk of hemorrhage. This often requires a multidisciplinary decision making process.
4. Brisk back bleeding thru the hub of the needle may require action before the needle is removed.
5. Treatment of subacute bleeding is usually immediately addressed with stopping and reversal of the anticoagulation or antiplatelet medications.
6. Treatment of acute bleeding includes good intravenous access, frequent evaluation of hemocrit/hemoglobin and coagulation status, and transfusion of blood products as needed, with a CTA of the area if there is persistent bleeding.
7. A post-biopsy patient who develops neurologic signs/symptoms that might indicate spinal cord compression requires immediate imaging and surgical evaluation in order to assess for the presence of an epidural hematoma as early spinal decompression is associated with better recovery.

References

Aguilar MI, Hart RG, Kase CS, Freeman WD, Hoeben BJ, Garcia RC, Ansell JE, Mayer SA, Norrving B, Rosand J, Steiner T, Wijdicks EFM, Yamaguchi T, Yasaka M. Treatment of warfarin-associated intracerebral hemorrhage: literature review and expert opinion. Mayo Clin Proc. 2007;82:82–92.

Ansell J, Hirsch J, Hylek E, Jacobson A, Crowther M, Palareti G. Pharmacology and management of the vitamin K antagonists: American College of Chest Physicians evidence-based clinical practice guidelines (8th ed.). Chest. 2008;133:160S–98S.

Baron TH, Kamath PS, McBane RD. Management of antithrombotic therapy in patients undergoing invasive procedures. N Engl J Med. 2013;368:2113–24.

Bijsterveld NR, Moons AH, Boekholdt SM, van Aken BE, Fennema H, Peters RJ, Meijers JC, Buller HR, Levi M. Ability of recombinant factor VIIa to reverse the anticoagulant effect of the pentasaccharide fondaparinux in healthy volunteers. Circulation. 2002;106:2550–4.

Bülent Ö, Madhvi R, Lusher JM. How do you treat bleeding disorders with desmopressin? Postgrad Med J. 2007;83:159–63.

Bux J. Transfusion-related acute lung injury (TRALI): a serious adverse event of blood transfusion. Vox Sang. 2005;89:1–10.

Cattaneo M. Advances in antiplatelet therapy: overview of new P2Y12 receptor antagonists in development. Eur Heart J Suppl. 2008;10(Suppl I):I 33–7.

Colucci G, Stutz M, Rochat S, Conte T, Pavicic M, Reusser M, Giabbani E, Huynh A, Thürlemann C, Keller P, Alberio L. The effect of desmopressin on platelet function: a selective enhancement of procoagulant COAT platelets in patients with primary platelet function defects. Blood. 2014;123: 1905–16.

Crockett MT, Moynagh MR, Kavanagh EC. The novel oral anticoagulants: an update for the interventional radiologist. AJR Am J Roentgenol. 2012;199[web]:W 376–9.

Desmurs-Clavel H, Huchon C, Chatard B, Negrier C, Dargaud Y. Reversal of the inhibitory effect of fondaparinux on thrombin generation by rFVIIa, aCCP and PCC. Thromb Res. 2009;123:796–8.

Diener H-C, Cunha L, Ce F, Sivenius J, Smets P, Lowenthal A. European Stroke Prevention Study 2: dipyridamole and acetylsalicylic acid in the secondary prevention of stroke. J Neurol Sci. 1996;143:1–13.

Douketis JD, Spyropoulos AC, Spencer FA, Mayr M, Ak J, Eckman MH, Dunn AS, Kunz R. Perioperative Management of Antithrombotic Therapy. Antithrombotic Therapy and Prevention of Thrombosis, 9th ed: American College of Chest Physicians evidence-based clinical practice guidelines. Chest. 2012;11: e326S–50S.

Hall R, Mazer CD. Antiplatelet drugs: a review of their pharmacology and management in the perioperative period. Anesth Analg. 2011;112:292–318.

Hunt BJ. Bleeding and coagulopathies in critical care. N Engl J Med. 2014;370:847–59.

Hursting MJ, Lewis BE, Macfarlane DE. Transitioning from argatroban to warfarin therapy in patients with heparin-induced thrombocytopenia. Clin Appl Thromb Hemost. 2005;11:279–87.

Jaffe T, Raiff D, Ho L, Kim C. Management of anticoagulant and antiplatelet medications in adults undergoing percutaneous interventions. AJR Am J Roentgenol. 2015;205:421–8.

Jneid H, Anderson JL, Wright RS, Adams CD, Bridges CR, Casey Jr DE, Ettinger SM, Fesmire FM, Ganiats TG, Am L, Peterson ED, Philippides GJ, Theroux P, Wenger NK, Zidar JP. 2012 ACC/AHA focused update of the guideline for the management of patients with unstable angina/non-ST-elevation myocardial infarction (updating the 2007 guideline and replacing the 2011 focused update). J Am Coll Cardiol. 2012;60:645–81.

Khan H, Belsher J, Yilmaz M, Afessa B, Winters JL, Moore SB, Hubmayr RD, Gajic O. Fresh-frozen plasma and platelet transfusions are associated with development of acute lung injury in critically ill medical patients. Chest. 2007;131:1308–14.

Kohi MP, Fidelman N, Behr S, Taylor AG, Kolli K, Conrad M, Hwang G, Weinstein S. Periprocedural patient care. Radiographics. 2015;35:1766–78.

Layton KF, Kallmes DF, Horlocker TT. Recommendations for anticoagulated patients undergoing image-guided spinal procedures. AJNR Am J Neuroradiol. 2006;27:467–71.

Lazo-Langner A, Lang ES, Douketis J. Clinical management of new oral anticoagulants: a structured review with emphasis on the reversal of bleeding complications. Crit Care. 2013;17:230–242

Lee SB, Manno EM, Layton KF, Wijdicks EF. Progression of warfarin-associated intracerebral hemorrhage after INR normalization with FFP. Neurology. 2006;67:1272–4.

Levi M, Vink R, de Jonge E. Prevention and treatment of bleeding by pro-hemostatic treatment strategies. Wien Med Wochenschr. 2003;153:421–5.

Lexicomp Online. Oral anticoagulant comparison chart. Lexi-Comp: Hudson; 2014a.

Lexicomp Online. Prothrombin complex concentrate (human) (factors II, VII, IX, X), protein C and protein S. Lexi-Comp: Hudson; 2014b.

Lexicomp Online. Dabigtran Etexilate (Lexi-Drug). Lexi-Comp: Hudson; 2014c.

Lexicomp Online. Cilostazol (Lexi-Drug). Lexi-Comp: Hudson; 2014d.

Makris M, Greaves M, Phillips WS, Kitchen S, Rosendaal FR, Preston EF. Emergency oral anticoagulant reversal: the relative efficacy of infusions of fresh frozen plasma and clotting factor concentrate on correction of the coagulopathy. Thromb Haemost. 1997;77:477–80.

Makris M, Watson HG. The management of coumarin-induced over-anticoagulation Annotation. Br J Haematol. 2001;114:271–80.

Mannucci PM, Aberg M, Nilsson IM, Robertson B. Mechanism of plasminogen activator and factor VIII increase after vasoactive drugs. Br J Haematol. 1975;30:81–93.

McCoy CC, Lawson JH, Shapiro ML. Management of anticoagulation agents in trauma patients. Clin Lab Med 2014;34:563–74 27.

Narouze S, Benzon HT, Provenzano DA, Buvanendran A, De Andres J, Deer TR, Rauck R, Huntoon MA. Interventional Spine and Pain Procedures in Patients on Antiplatelet and Anticoagulant Medications. Guidelines from the American Society of Regional Anesthesia and Pain Medicine, the European Society of Regional Anaesthesia and Pain Therapy, the American Academy of Pain Medicine, the International Neuromodulation Society, the North American Neuromodulation Society, and the World Institute of Pain. Regional Anesthesia Pain Med. 2015;40:182–212.

Patel IJ, Davidson JC, Nikolic B, Salazar GM, Schwartzberg MS, Walker TG, Saad WE. Consensus guidelines for periprocedural management of coagulation status and hemostasis risk in percutaneous image-guided interventions. J Vasc Interv Radiol. 2012;23:727–36.

Patel IJ, Davidson JC, Nikolic B, Salazar GM, Schwartzberg MS, Walker TG, Saad WE. Addendum of newer anticoagulants to the SIR consensus guideline. J Vasc Interv Radiol. 2013;24:641–5.

Stangier J, Rathgen K, Stahle H, Gansser D, Roth W. The pharmacokinetics, pharmacodynamics and tolerability of dabigatran etexilate, a new oral direct thrombin inhibitor, in healthy male subjects. Br J Clin Pharmacol. 2007;64:292–303.

Yorkgitis BK, Ruggia-Check C, Dujon JE. Antiplatelet and anticoagulation medications and the surgical patient. Am J Surg. 2014;207:95–101.

Vanermeulen EP, Van Aken H, Vermylen J. Anticoagulants and spinal-epidural anesthesia. Anesth Analg. 1994;79:1165–77.

Wun T, Paglieroni TG, Lachant NA. Desmopressin stimulates the expression of P-selectin on human platelets in vitro. J Lab Clin Med. 1995;126:401–9.

Zareh M, Davis A, Henderson S. Reversal of warfarin-induced hemorrhage in the emergency department. West J Emerg Med. 2011;12:386–92.

Image-Guided Percutaneous Spine and Rib Biopsy: Tools and Techniques

3

A. Orlando Ortiz and Joel Marden

Learning Objectives

1. To introduce tools that can be used for image-guided percutaneous spine and rib biopsy procedures
2. To learn when and how to use these instruments
3. To learn techniques that can be applied with these tools to improve their diagnostic utility
4. To learn the basic technical aspects of CT guidance in order to perform these procedures

3.1 Introduction

In order to properly and safely perform an image-guided percutaneous spine or rib biopsy procedure, the operator must select and correctly utilize the instruments that are necessary to perform that procedure. The operator must have a solid comfort level with a specific biopsy instrument and must understand how to use the tool. All of these instruments are packaged with product specifications and instructions for use. An operator is required to know the product specifications and to review the instructions for use prior to using the instrument. When an operator knows specific details about the instrument such as inner and outer diameter and length of a needle, then the operator will be able to easily utilize the instrument especially when deploying it with coaxial technique. If the operator is uncertain about which coaxial instrument matches or is compatible with another, then they should examine the tools and decide upon their use before the procedure. The operator should understand the advantages and disadvantages of each tool and be able to exploit the advantages of a given tool for a specific situation. For example, if the operator encounters a lytic osseous lesion and is not successful in retrieving tissue with a bone biopsy needle, then the operator can switch to a fine needle aspiration technique or use a soft tissue cutting needle instead (Fig. 3.1). In other words, the use of the correct tool can turn a nondiagnostic biopsy procedure into a procedure that not only yields a biopsy specimen but also the correct pathologic diagnosis.

Disclaimer

The demonstration of the instruments in this chapter does not constitute an endorsement of the product or the manufacturing company. Furthermore, the authors have absolutely no financial relationships with the manufacturers of these products, and no corporate entity has contributed to this endeavor. As the emphasis of this chapter is on the product type and the principles of application for a given product type, we have refrained from disclosing actual product names. Indeed, a large variety of

A.O. Ortiz, *Image-Guided Percutaneous Spine Biopsy*, DOI 10.1007/978-3-319-43326-4_3

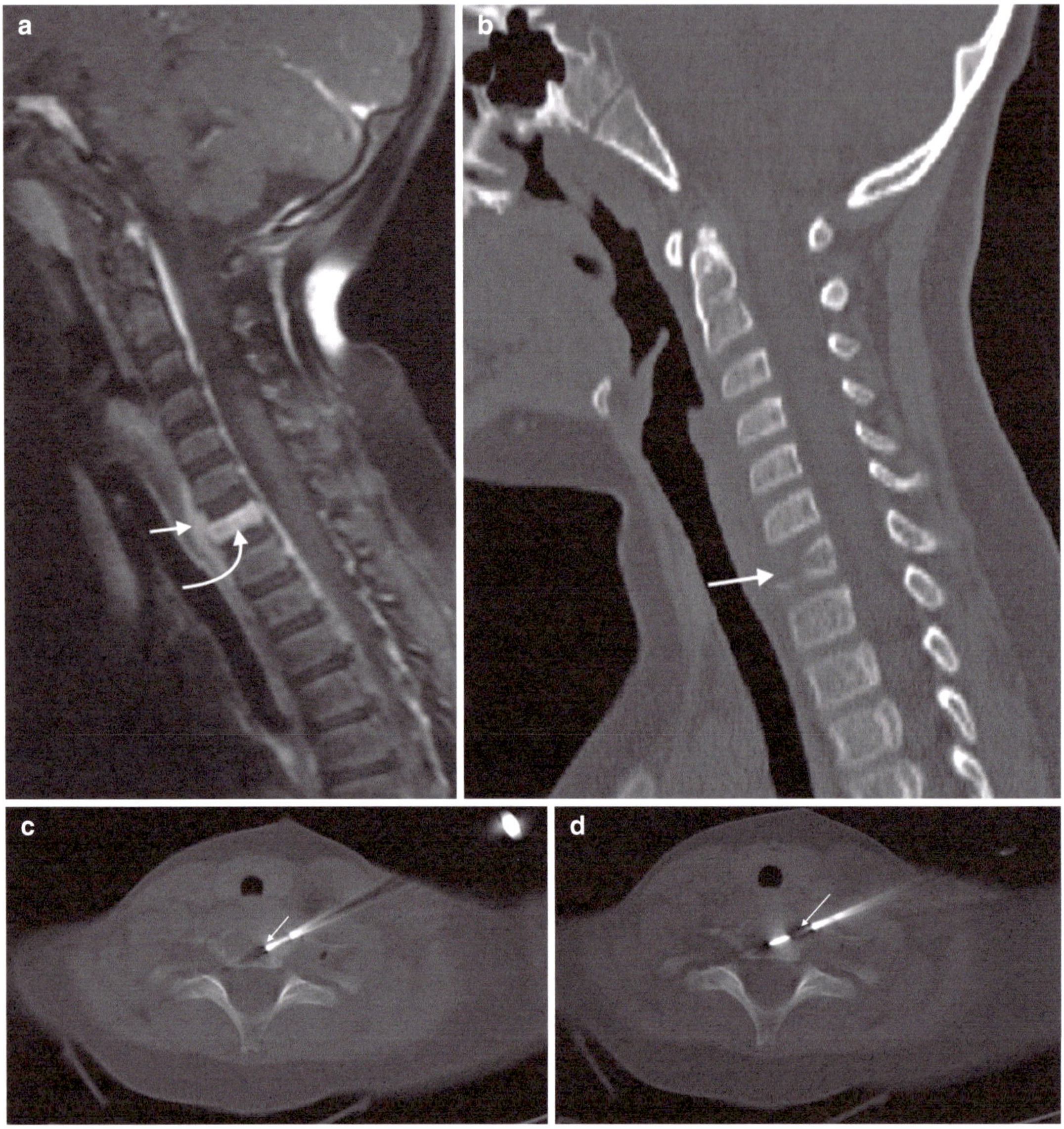

Fig. 3.1 A 5-year-old male with neck pain. Fat-suppressed contrast-enhanced T1-weighted sagittal image (**a**) shows a partial C7 vertebral compression deformity that is associated with diffuse contrast enhancement (*curved arrow*) and focal prevertebral soft tissue enhancement (*arrow*). Sagittal CT reformation in bone window algorithm (**b**) shows a partially lytic lesion (*arrow*) at C7. Axial CT image (**c**) from biopsy procedure shows coaxial insertion of a 14 gauge trephine bone needle (*arrow*) into the C7 vertebral body. Despite multiple attempts and maneuvers, a specimen could not be obtained. Axial CT image (**d**) shows that the bone needle has been exchanged coaxially for a 16 gauge soft tissue core biopsy needle (*arrow*). Two soft tissue cores were obtained and showed a pathologic diagnosis of Langerhans cell histiocytosis

percutaneous biopsy products are commercially available. Prospective users of these products can easily locate and purchase the necessary instruments in order to perform these biopsy procedures.

3.2 The Tools

Prior to performing image-guided percutaneous spine or rib biopsy, the operator should become familiar with spine and rib biopsy instruments and techniques. It is best for the operator to develop a fundamental understanding and

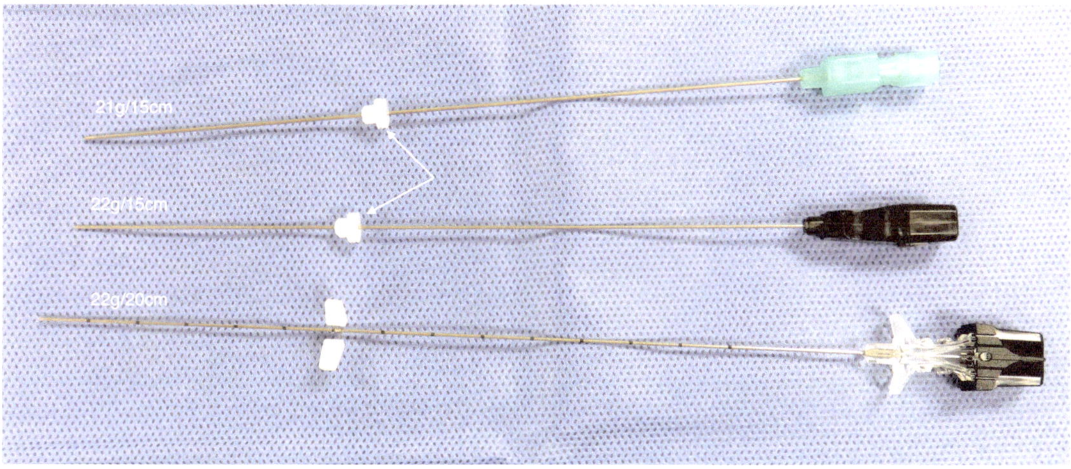

Fig. 3.2 Examples of FNA needles. The 21 gauge and 22 gauge 15 cm long needles have small adjustable depth markers (*arrows*). The 22 gauge 20 cm needle also has 1 cm markings

experience with a few basic tools of each type: fine needles, soft tissue cutting needles, and bone biopsy needles. This will enable the operator to develop sound techniques and understand which biopsy scenarios require specific instruments and in which order to utilize, integrate, or exchange these instruments.

Tools

1. Fine needle
2. Soft tissue core or cutting needle
3. Bone needle

3.2.1 Fine Needle Aspiration

Fine needle aspiration (FNA) is a relatively quick procedure to learn and perform, yet it takes a very long time to master this procedure. In the majority of cases, the needles that are used for the spine or rib biopsy procedure range in length from 10 to 20 cm (Fig. 3.2). The objective of this procedure is to make short to-and-fro excursions with a lengthy but small-bore cutting needle, in the range of 25–18 gauge, while applying continuous suction, with a small Luer-Lok syringe attached to the hub of the needle (Fig. 3.3). The suction is stopped immediately prior to removal of the needle tip from the lesion so as not to aspirate cells from normal tissue and to avoid aspiration of hemorrhagic fluid. The latter phenomena, unfortunately, is not an uncommon occurrence that confounds if not prevents a cytologic diagnosis. Lesions which may be amenable to FNA include soft tissue masses that are solid or composed of variable matrix, such as mixed solid cystic lesions (Table 3.1). FNA may be attempted on purely cystic masses in order to sample the cyst wall. When there is either a breach in the osseous cortex or a bone needle has penetrated into the marrow space of the vertebra or rib, it may be possible to perform FNA using a coaxial approach.

The key to performing a successful FNA procedure is preparation. After lesion analysis, for both matrix and measurement, the operator decides upon an approach that will safely access the lesion and provide the best opportunity for specimen yield. Factors that impact on maximizing specimen yield for sampling potentially neoplastic lesions include choosing a solid, non-necrotic portion of the lesion. This may consist of an area that shows contrast enhancement or avid FDG uptake on a pre-procedure examination. Choose a trajectory that maximizes the possibility of passes and the excursion distance of the biopsy needle inside of the lesion. Literally, try to get into the “meat” of the lesion with your biopsy passes and avoid the ill-defined areas where there may be necrosis, cyst fluid, or a possibility of sampling normal tissue. For infection, however, do sample the fluid-containing areas as these might be abscess collections. Given the

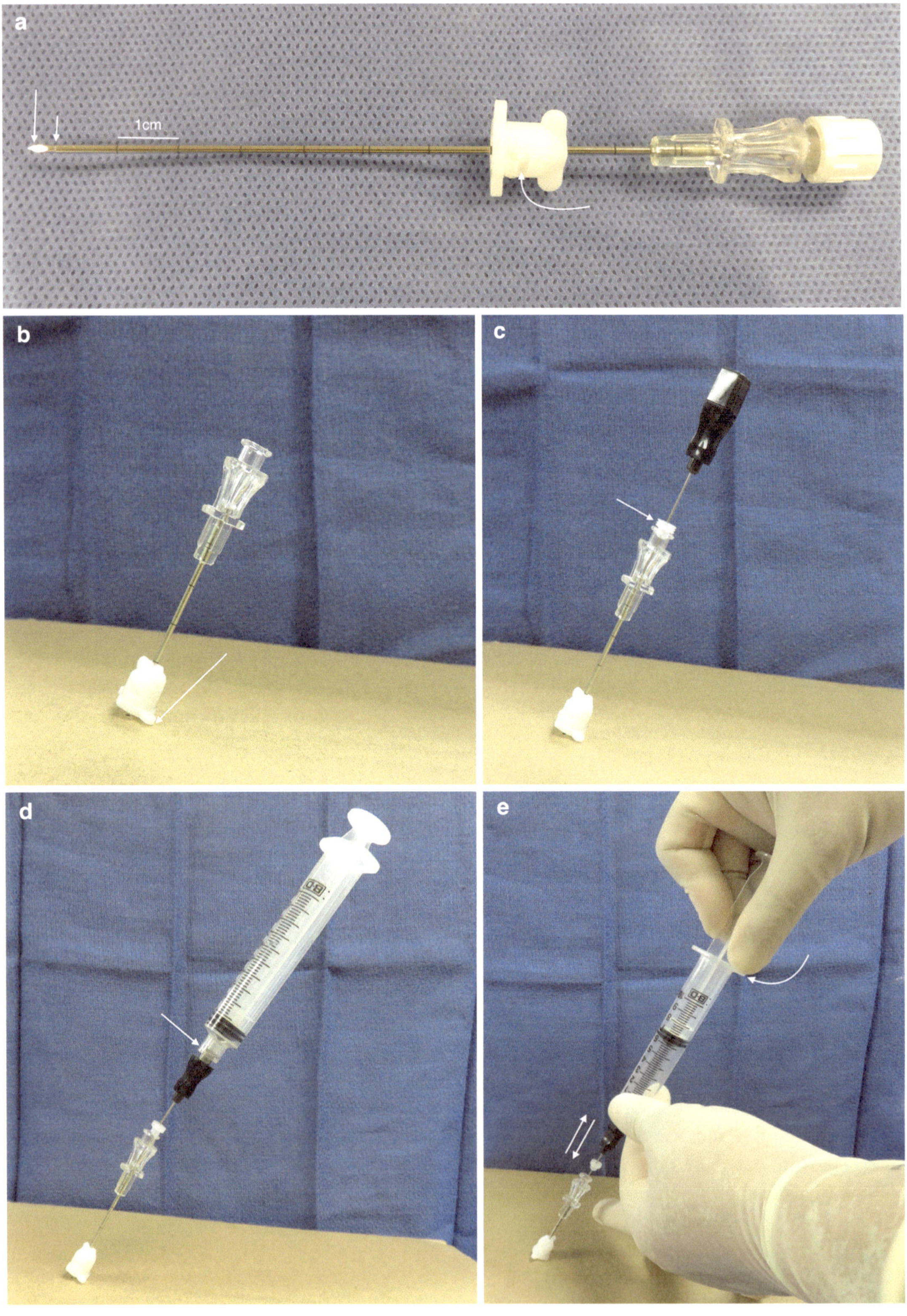
a
1cm
b
c
d
e

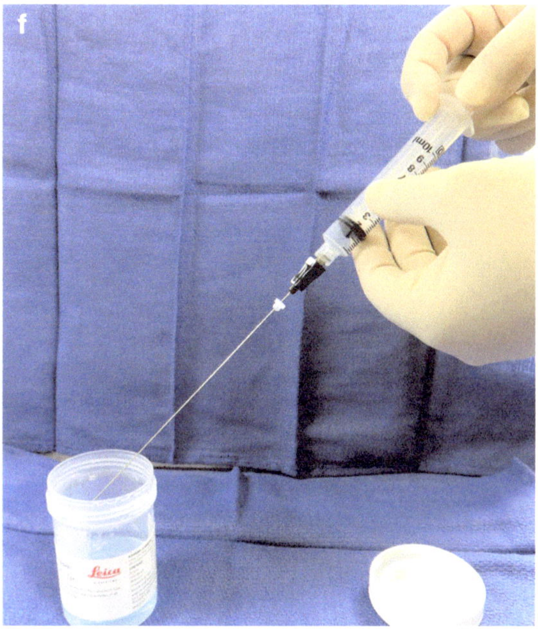

Fig. 3.3 (continued)

Table 3.1 Biopsy Techniques

1. Fine needle aspiration
Neoplasm
Solid soft tissue mass
Soft tissue mass composed of variable matrix
Hypervascular soft tissue mass (e.g., renal carcinoma metastasis)
Lesion involves the marrow cavity of the vertebra or rib
Infection
Disk
Paraspinal abscess
Facet joint
2. Soft Tissue Core Biopsy
Neoplasm
Extraosseous soft tissue mass
Intraosseous soft tissue mass: lytic lesion or marrow space occupying soft tissue lesion
Infection
Soft tissue phlegmon
Disk – may require an automated percutaneous diskectomy device
3. Bone Biopsy
Neoplasm
Vertebra or rib lesion (lytic, sclerotic, mixed lytic-sclerotic)
Infection
Disk-vertebral end plate
Facet joint

increased viscosity of the purulent abscess material, large gauge needles, such as 18 gauge or larger, should be considered for use when aspirating a suspected abscess collection.

When sampling a soft tissue mass with an FNA procedure, the objective is to separate a small cell cluster from the mass by using the cutting properties of the needle and then aspirate this cell cluster into the needle bore (Gupta et al. 2002). The to-and-fro or back-and-forth excursions of the FNA needle within the lesion should be short, quick, and choppy. Slight rotations of the needle within the lesion matrix help to exploit the cutting properties of the needle. Also, mild angulations of the needle as it is moved forward help to separate and break up the tissue planes along the needle trajectory. Consistent aspiration with the syringe, by pulling back on the plunger, is applied when the needle tip is within the lesion matrix. Small syringes, 5–10 mL, can be used with smaller gauge needles, such as 25 and 22 gauge needles. A 20 gauge syringe can be used with larger gauge needles, such as an 18 gauge needle, especially when attempting to aspirate an abscess collection. Some

Fig. 3.3 Photographs of step-by-step simulated demonstration of an FNA procedure; FNA can be used for soft tissue components of vertebral or rib lesions. A 17 gauge 10 cm guide needle (**a**) has a beveled tip (*large arrow*) that projects a few millimeters distal to the guide cannula tip (*small arrow*). The guide cannula has 1 cm markings which help guide and control advancement of the guide cannula. A plastic depth gauge has an adjustable lock (*curved arrow*) that prevents the guide cannula from being advanced further than this set point and helps to secure the guide cannula at the skin entry site. After guide needle placement (**b**) to the desired depth (*arrow*), the stylet is removed. A 22 gauge needle (**c**) is coaxially inserted through the guide needle to the desired depth (*arrow*). After the FNA needle is inserted into the lesion (**d**), the stylet is removed, and a 10 mL Luer-Lok syringe is attached to the needle hub (*arrow*). Aspiration (**e**) is performed by maintaining continuous suction (*curved arrow*) on the needle as it is moved slightly back and forth (*arrows*) within the lesion. After stopping the aspiration within the lesion, the needle is removed, and the specimen is either transferred to a slide or to the appropriate cytologic media (**f**) commercially available syringes and FNA systems have a locking mechanism that is activated by twisting the retracted plunger in order to provide continuous suction during the aspiration phase of the biopsy. The main property of the syringe is that it should have a Luer-Lok technology that allows for a good twist-on connection to the needle hub. This will prevent an air leak, which would otherwise foil the aspiration. After the operator completes the aspiration, the syringe plunger can be released in order to cease the aspiration. With a basic syringe and fine needle, this can occur with the needle tip still located within the lesion. The FNA needle is then withdrawn, and the sample is expressed either onto a slide or into a cytologic alcohol medium for subsequent microscopic analysis. In other FNA biopsy systems, the syringe plunger remains withdrawn until the operator is ready to deposit the sample, as pushing the plunger ejects the specimen (Fenton and Czervionke 2003). The presence of a cytotechnologist or pathologist greatly enhances the efficiency of the FNA process as these individuals can confirm whether or not the operator has obtained adequate specimens.

The FNA procedure becomes even safer and more efficient with the use of coaxial technique and CT guidance (Table 3.2). With the use of coaxial technique, a guide needle is advanced to the margin of the lesion. This avoids reentry injury to the skin and subcutaneous tissues and enhances patient comfort during the procedure. Coaxial technique provides a safe conduit to the lesion, subjecting adjacent critical structures to fewer chances of needle injury that might otherwise result from multiple needle passes. Once the guide needle is positioned, a CT image is obtained to confirm the position of the guide needle. The guide needle stylet is removed, and multiple sequential FNA passes can be made through the guide needle. The length of the FNA or insert needle should be greater than the length of the guide needle so as to allow for the appropriate movement or excursion of the insert needle within the lesion. The FNA needle is advanced into the margin of the lesion using CT guidance. The FNA needle stylet is removed, and a syringe is connected to the FNA needle hub. By analyzing the CT image, the operator will know how long to make the needle excursions and in which directions. An aspiration is performed, and the needle is removed and replaced by another needle in order to repeat the process. With each needle exchange, a CT image is studied in order to assess the position of the guide needle and the FNA needle relative to the lesion and the adjacent critical structures. By moving and angling the guide cannula hub slightly, the operator is able to redirect the FNA needle in a slightly different trajectory within the lesion. At least three FNA passes should be performed or more if necessary and possible. If specimen is obtained upon the initial passes and the cytopathologist is confident about the diagnosis, then the procedure can be stopped at the discretion of the operator and the pathologist.

Table 3.2 FNA CT-guided percutaneous spine or rib biopsy

Step	Comment
Localize	Use CT and a skin grid to localize the lesion Mark the skin entry site
Sterilize	Prep and drape the area of the skin entry site
Anesthetize	Use local anesthetic agent at the skin entry site and adjacent to the periosteal surface or lesion margin; use intravenous sedation or analgesia or anesthesia
Advance	Guide needle to the margin of the lesion under CT guidance
Confirm	Guide needle position, lesion dimensions to determine excursions of the fine needle within the lesion, relative to nearby critical structures
Insert	Fine needle
Prepare	Remove fine needle stylet and carefully attach an aspiration syringe
Aspirate	Use continuous suction within the lesion as the fine needle is moved within the lesion; cease aspiration when retrieving the fine needle from the lesion
Specimen delivery	Onto slide or cytologic alcohol media
Repeat FNA	Ideally, three passes or as many as safely possible

A soft tissue core biopsy can be performed after the FNA passes. These soft tissue cores provide additional specimen that might be helpful in the event that special stains are required for further analysis of the tissue in question. The FNA procedure should be performed first because soft tissue core biopsy tends to cause intralesional hemorrhage, and this blood contaminates the cytologic specimen and compromises the cytologic diagnosis.

3.2.2 Soft Tissue Core Biopsy

Soft tissue core biopsy is very helpful in the evaluation of soft tissue masses (Ray-Coquard et al. 2003). This procedure is frequently performed for the evaluation of spine and rib lesions. Initially, this statement appears to be counterintuitive. Many operators assume that this procedure will have no utility in the sampling of osseous structures but, with experience, realize that there are a plethora of destructive lesions that breach the osseous margins of the spine or rib and, therefore, are amenable to soft tissue sampling techniques (Fig. 3.1). A few different types of core biopsy needles are available for soft tissue biopsy. The majority of these, as evidenced by their bulky design, have been developed for use elsewhere in the body. Nevertheless, there are a few of these core biopsy systems that can be used for spine or rib biopsy (Figs. 3.4 and 3.5). The critical aspect of core soft tissue biopsy is a combination of the furthest distance which the needle tip travels within the lesion and the length of the coring chamber that can be deployed within the lesion matrix. In some needle systems, the needle is placed at the proximal margin of the lesion, and the cutting mechanism is activated such that the needle travels a preset distance within the lesion in order to obtain a sample (Fig. 3.6). In other systems the needle tip is advanced deep enough into the lesion in order to subsequently expose the biopsy chamber within the matrix of the lesion so as to then obtain a soft tissue core sample (Fig. 3.4). Yet in another system, the needle is advanced into the lesion, and the biopsy chamber is temporarily exposed within the lesion and then retracted when the biopsy device is fully loaded; when the device is activated or fired, it sends the core needle back into its original position within the lesion with immediate, near simultaneous deployment of the cutting cannula (Fig. 3.7). The practical aspect of soft tissue core biopsy is to be aware of when these needles can be used during the biopsy process. Key factors that influence this decision are the presence of a large soft tissue mass and absence of osseous matrix along the needle trajectory. These are soft tissue cutting needles, not bone cutting needles, and their use for osseous lesions or in the setting of osseous material requires careful and thoughtful preparation. The use of a soft tissue cutting needle within the bone may result in bending or breakage of the needle tip; the needle may get stuck within the lesion which then will require a very extensive conversation with the patient and may require a surgical procedure to remove the device (Fig. 3.8). Only when there is a breach in the osseous margin of a lesion, or a coaxial channel has been made with a larger gauge bone needle, should the operator consider the possibility of approaching a lytic lesion or a marrow space lesion with a soft tissue core biopsy needle.

Soft tissue core needle biopsy is best performed using coaxial technique with a guide needle and CT guidance (Table 3.3). This will facilitate multiple safe biopsy needle passes and maximize the harvest of biopsy specimen. The use of large diameter biopsy needles (e.g., 14 gauge) is desirable, but this is determined by the lesion size and location relative to critical structures and balanced against the risk of hemorrhage. The larger diameter needles are able to obtain larger soft tissue cores, and this in turn improves the likelihood of obtaining a pathologic diagnosis. The guide needle and the soft tissue cutting needle are usually packaged in the same kit; the working diameter of these needles is therefore preset to facilitate coaxial technique. The guide needle is advanced to the margin of the lesion under CT guidance; the stylet of the guide needle is removed prior to insertion of the biopsy needle. Measurements are then made along the trajectory from the guide needle to the opposite margin of the lesion. This enables the operator to determine the optimal length of the biopsy "throw," or core length, within the lesion matrix. Most soft tissue core biopsy needles have preset "throw" lengths (penetration or depth settings) that can be selected; the length of the "throw" should be less than the diameter of the lesion along the needle trajectory. Once the biopsy needle sample length is selected and set, then the biopsy needle is "loaded" or armed. The biopsy needle can now be deployed at the operator's discretion in order to obtain a soft tissue core. Some biopsy needles can be loaded prior to coaxial

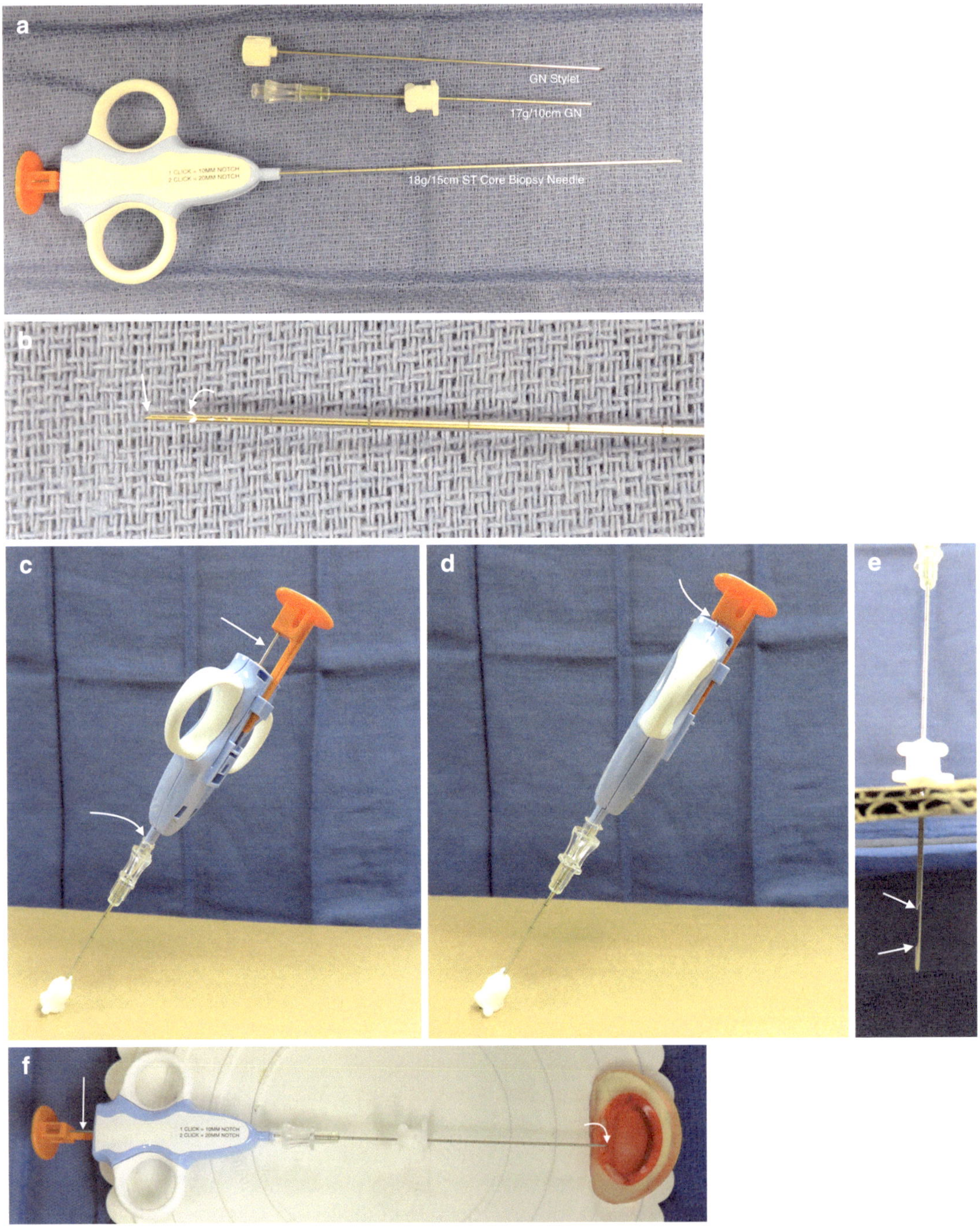

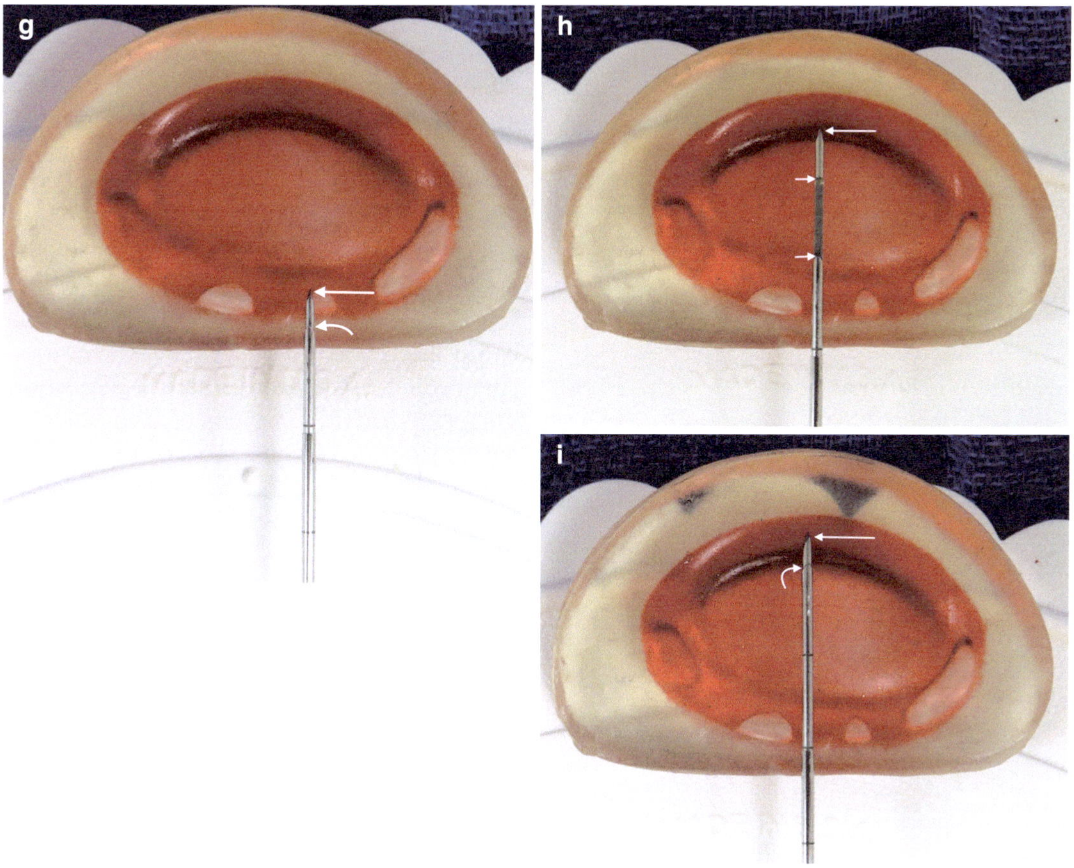

Fig. 3.4 (continued)

Fig. 3.4 Photographs of a semiautomated soft tissue core biopsy needle. The 18 gauge 15 cm length soft tissue core biopsy needle (**a**) fits coaxially through the 17 gauge 10 cm length guide needle. Close-up of needle (**b**) shows that the diamond tip needle stylet (*arrow*) projects a few millimeters beyond the cutting edge of the outer cannula (*curved arrow*). Once the guide cannula is positioned and its stylet removed (**c**), the core biopsy needle is inserted (*curved arrow*) into the guide cannula. The needle can be loaded (*arrow*) prior to or during the insertion; in this case the size of the core biopsy chamber can be set to either 1 or 2 cm. After imaging confirmation of the position of the core biopsy needle within the proximal lesion margin (**d**), the needle plunger is pushed forward, but not activated, as seen by the small gap (curved arrow). This exposes the needle's biopsy chamber (*arrows*) within the lesion (**e**); this step would also require imaging confirmation. Simulation (**f**) of these maneuvers shows loaded or primed core needle (*arrow*) with the needle tip at the margin of the lesion (*curved arrow*). Closeup view of the needle (**g**) shows the stylet tip within the proximal lesion (*arrow*) and the biopsy cannula edge (*curved arrow*) at the lesion margin. By pushing the plunger forward (**h**), but not activating the cutting mechanism, the core biopsy chamber (*small arrows*) is exposed (in this case for a distance of 1 cm) within the lesion, while the needle tip (*large arrow*) extends toward the distal lesion margin. Additional forward pressure on the plunger (**i**) triggers the cutting mechanism, and the cutting edge of the cannula (*curved arrow*) slides over the biopsy chamber to sequester tissue within it; the tip of the needle stylet (*arrow*) remains in position near the distal lesion margin

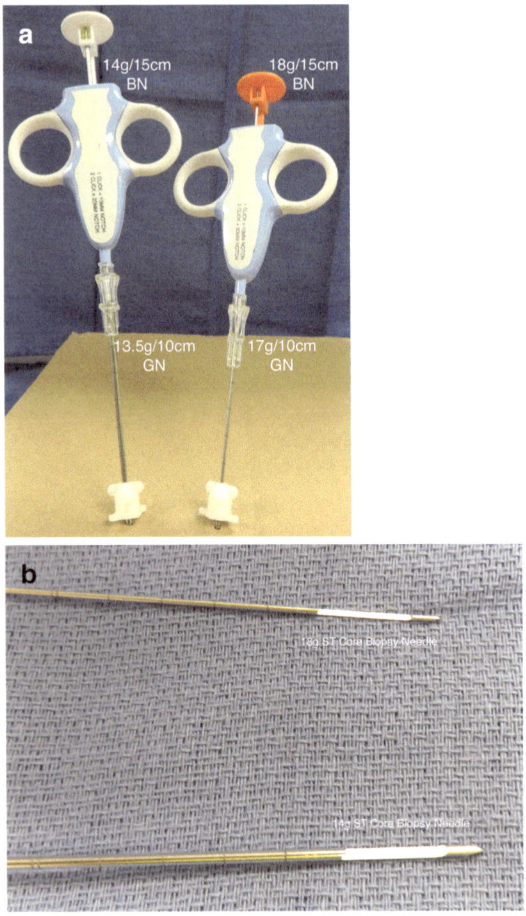

Fig. 3.5 Comparison of two soft tissue core biopsy needle sizes. The 14 gauge biopsy needle is not only larger than the 18 gauge biopsy needle (**a**) but also has a larger core biopsy chamber (**b**). A larger needle is able to harvest more tissue

insertion into the guide cannula, and some may require arming after coaxial insertion. CT guidance is required to monitor coaxial needle insertion. A specific semiautomated biopsy system with a lightweight handle allows the core chamber to be exposed within the substance of the lesion prior to firing or activating the cutting mechanism of the needle. This can be imaged with CT in order to show the exposed core chamber within the lesion and confirm the accuracy and safety of the biopsy needle location. The position and the throw length of other soft tissue core needle biopsy systems should always be confirmed using CT guidance. By activating the firing mechanism of the biopsy needle, a core sample is promptly obtained. The firing mechanism is activated by either pressing or sliding a button on the top or side of the needle handle or pressing on the plunger of the needle handle. The cutting needle is removed from the biopsy needle, and the stylet is placed within the guide needle to secure it and minimize back-bleeding. The soft tissue core is then removed from the core biopsy needle and placed in the appropriate transport medium for subsequent pathologic analysis. This often requires some form of manipulation of the soft tissue core with a small needle or a scalpel in order to dislodge the sample from the biopsy chamber. The biopsy needle can be reused if sterile technique has been maintained, or perhaps a different biopsy needle can be used, with a different diameter depending on the lesion in question. An attempt should be made to obtain four soft tissue cores, if possible, in order to optimize the diagnostic yield (Wu et al. 2008).

It should be kept in mind that some of the soft tissue core biopsy needles, which are used for biopsy applications in other body parts, are somewhat "top heavy" with respect to the needle handle. A bulky needle handle may cause the biopsy needle to bend just outside the guide cannula with resultant needle tip deflection from the intended target. The spine and ribs are not located that far from the skin surface, thus deeper placement of the guide cannula (a method used to stabilize the biopsy needle) in these cases is not always feasible. In these situations, the operator can either choose a soft tissue core biopsy system with a lightweight handle or they can hold the biopsy needle handle with a long clamp in order to perform the biopsy under CT guidance. The latter maneuver entails some radiation exposure to the operator.

3.2.3 Intervertebral Disk Biopsy

Soft tissue core biopsy of the intervertebral disk is performed to evaluate for the presence of infection (Table 3.4). Attempting to obtain disk

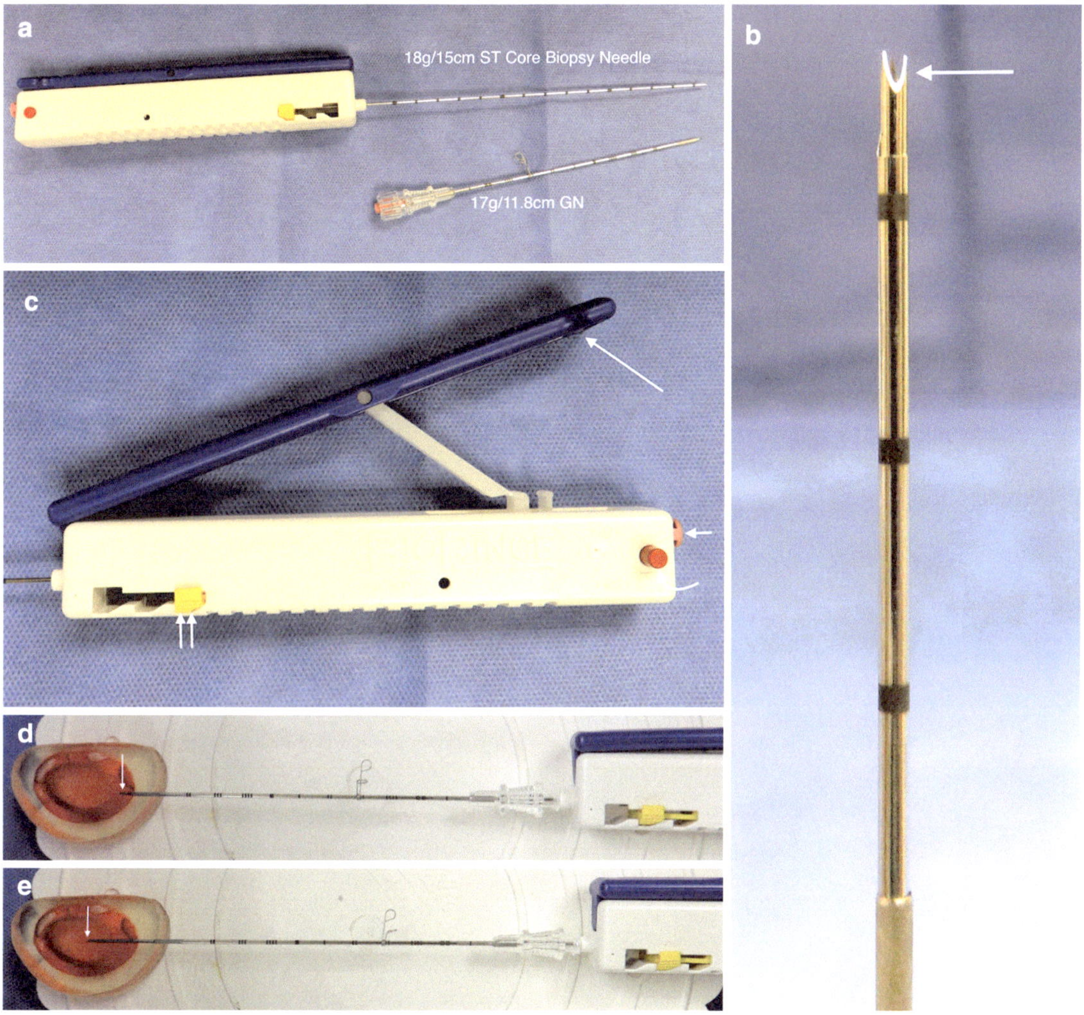

Fig. 3.6 Photographs of a soft tissue core biopsy needle. This 18 gauge 15 cm length (**a**) soft tissue core biopsy needle is used with a 17 gauge 11.8 cm guide needle. Closeup view (**b**) of the cutting tip (*arrow*) of the needle. This biopsy needle (**c**) is loaded by cocking the side handle (*arrow*); a side safety button (*curved arrow*) must be adjusted prior to activating the cutting mechanism by pressing the back button (*small arrow*). Simulation (**d**) of the positioning of the needle (*arrow*) relative to the proximal lesion margin prior to biopsy. After triggering the cutting mechanism (**e**), the needle moves forward within the lesion (*arrow*) a preset distance of 13, 23, or 33 millimeters. The needle would then be removed from the lesion out of the guide cannula in order to then harvest the specimen

material with FNA or soft core techniques is quite challenging. Due to its intrinsic annulus fibrosis architecture, disk tissue is quite adherent. Infected disk material is also adherent and very viscous. Small bore needles have shown limited success in obtaining biopsy material from the disk. Many operators end up injecting a small amount of sterile saline or anesthetic agent in order to obtain a disk lavage. This traditional approach may account for many false negative or "no growth" disk biopsy procedures for suspected infection. Many soft tissue core needles possess penetration lengths that are not suitable or safe for disk biopsy. Furthermore, the possibility of needle damage may occur when the biopsy needle is fired and strikes the vertebral

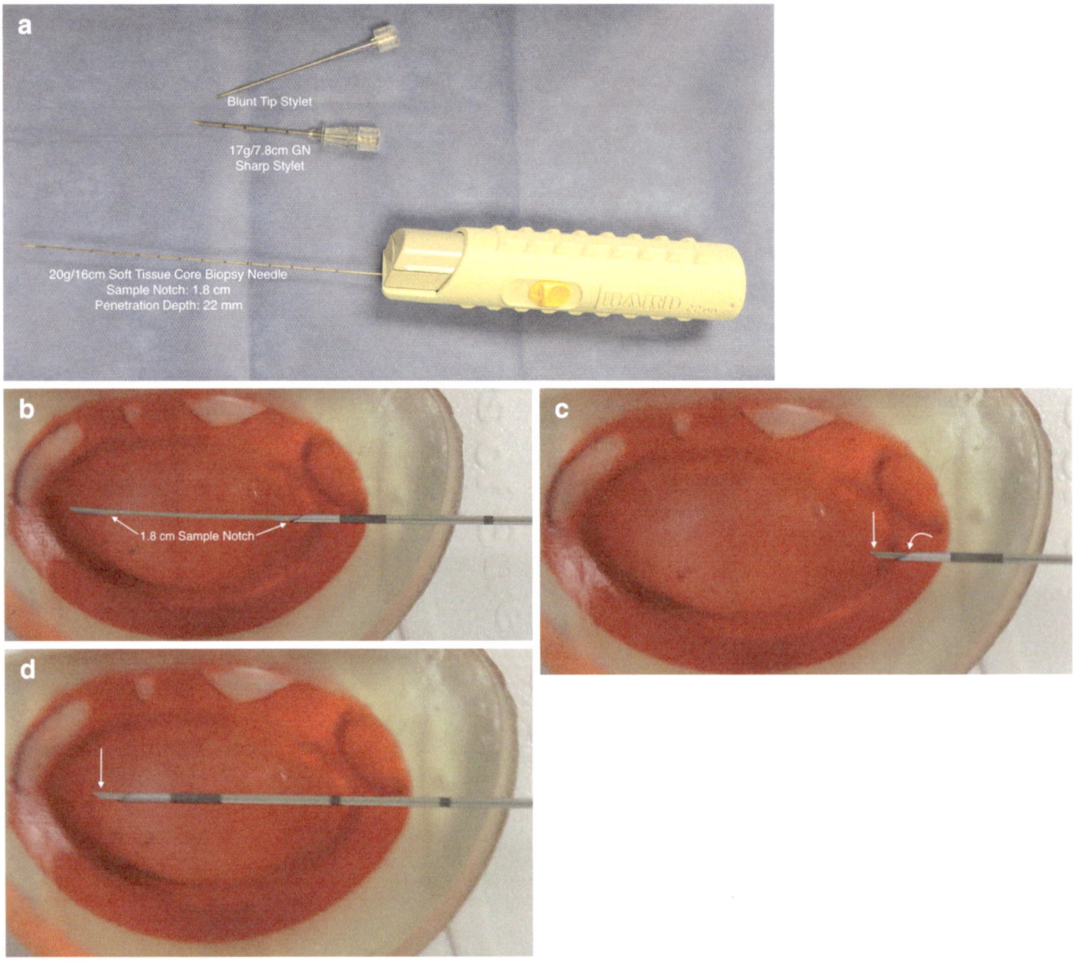

Fig. 3.7 Photographs of a soft tissue core biopsy needle. This 20 gauge 16 cm soft tissue core biopsy needle (**a**) is used coaxially with a 17 gauge 7.8 cm guide needle. Simulation (**b**) shows that the initial loading of this needle exposes the biopsy chamber within the lesion for a distance of 1.8 cm (*arrows*). The needle (**c**) is now set to biopsy and retracts to the proximal lesion margin; there is a 4 mm offset between the needle stylet tip (*arrow*) and the cutting outer cannula (*curved arrow*). After the cutting mechanism is activated (**d**), the needle extends forward into the lesion (*arrow*) to obtain the soft tissue core

end plate. In this latter situation, it is possible that the needle may get stuck within the disk space or its somewhat fragile tip may fracture. Since the goal of any biopsy procedure is to obtain diagnostic tissue or specimen, it is reasonable to perform removal of a small amount of diagnostic disk tissue using a percutaneous diskectomy device (Yu et al. 1991) (Fig. 3.9). This procedure is best performed with fluoroscopic guidance in order to monitor the position of the device at all times throughout the diskectomy procedure. These devices reliably obtain tissue from the disk (Wattamwar and Ortiz 2010).

3.3 Bone Biopsy

Three basic bone biopsy techniques

1. Single needle
2. Tandem needle
3. Coaxial needle

3.3.1 Vertebra or Rib

There are essentially three basic techniques that have been developed to perform image-guided

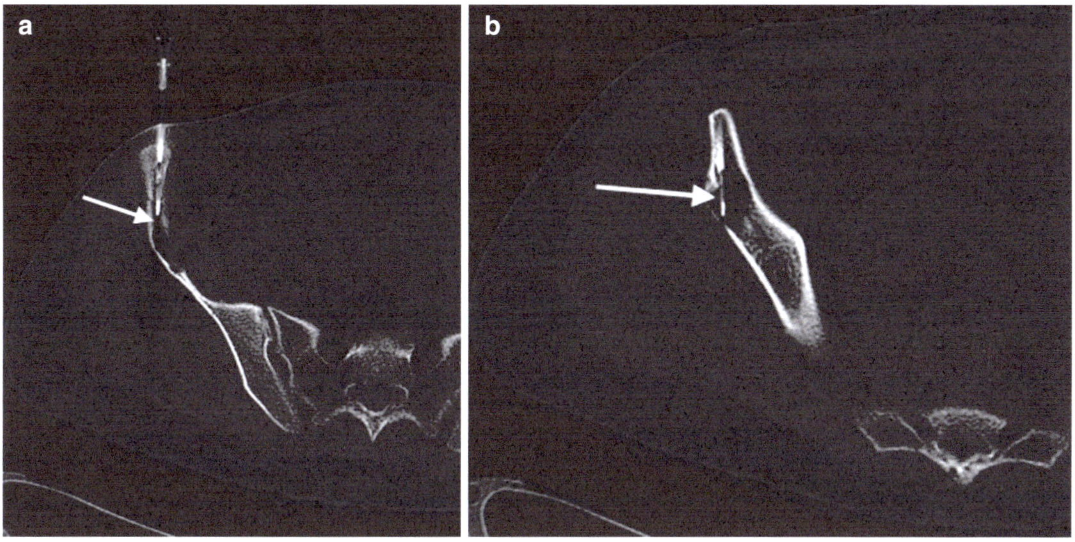

Fig. 3.8 Biopsy complication: broken needle. Axial CT image (**a**) shows guide cannula in place within the iliac crest. An attempt was made to biopsy the lytic lesion (*arrow*) with a soft tissue core biopsy needle. Axial CT image (**b**) shows the distal tip of the needle (*arrow*) lodged within the lesion. This was left within the lesion and the patient was informed of the complication

Table 3.3 Soft tissue core biopsy in CT-guided percutaneous spine or rib biopsy

Step	Comment
Localize	Use CT and a skin grid to localize the lesion
	Mark the skin entry site
Sterilize	Prep and drape the area of the skin entry site
Anesthetize	Use a local anesthetic agent at the skin entry site and adjacent to the periosteal surface or lesion margin; use intravenous sedation and/or analgesia or anesthesia
Advance	Guide needle to the margin of the lesion under CT guidance
Confirm	Guide needle position, lesion dimensions to determine excursions of the biopsy needle within the lesion and its proximity to critical structures
Insert	Biopsy needle
Prepare	Load the firing mechanism of the biopsy needle; this is done either before or after needle positioning based upon the biopsy needle specifications
Position	Position the tip of the biopsy needle such that the ultimate location of the biopsy chamber falls within the lesion matrix
Confirm	Biopsy needle position under CT guidance
Activate	The cutting mechanism of the biopsy needle to obtain a soft tissue core
Specimen delivery	Into a specimen container
Repeat core biopsy	Ideally four soft tissue cores or as many as safely possible

percutaneous bone biopsy (Fenton and Czervionke 2003). These are (1) single needle technique, (2) tandem needle technique, and (3) coaxial needle technique. These techniques are listed in this specific order as this represents the practical evolution of bone biopsy techniques with advances in both the tool and imaging technologies. As the term implies, single needle technique entails the use of one needle that is advanced to the target under imaging guidance (Fig. 3.10). The stylet of the needle is removed prior to advancing the bone needle through the lesion in order to obtain a core specimen. The bone needle is removed, and the specimen is then transferred from the needle, by using an obturator to eject the specimen from the bone needle

Table 3.4 Fluoroscopy-guided intervertebral disk biopsy

Step	Comment
Localize	Use fluoroscopy to identify the target disk
	Position the fluoroscope
	Align the target disk – use a "Scotty dog" orientation
Sterilize	Prep and drape the area of the skin entry site
	Mark the skin entry site
Anesthetize	Use local anesthetic agent at the skin entry site and adjacent to the disk margin Use intravenous sedation and/or analgesia or anesthesia
Advance	Guide needle to the margin of disk
Confirm	Use multidirectional fluoroscopy to check the needle position and direction with frontal, lateral, and oblique projections
Advance	Guide needle into the disk
Confirm	Position of the guide needle within the periphery of the disk with fluoroscopy
Insert	Percutaneous diskectomy device after removing the guide needle stylet
Confirm	Location of the tip of the diskectomy probe with fluoroscopy
Activate	Percutaneous diskectomy device and maneuver it within the disk under fluoroscopic guidance
Specimen delivery	Remove specimen from the device and transfer it into a specimen container
Repeat	At least three passes
Exchange	For a bone biopsy system to biopsy the disk end plate complex
	Use an over-the-wire needle coaxial technique (recommended) or insert a separate bone needle
Confirm	Position of the coaxial system or bone needle with imaging guidance
Perform biopsy	Obtain core tissue sample(s) and place in the appropriate transport media
Repeat	Will need at least two cores – one for pathology and one or more for microbiology, hence the value of coaxial technique

lumen, into the appropriate transport media (Fig. 3.11). This was the technique with which percutaneous bone biopsy procedures were first performed (Robertson and Ball. 1935). This was and remains a single-pass procedure. Once the needle is removed from the biopsy tract, then in order to make a second pass, the operator must essentially start the majority of the procedure over again. Because the bone needle is passing through critical structures, the potential for a complication is greater with this type of technique.

Tandem needle techniques were developed in order to improve the accuracy of biopsy needle placement. A small-gauge needle is initially placed along the intended biopsy trajectory using imaging guidance. This first needle can also be used to administer an anesthetic agent. The first needle helps to guide subsequent bone biopsy needle placement with improved targeting and also helps to avoid critical structures along the biopsy trajectory (Fig. 3.12). The second or bone biopsy needle is inserted in close proximity to the first needle and advanced along a parallel or tandem trajectory under imaging guidance. The bone needle is then used, as with single needle technique, to obtain one bone core. The bone needle is removed, but the first needle is left in place to maintain the desired trajectory should a subsequent bone biopsy needle pass be attempted. Tandem needle technique is an improvement upon single needle technique and is still used by some operators.

Coaxial needle technique reflects the benefits of improved bone biopsy needle technology. The objectives of these techniques are to collect multiple bone cores while minimizing access site trauma. These techniques are useful for both spine and rib biopsy procedures. A crosshair

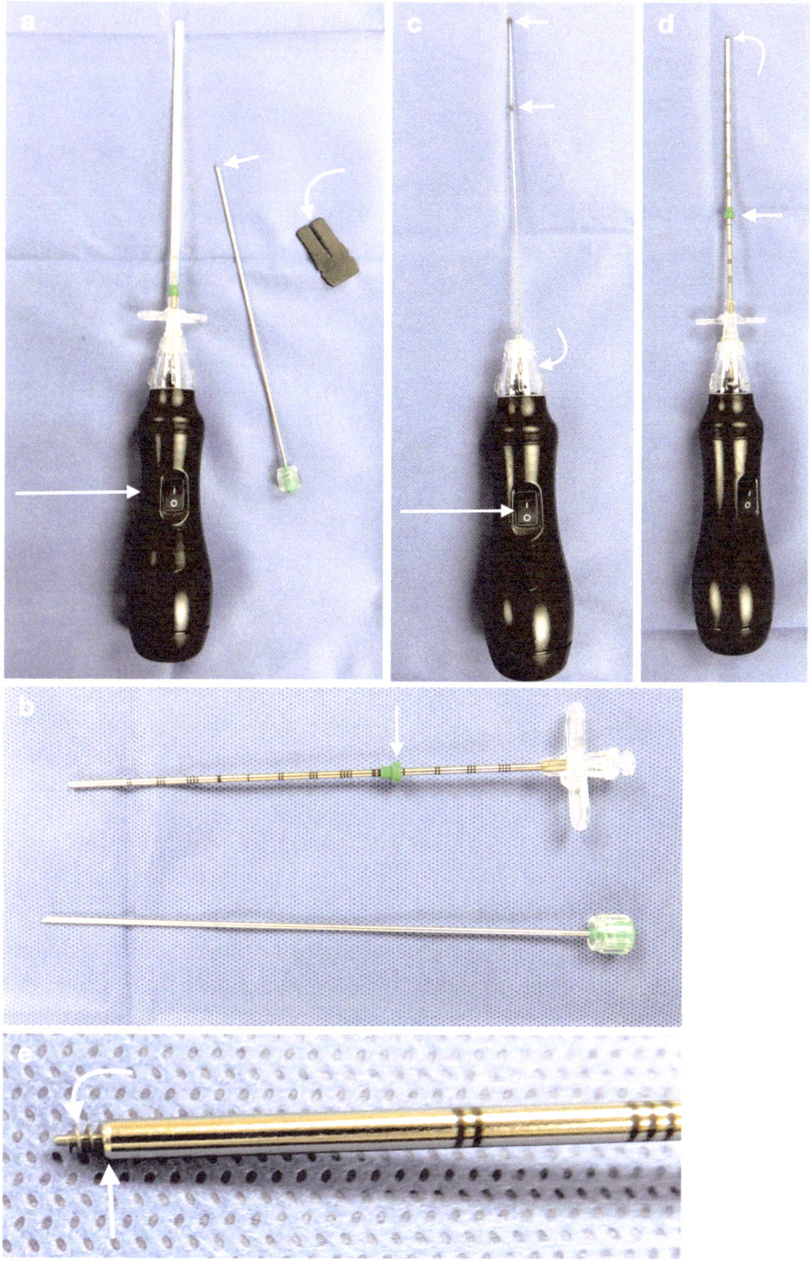

Fig. 3.9 Photographs of a percutaneous diskectomy device (**a**). This device (*large arrow*) is used coaxially with a 13 gauge 6 inch cannula that is first advanced with a beveled tip stylet (*small arrow*); the probe cleaner (*curved arrow*) is used to obtain the specimen. A depth marker (*arrow*) is located on the guide cannula (**b**). The battery operated diskectomy probe (**c**) has an on/off switch (*large arrow*), a collection chamber (*curved arrow*) and proximal and distal (*small arrows*) augers on the auger shaft. When the guide cannula is within the disk (**d**), the diskectomy probe is inserted into the guide cannula; the depth marker (*arrow*) will allow the operator to visually monitor the maximal insertion distance of the probe (*curved arrow*) into the disk. Closeup view of cannula/diskectomy probe (**e**) shows distal auger (*curved arrow*) protruding just beyond the guide cannula (*arrow*). Closeup view of distal auger shaft (**f**) shows proximal and distal augers; the probe cleaner (*curved arrow*) is used to clear specimen from the auger shaft and augers

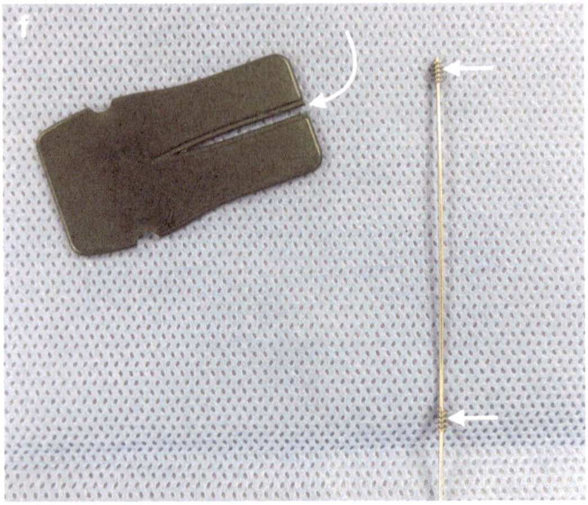

Fig. 3.9 (continued)

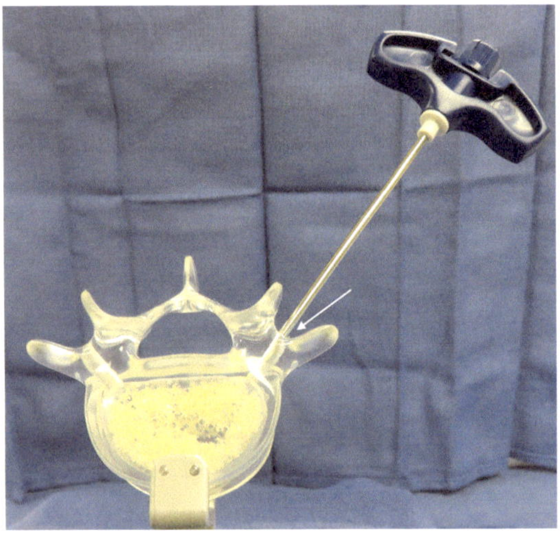

Fig. 3.10 Photograph of single needle technique for bone biopsy. An 11 gauge 10 cm long bone needle has been inserted into vertebral body using a transpedicular approach (*arrow*)

incision with a small scalpel at the skin entry site helps to facilitate the initial needle punctures and the advancement of the bone needle cannula. With this technique, a larger diameter needle or cannula is advanced either to the periosteal margin or within the proximal aspect of the vertebra or rib. This larger diameter cannula serves as a guiding cannula for the placement of smaller diameter but longer length, biopsy needles. There are two major methods for performing coaxial technique: (1) use of over-the-wire biopsy systems and (2) use of a larger guiding bone needle cannula (Table 3.5). Some bone biopsy kits come with an introducer or guide needle that has a removable hub (Geremia et al. 1992). Alternatively, some operators will use a long introducer needle and cut the hub (Yaffe et al. 2003). With the former technique, this introducer or guide needle is advanced to the periosteal margin (Fig. 3.13). The introducer needle is used to administer an anesthetic agent over the periosteal surface. The hub of the introducer needle is then removed, and this guide needle now serves as a guidewire for the subsequent insertion and advancement of a combined guide cannula and tapered introducer (Fig. 3.14). This combined needle set consists of an inner tapered introducer or blunt dissector and an outer guide cannula. The blunt-tipped guide cannula introducer facilitates the passage of the guide cannula over the guidewire and minimizes any traumatic injury to the underlying soft tissues. Once the guide cannula reaches the periosteal surface, then the guidewire and blunt-tipped introducer are removed and exchanged for a bone biopsy needle. It is important for the operator to hold the guide cannula in place with one hand, stabilizing it against the periosteal surface, while performing the bone biopsy needle exchange with the other hand. The bone biopsy needle is then advanced into the bone by a combination of forward pressure and rotation of the biopsy needle handle. Another form of coaxial technique entails the initial placement of a bone needle with imaging guidance (Figs. 3.15, 3.16, and 3.17). The bone needle stylet is removed, and smaller diameter bone needles of a length longer than the first or guiding bone cannula can be inserted in coaxial fashion. These maneuvers along with all needle exchanges are carefully and sequentially monitored with imaging guidance (Fig. 3.18). The sequential bone biopsy needle placements can increase the specimen yield (Fig. 3.18). Another method that can be used to obtain more specimen entails angling the

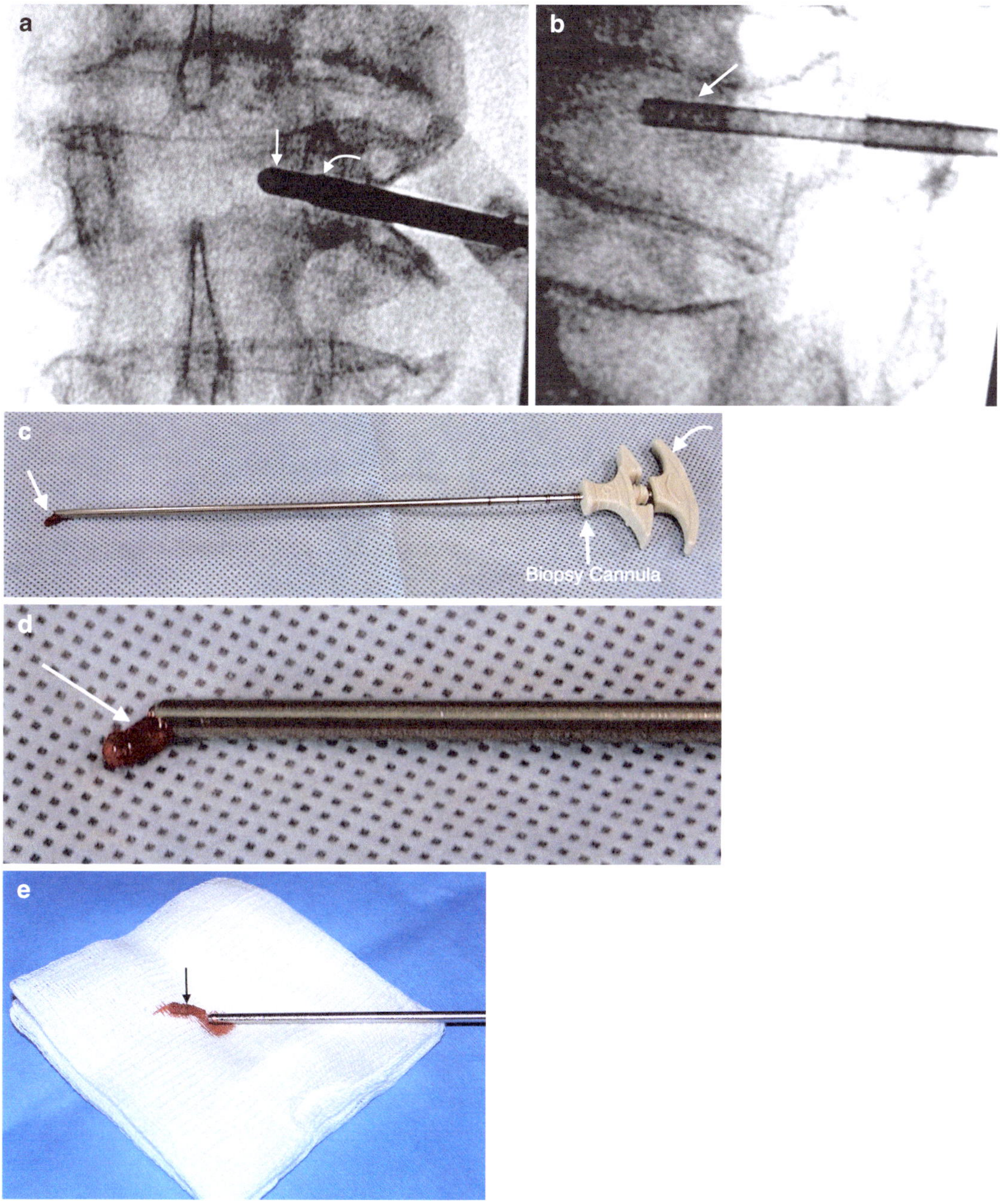

Fig. 3.11 An 84-year-old male with prior history of prostate cancer and a painful vertebral compression fracture. Frontal (**a**) and lateral (**b**) fluoroscopic images show transpedicular placement of an 8 gauge guide cannula (*curved needle*) and bone biopsy needle (*arrow*) into the vertebral body. The specimen (*arrow*) is expressed from the biopsy cannula (**c**) with an obturator (*curved arrow*). A closeup view (**d**) of the specimen (*arrow*). This large bone biopsy needle (**e**) is able to yield large biopsy specimens (*arrow*)

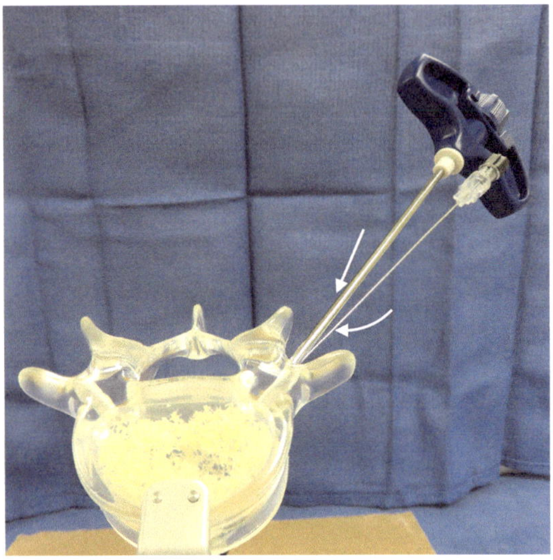

Fig. 3.12 Photograph of tandem needle technique for bone biopsy. The 22 gauge spinal needle (curved arrow) is used to not only administer a local anesthetic agent but also serve as a guide for subsequent bone biopsy needle (*arrow*) placement

Table 3.5 Image-guided percutaneous bone biopsy

Over the wire (OTW)	Non-OTW
Place the introducer needle under imaging guidance, anesthetize, remove needle hub	Anesthetize deep soft tissues and periosteum using a 22 or 20 gauge spinal needle
Advance the combined blunt dissector/guide cannula over the now hub-less guidewire under imaging guidance	Advance the bone needle into the periosteum under imaging guidance
Remove the guidewire and blunt dissector while stabilizing the guide cannula with the other hand	Bone needle is "parked" within the osseous cortex
Exchange immediately for a bone biopsy needle that fits coaxially into the guide cannula	Exchange the bone needle stylet for a bone biopsy needle that fits coaxially into the bone cannula
Perform sequential bone biopsies under imaging guidance	Perform sequential bone biopsies under imaging guidance
Obtain three or more bone cores whenever possible	Obtain three or more bone cores whenever possible

guide cannula and bone needle slightly in order to redirect the trajectory and sample another area within the bone (Fig. 3.19). Using larger gauge bone biopsy needles also facilitates increased specimen yield (Fig. 3.11). Whenever possible, the operator should attempt to collect at least three bone cores (Wu et al. 2008).

Stylet-bearing bone needles can have differ-

> The application of coaxial biopsy techniques improves the efficiency and safety of spine and rib biopsy procedures and contributes favorably to patient comfort. There are two major methods for performing coaxial technique:
>
> 1. Use of an over-the-wire biopsy system
> 2. Use of a larger guiding bone needle/cannula

tion. Always remember that a bone needle can be advanced quite easily through bone that has been damaged or weakened by pathologic processes such as infection or tumor. Therefore, careful needle advancement should be monitored with imaging guidance at all times. In order to obtain specimen, the operator must remove the bone needle stylet and advance the bone needle cannula through the lesion. Alternatively, with coaxial technique, a bone cannula is advanced through the guide cannula and into the lesion. The presumably abnormal bone tissue within the path of the bone needle cannula accumulates with the bone needle lumen as the cannula is advanced under imaging guidance. After the bone cannula has been advanced at least 3–4 mm, it can be removed; this is quite dependent on the lesion size and the ease of needle advancement. There are different methods that are used to retain the accumulated tissue within the bone needle lumen. One method entails removing the bone needle directly. Sometimes, this maneuver does not retain the bone tissue, and this situation may require reinsertion of the bone needle with additional advancement of the bone needle in order to secure a sample of tissue. Another method for securing the specimen within the biopsy cannula entails placing continuous suction on the bone needle with a Luer-Lok syringe that is attached to the hub of the bone

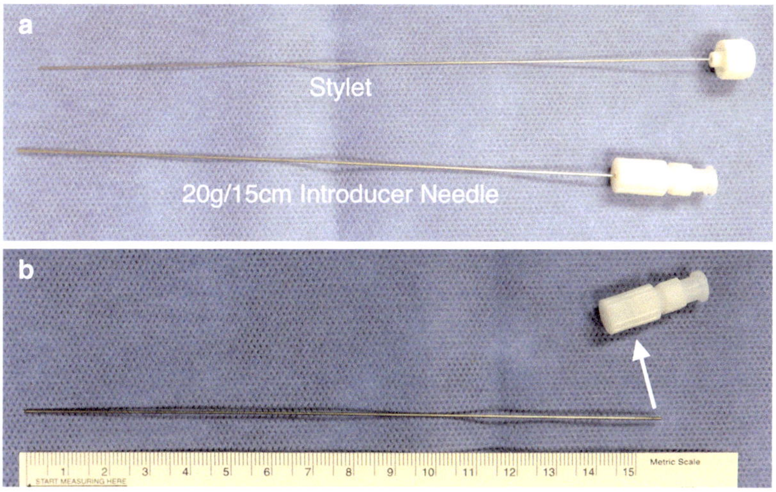

Fig. 3.13 Photograph of an introducer needle that can be converted to a guidewire. The 20 gauge 15 cm needle is shown (**a**) with its stylet. The needle hub (*arrow*) can be detached (**b**)

needle (Fig. 3.21). In certain instances, this maneuver will yield an aspirate of blood, with possible marrow elements. When this occurs, do not discard this specimen and instead submit it for pathologic evaluation as the specimen may contain diagnostic material (Hewes et al. 1983). Still another method for obtaining the biopsy specimen entails the use of an inner coaxial thin stylet that traps the bone tissue within the lumen of the bone needle (Fig. 3.21). An obturator is used to remove the bone core from the bone needle lumen. Some bone biopsy kits contain twist drills that can be used to advance the bone needle, especially through thick or sclerotic bone (Figs. 3.16 and 3.17). The drill is advanced for a short distance under imaging guidance. After removing the drill, always examine the drill tip for osseous or soft tissue fragments which can also be submitted for pathologic analysis.

Two biopsy dilemmas are sometimes encountered during bone biopsies. First, it can be challenging to obtain specimens from sclerotic bone lesions. In our experience, we have found that trephine bone needles can obtain small sequential samples from sclerotic lesions. Second, it can be deceptively difficult to sample lytic lesions with a bone needle. In these situations, attempting to sample the lesion margin which has some bone material may sometimes yield a specimen. Applying suction to the needle hub is sometimes helpful. Alternatively, the bone needle can be used as a guide cannula, and FNA or soft tissue core biopsy techniques can then be used to access the abnormal soft tissue within the vertebra or rib. This sequence of needle-type (i.e., FNA, soft tissue core biopsy, bone biopsy) usage may have to be altered when the soft tissue component of a vertebral or rib lesion is encountered prior to the osseous component (Fig. 3.22).

Care must be taken when advancing sharp biopsy needles within damaged osseous structures. This should be performed with meticulous imaging surveillance.

3.3.2 Vertebra and Disk

Coaxial needle technique can also be used to simultaneously sample the disk endplate complex in patients with suspected spine infection (Table 3.4). A common method for performing this procedure entails the use of a spinal needle to first attempt aspiration of the disk under fluoroscopic guidance with an oblique projection of the spinal axis ("Scotty dog" view). An 18 gauge spinal needle can be used for this first pass. A 20 gauge 25 cm needle with a removable hub can then be

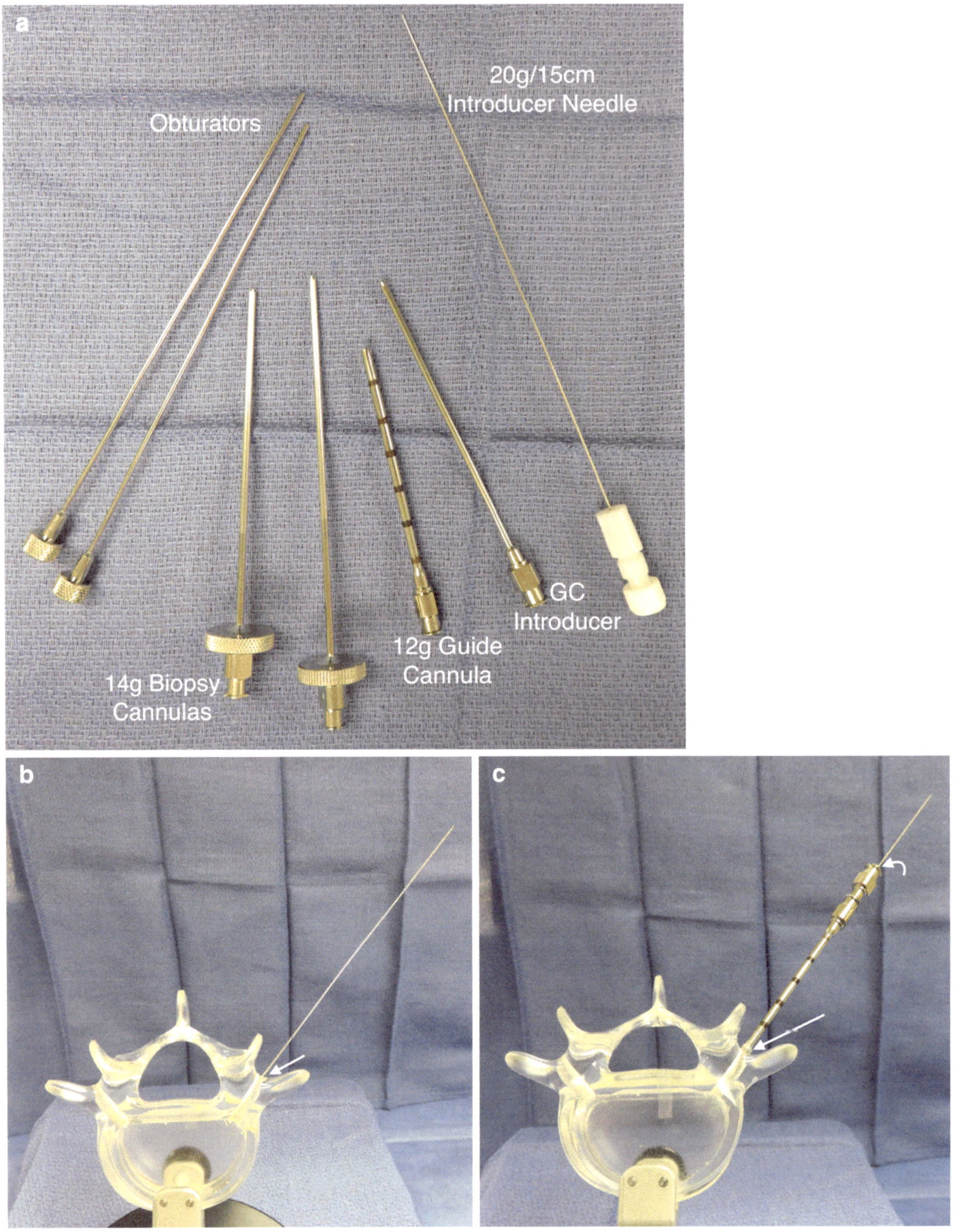

Fig. 3.14 Photograph of a coaxial over-the-wire bone biopsy needle system (**a**); *GC* guide cannula. After the introducer needle is advanced with imaging guidance to the periosteal surface (**b**) and local anesthetic is administered around the pedicle (*arrow*), the hub of the needle is removed – it is now a guidewire. The tapered guide cannula introducer and guide cannula (**c**) are advanced over the guidewire (*curved arrow*) to the periosteal surface (*arrow*). The introducer cannula and guidewire are removed (**d**) leaving the guide cannula in place (*arrow*). A bone biopsy needle (*small arrow*) is advanced coaxially (**e**) through the guide cannula (*large arrow*) and into the vertebral body (*curved arrow*). This type of trephine needle is advanced by rotational movements and forward pressure. After a specimen is obtained, the bone biopsy needle (**f**) is exchanged for a longer bone biopsy needle (*curved arrow*) in order to obtain more specimens. The specimen can be expressed (**g**) from the bone needle (*curved arrow*) with an obturator (*arrow*). Sometimes it is necessary to use the palm of the hand (*arrow*) to express the bone specimen (**h**) from the bone needle (*curved arrow*). Close-up view (**i**) shows simulated 3 mm biopsy specimen (*arrow*) removed from the trephine biopsy cannula (*curved arrow*)

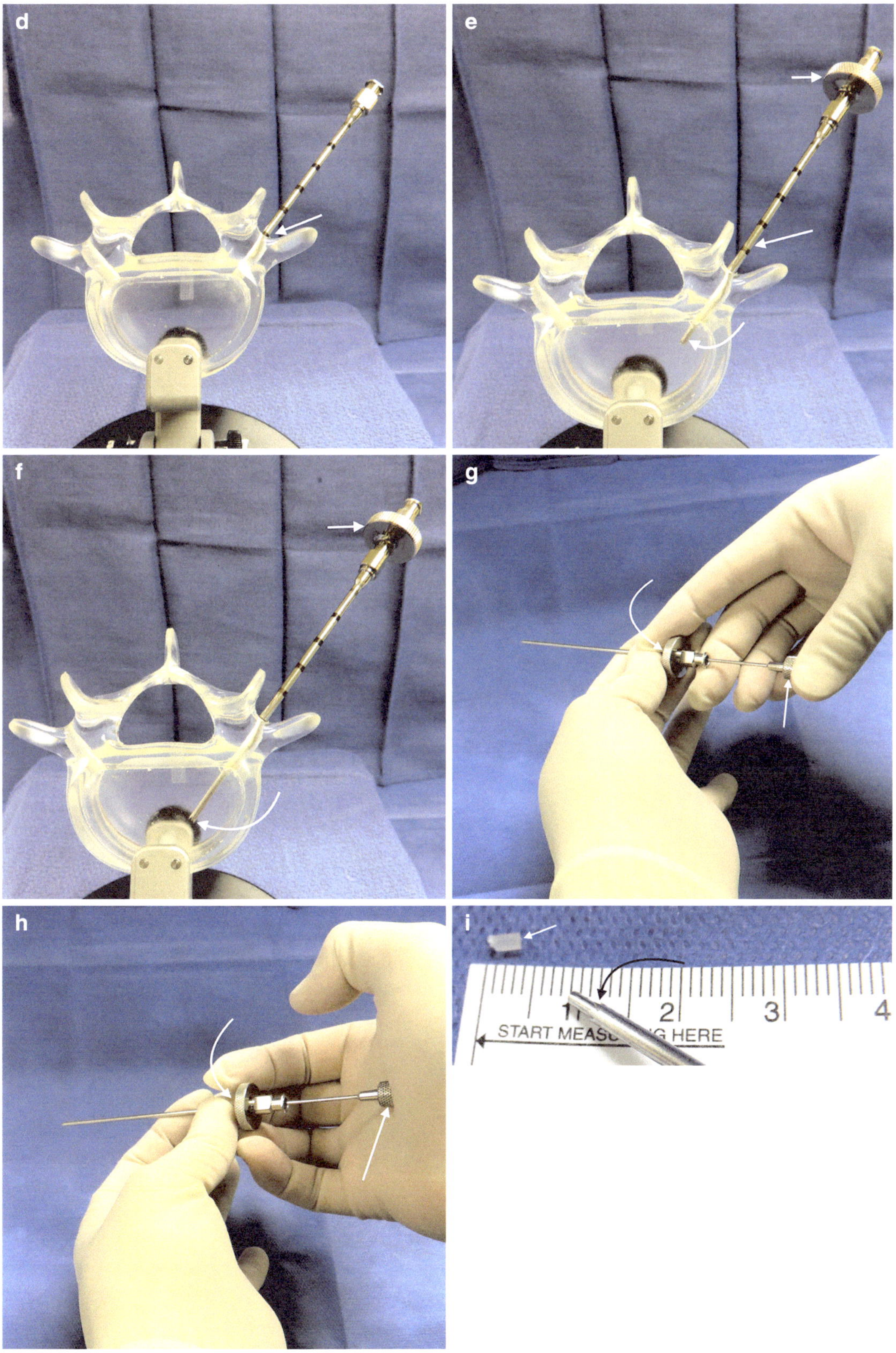

Fig. 3.14 (continued)

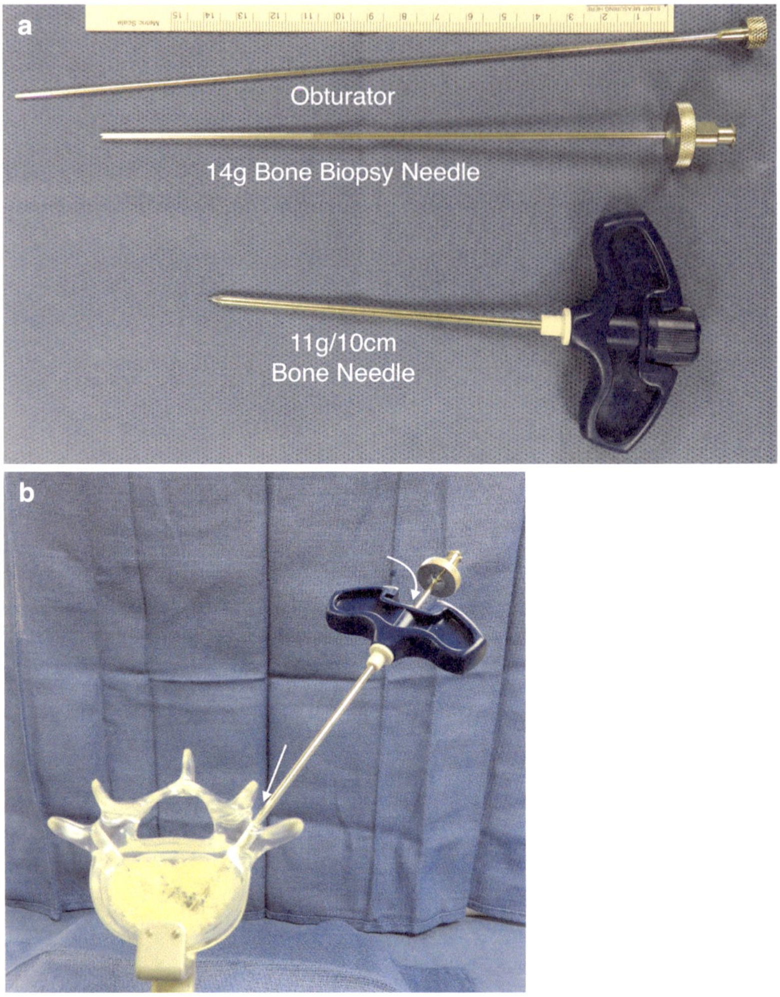

Fig. 3.15 Photographs of a non-over-the-wire bone biopsy approach. An 11 gauge 10 cm bone biopsy needle (**a**) can be used as a guide cannula for a 14 gauge bone biopsy needle. Once vertebral access is achieved with the larger bone biopsy needle (**b**), the stylet is removed, and the cannula (*arrow*) serves as a coaxial conduit for the smaller gauge bone biopsy needle (*curved arrow*)

used to exchange the 18 gauge spinal needle for either a bone needle or a coaxial introducer and guide cannula system. With either variation of this technique, the bone needle is angled cephalad or caudad into the disk endplate margin in order to obtain tissue samples from this location. Another approach to this type of procedure is to first use a percutaneous diskectomy device to obtain disk tissue and then perform a coaxial exchange for a bone biopsy needle system (*Refer to the* Chap. 9). While disk endplate biopsies can be performed with CT guidance, this type of biopsy is readily and efficiently performed with fluoroscopic guidance, especially within the lumbar spine.

3.4 Imaging Guidance

Image-guided percutaneous biopsy of the spine or ribs can be performed with accuracy and safety using CT or fluoroscopic guidance (Jelinek et al. 2002; Omura et al. 2011; Puri et al. 2006). The use of CT guidance for the performance of spine biopsy was initially reported in 1981 (Adapon et al. 1981). A diagnostic specimen was obtained in 18/22 cases for a diagnostic yield of 82 %. One patient suffered transient quadriparesis for a complication rate of 4.5 %. This led to increased use of this modality for performing spine biopsy procedures, especially in the thoracic spine where many operators previously deferred to open biopsy in order to avoid lung injury. CT guidance is particularly helpful in certain specific situa-

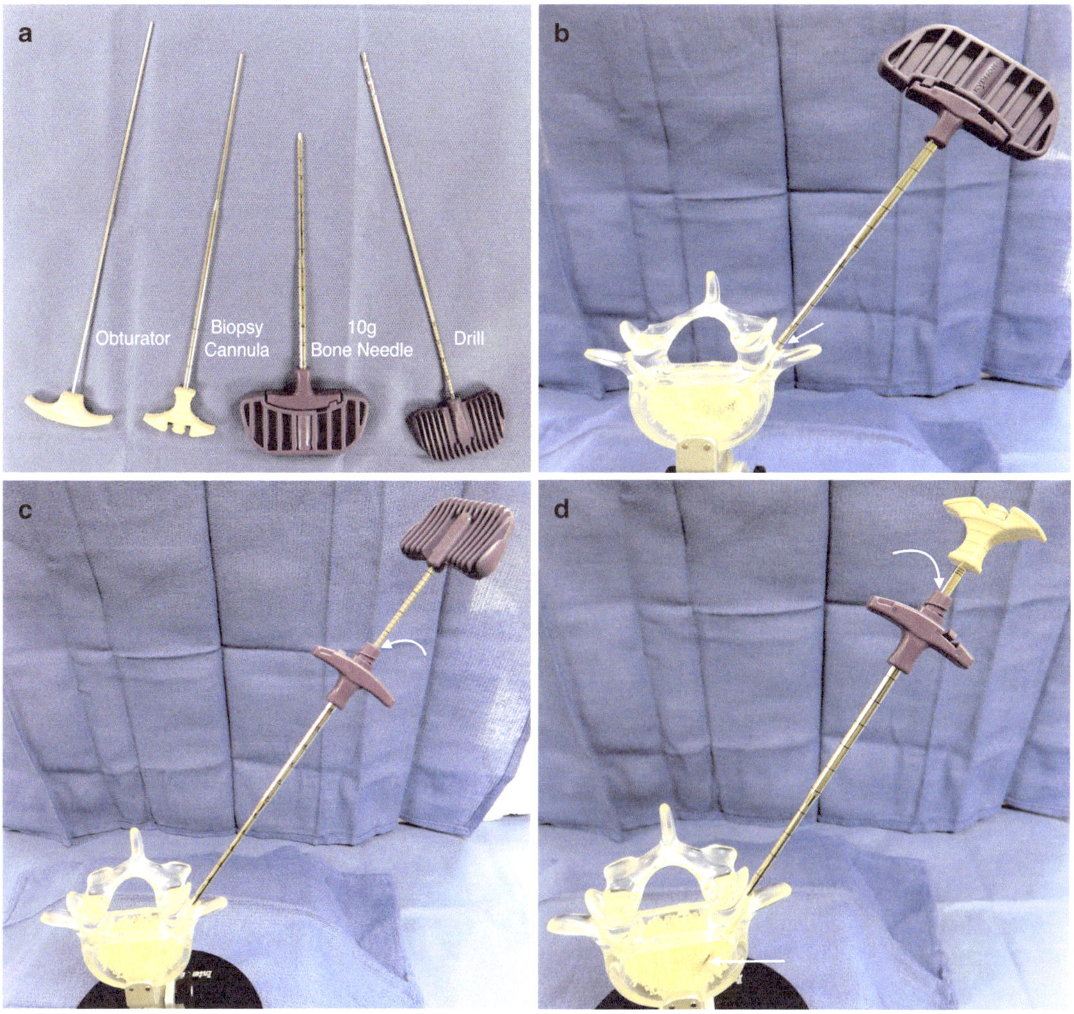

Fig. 3.16 Photographs of a 10 gauge bone biopsy system (**a**) with a twist drill and biopsy cannula. This is a non-over-the-wire coaxial system. The bone needle accesses the vertebral cortex (**b**) through either a transpedicular (*arrow*) or extra-pedicular approach. A drill (*curved arrow*) is inserted to facilitate advancement of the bone cannula (**c**). The drill can also be used to redirect the cannula. Once the cannula is deemed to be in an appropriate location (**d**), the bone biopsy needle (*arrow*) is inserted through guide cannula (*curved arrow*) in order to obtain a biopsy specimen

tions. These include the sampling of small vertebral or paraspinal lesions, posterior element biopsy, paraspinal soft tissue mass biopsy, neural foramen, and epidural space lesions. CT is also a modality that is well suited for rib biopsy (Jakanani and Saifuddin 2013). One of the earliest reports on CT-guided rib biopsy showed a favorable diagnostic efficacy in 10 out of 11 patients (Hardy et al. 1987). The addition of CT fluoroscopy with its real-time capability enhances the speed of the CT-guided biopsy procedure. The use of CT fluoroscopy is our scanning technique of choice when performing CT- guided spine and rib biopsies. By pressing on the foot pedal, the operator is able to simultaneously obtain and view three axial images in 4.8 mm slice thickness starting from the head to the foot. CT fluoroscopy enables minimal amounts of radiation to be used to acquire adequate images thereby helping to reduce procedure-related patient radiation dose. While radiation exposure to both the patient and the operator is associated with this procedure, it can be minimized by sound pre-procedure preparation, using low-dose tech-

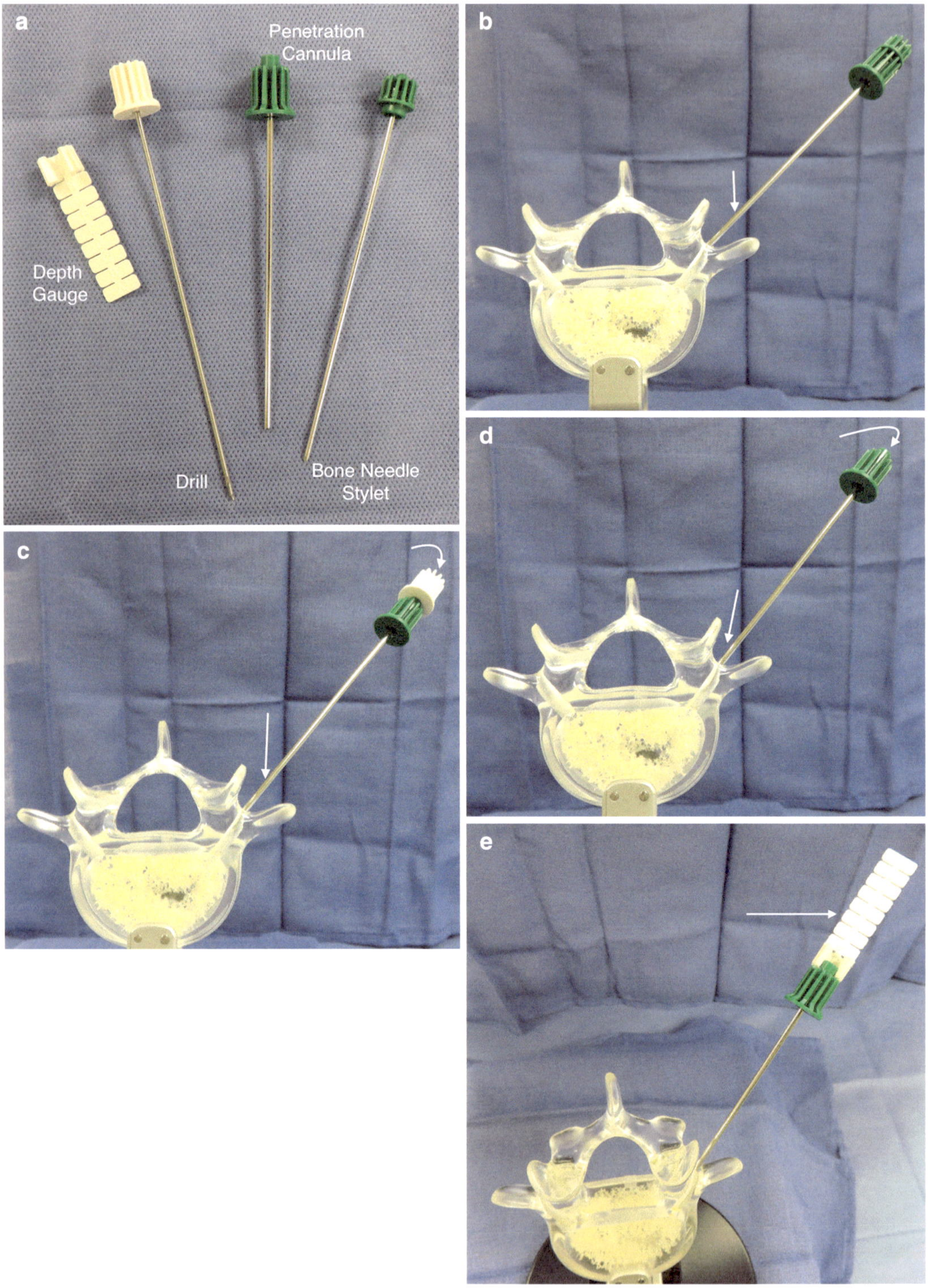
a
Penetration Cannula
Depth Gauge
Drill
Bone Needle Stylet
b
c
d
e

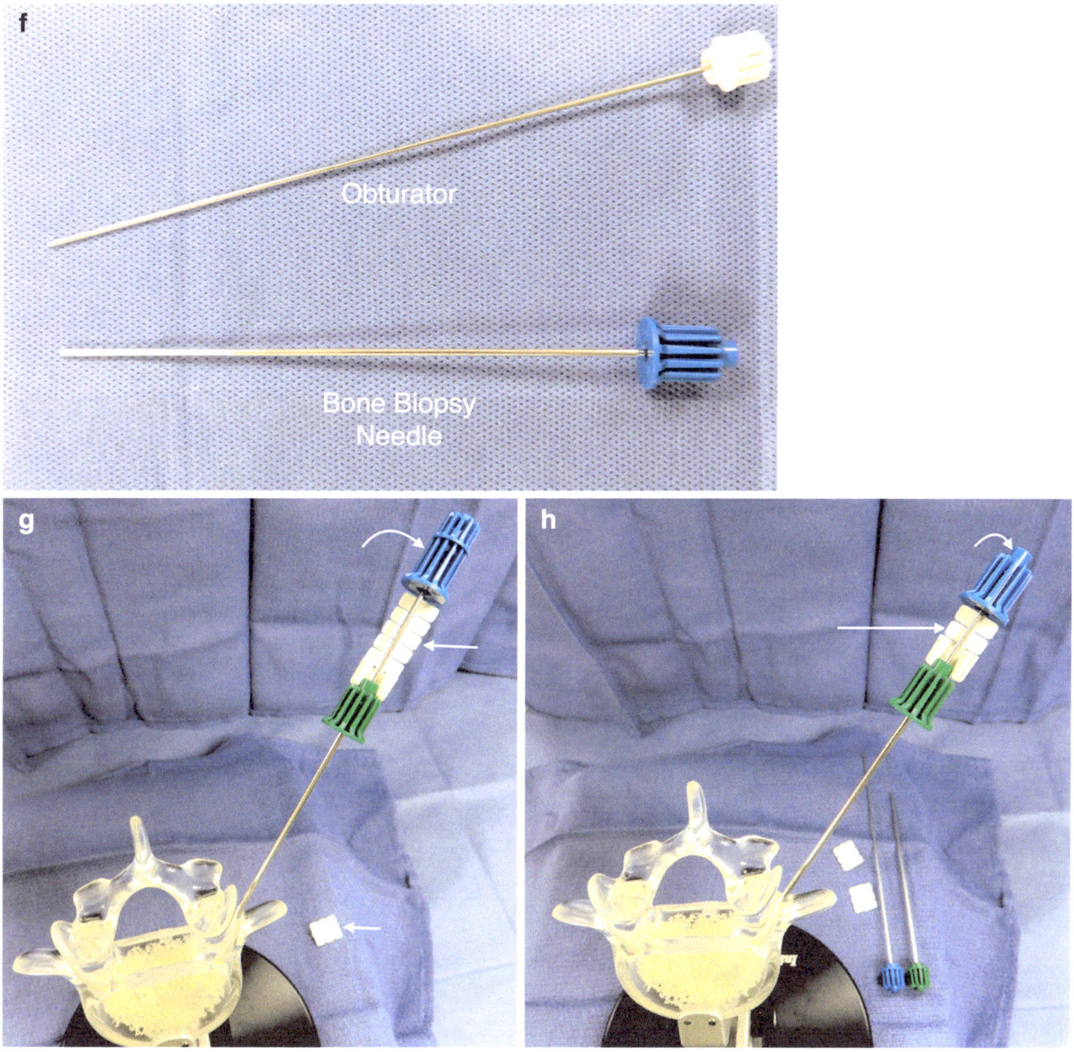

Fig. 3.17 (continued)

Fig. 3.17 Photographs of a coaxial bone biopsy system that uses a depth gauge to assist in the bone biopsy procedure (**a**). The 9.5 cm long penetration cannula (*arrow*) with an inner diameter of 1.8 mm is advanced into the vertebra (**b**). A twist drill (*curved arrow*) is inserted into the penetration cannula (*straight arrow*) after removal of the stylet in order to advance the guide cannula further into the vertebra (**c**). Once the penetration cannula (*arrow*) is advanced into the vertebral body (**d**), the drill is removed and the cannula can be prepared for the biopsy portion of the procedure (*curved arrow*). The depth gauge (*arrow*) is attached to the hub of the penetration cannula (**e**). The 13 cm bone biopsy needle (**f**) has an outer diameter of 1.7 mm and an inner diameter of 1.3 mm. In this example (**g**) three 5 mm tabs (*small arrow*) have been removed from the depth gauge (*large arrow*); this allows the biopsy cannula (*curved arrow*) to be advanced 15 mm beyond the penetration cannula. The needle position will also be monitored with imaging guidance. After acquiring one specimen, the biopsy cannula can be reinserted (**h**); this time an additional 3 tabs (*arrow*) have been removed allowing for further penetration of the biopsy cannula (*curved arrow*) into the target lesion

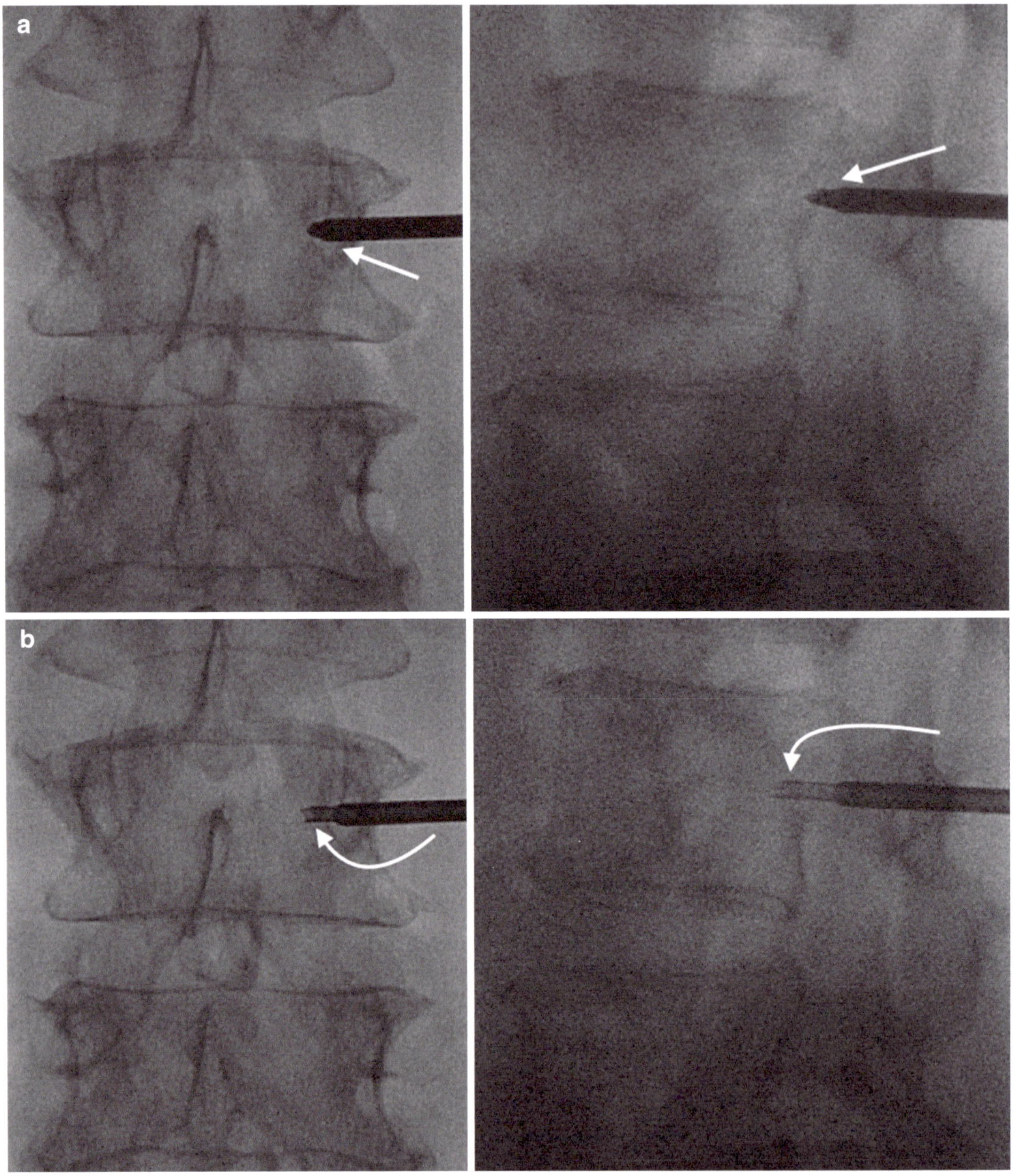

Fig. 3.18 A 63-year-old female with a prior history of breast cancer, low back pain, and an L3 bone lesion detected with an MRI study. Frontal and lateral fluoroscopic images of the lumbar spine (**a**) show transpedicular bone needle placement with advancement toward the posterior vertebral body (*arrows*). A bone biopsy is performed (**b**) at the posterior vertebral body (*arrows*) with a biopsy cannula using coaxial technique. Continuous sequential fluoroscopic monitoring shows advancement of the bone needle for a second pass (**c**) within the posterior vertebral body (*arrows*). The third pass (**d**) extends into the middle of the vertebral body (*arrows*). This was the maximal distance that the biopsy cannulas could traverse within the guide cannula, with the guide cannula located in the most anterior aspect of the pedicle. Therefore, a stylet was inserted into the guide cannula (**e**), and the bone needle was advanced from the anterior pedicle into the posterior vertebral body. This simple maneuver allowed for additional passes (**f**) into the anterior vertebral body and the opportunity to obtain additional specimens

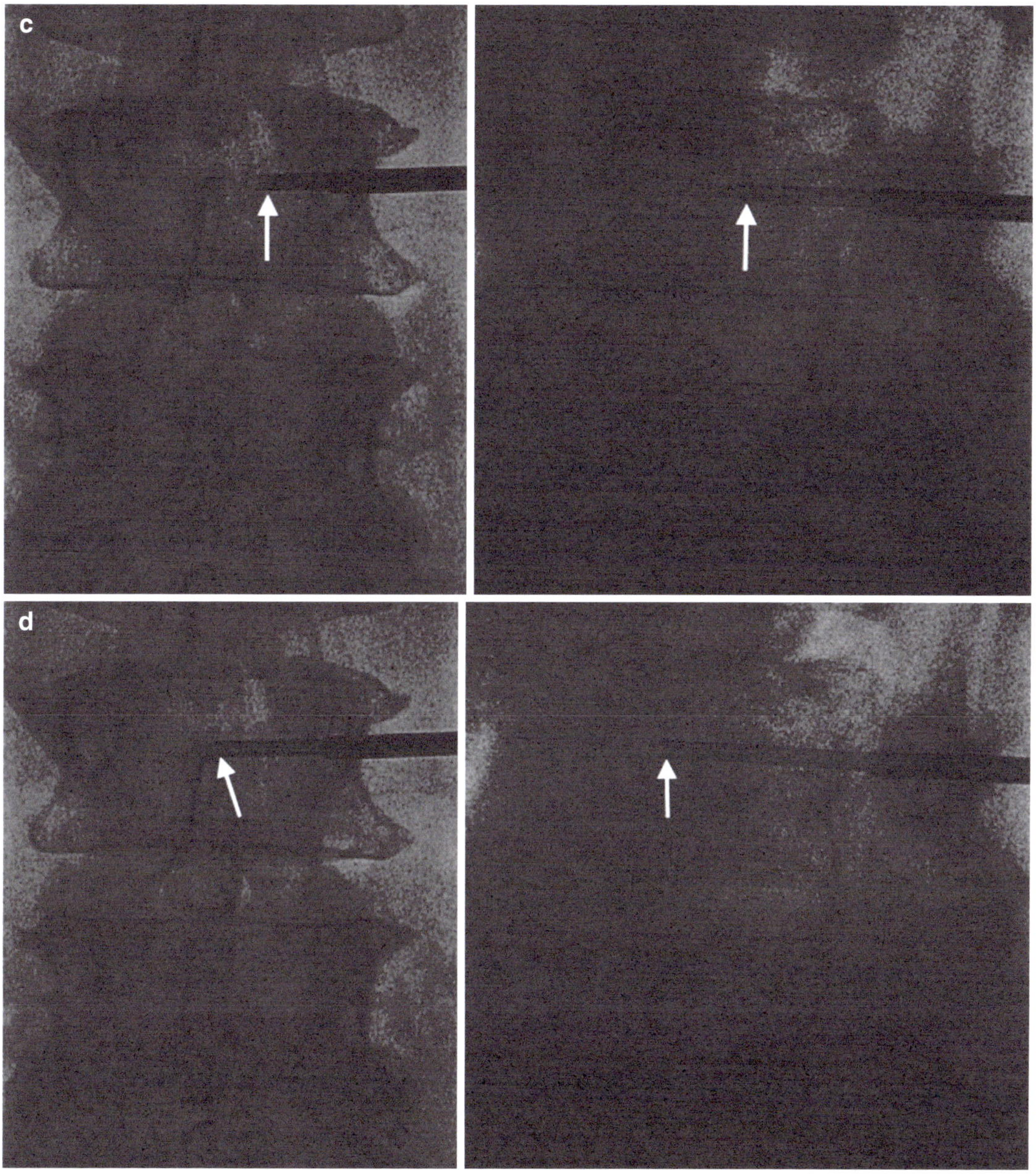

Fig. 3.18 (continued)

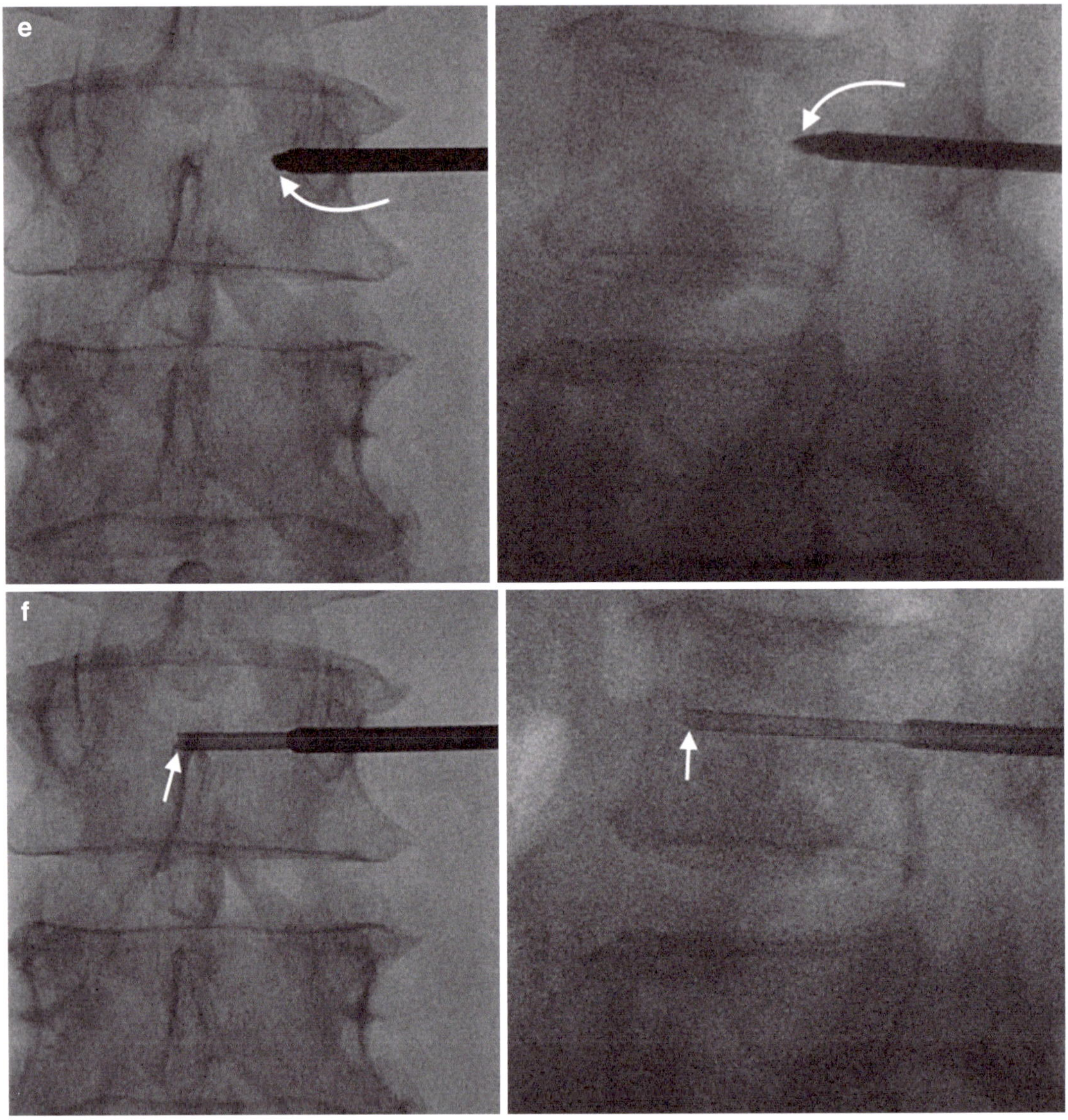

Fig. 3.18 (continued)

niques on the CT scanner, limiting the area of coverage, and active monitoring of radiation exposure (Shpilberg et al. 2014). The operator is also able to minimize their radiation exposure by standing behind a lead shield during the fluoroscopic acquisitions. Lastly, with increasing operator experience with these CT-guided biopsy procedures, the overall amount of radiation used per case decreases over time.

Imaging guidance can also be performed with fluoroscopy. Fluoroscopic guidance provides real-time monitoring of the needle position, the needle tip location, and the biopsy target. Needle angulation or redirection is easily performed with fluoroscopic monitoring. Transient, minor patient motion does not adversely affect fluoroscopy-guided procedures as the fluoroscope and/or table are slightly adjusted to compensate for a slight change in patient position. Fluoroscopic guidance can be utilized for transpedicular thoracic or lumbar vertebral body biopsies of large or diffuse vertebral body lesions. Intervertebral disk biopsies can be performed anywhere along the spinal axis using fluoroscopic guidance. The fluoroscopic procedure does expose the patient, the operator, and the staff to radiation. The radiation exposure can be reduced by careful case preparation and patient selection, use of radiation-reducing functions of the fluoroscopy equipment (such as pulsed fluoroscopy, low-dose technique, shielding and collimation, fluoroscopy time

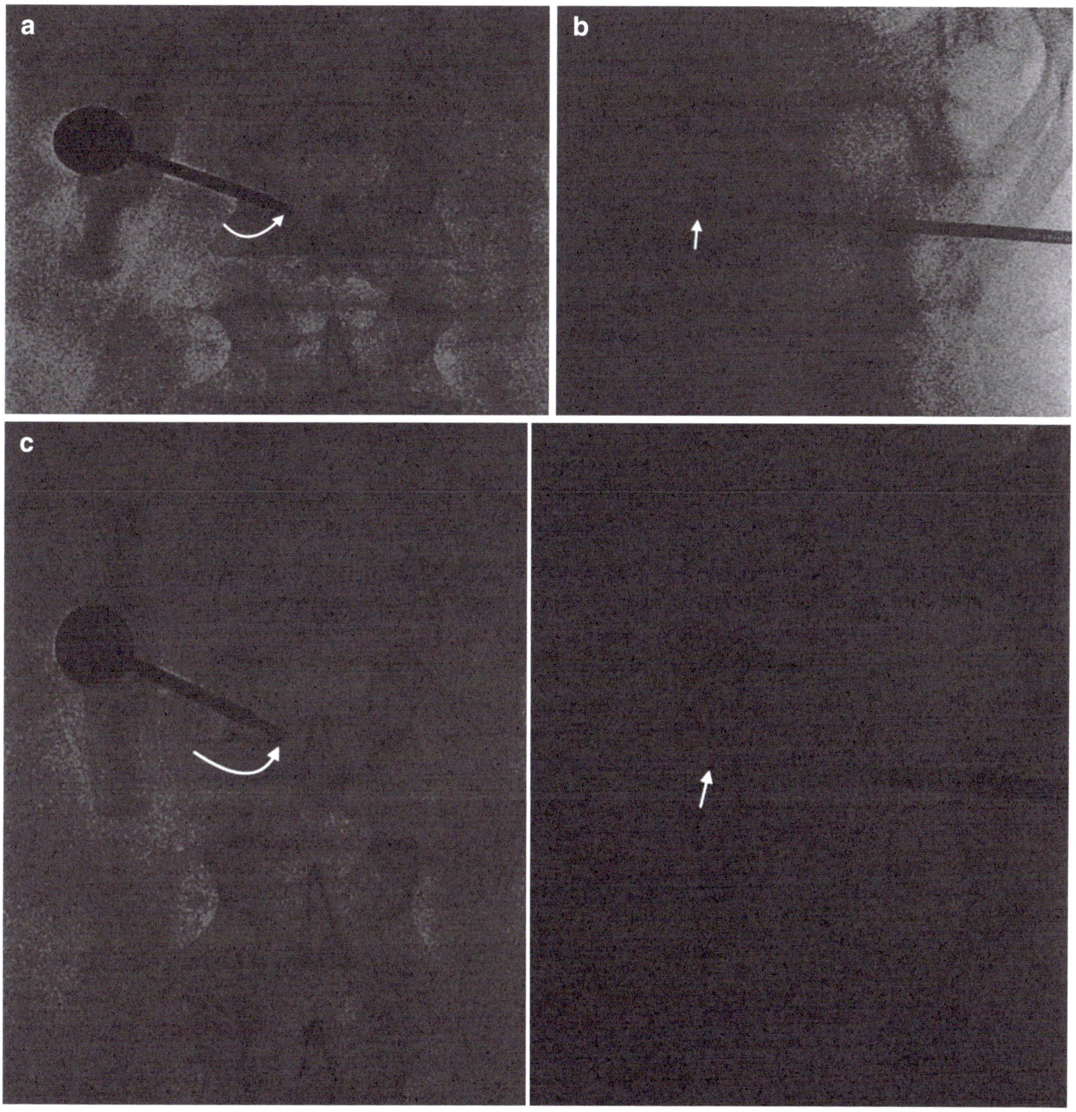

Fig. 3.19 A 76-year-old male with lung cancer and a PET/CT study that showed an abnormal L1 vertebral body. Frontal (**a**) and lateral (**b**) fluoroscopic images at the L1 level show coaxial insertion of a 14 gauge bone biopsy needle (*arrows*) through an 11 gauge guide needle (see Fig. 3.15); the 11 gauge guide needle was previously inserted via a transpedicular approach. The bone biopsy needle (arrows) was advanced into the anterior vertebral body as shown on the frontal and lateral fluoroscopic images (**c**). With the guide needle docked in the posterior vertebral body, it was possible to redirect the smaller 14 gauge bone biopsy needle (*arrows*) in order to obtain additional specimen as shown on the frontal and lateral fluoroscopic images (**d**). It is possible to use a coaxial system to reposition and redirect the biopsy tools along trajectories that will increase the specimen yield

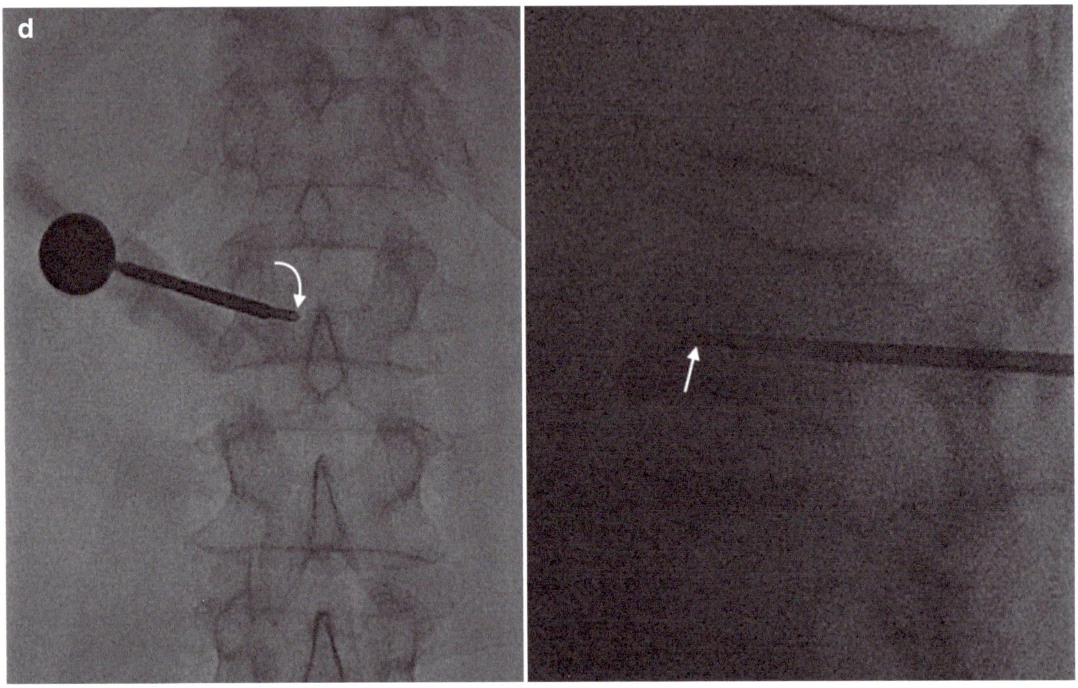

Fig. 3.19 (continued)

alarms), and appropriate use of distance from the x-ray tube.

3.5 Optimizing the CT-Guided Spine or Rib Biopsy Procedure

Quite a bit of planning and strategic activity must occur prior to, during, and after a successful CT-guided spine or rib biopsy procedure (*refer to* Chap. 1). The CT biopsy team often consists of the operator, the nurse, and the CT technologist. Each of these individuals has a critical role in the care of the patient and the performance of the procedure. A successful biopsy procedure is one in which the patient is recovered back to their baseline health status, and the biopsy is accomplished. Each team member in the procedure suite is a stakeholder in the patient's care and outcome. The team must function as a professional unit in order to earn the confidence and trust of the patient and their family members. This in turn will decrease the patient's anxiety level and will facilitate patient cooperation throughout the procedure.

Preparation
Pre-biopsy evaluation
Patient selection
Lesion selection
Approach
Imaging guidance method
Biopsy instruments

The nurse is immersed in the patient's care, and an excellent nurse will be the patient's advocate. The nurse assesses and confirms all pertinent aspects of the patient's health record, including medical and medication history, medical allergies, laboratory values, and NPO status. By discussing the procedure ahead of time with the nurse, the operator will assist the nurse in

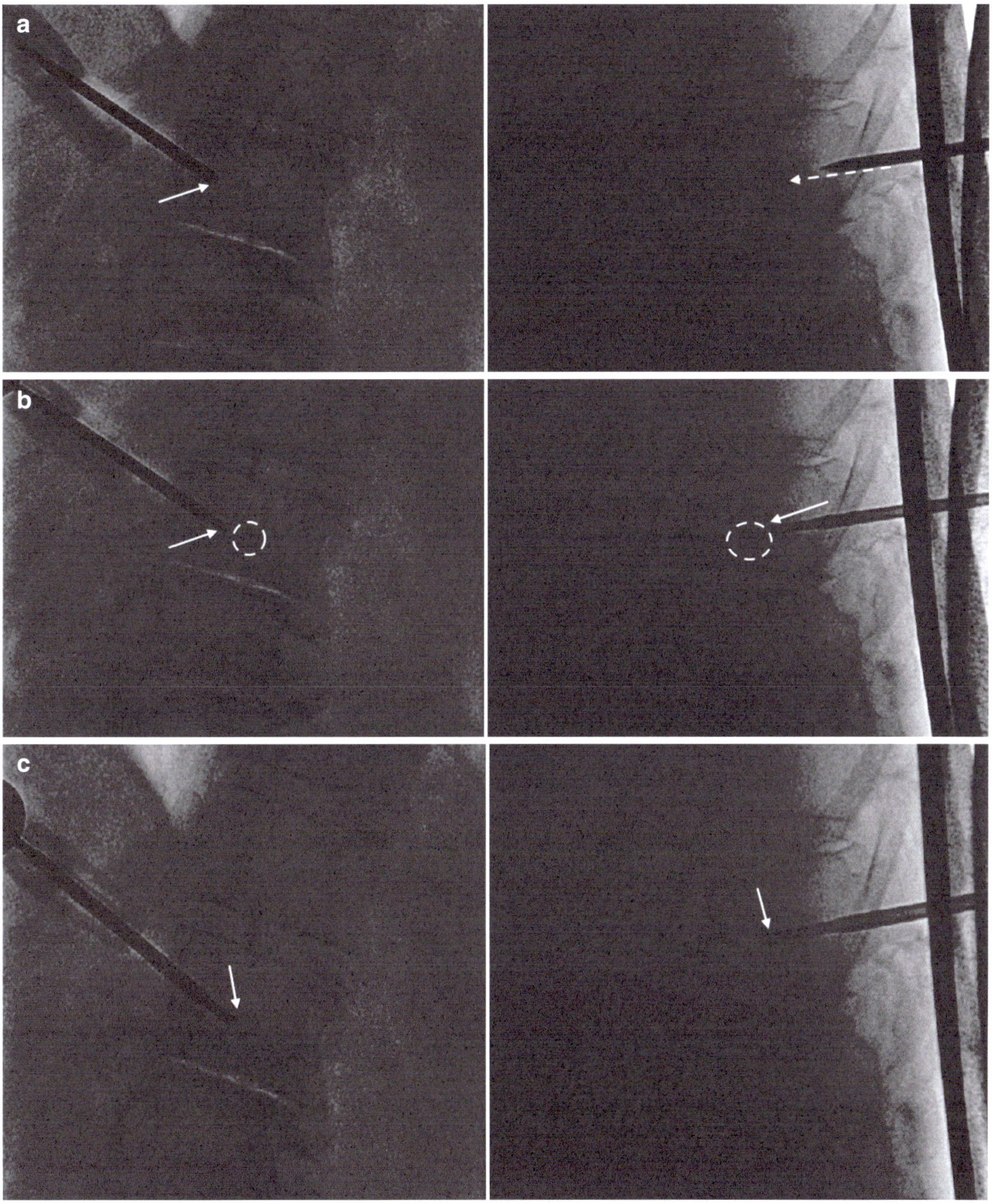

Fig. 3.20 An 83-year-old female with breast cancer and thyroid cancer and an L1 bone lesion on an MRI examination. Frontal and lateral fluoroscopic images (**a**) show transpedicular placement of a bone needle. Frontal and lateral fluoroscopic images (**b**) show coaxial insertion of a biopsy cannula (*arrows*) that is directed towards a sclerotic lesion (*oval*). Frontal and lateral fluoroscopic images (**c**) show coaxial advancement of the bone biopsy cannula into the lesion (*arrows*) which was pathologically shown to be a breast metastasis

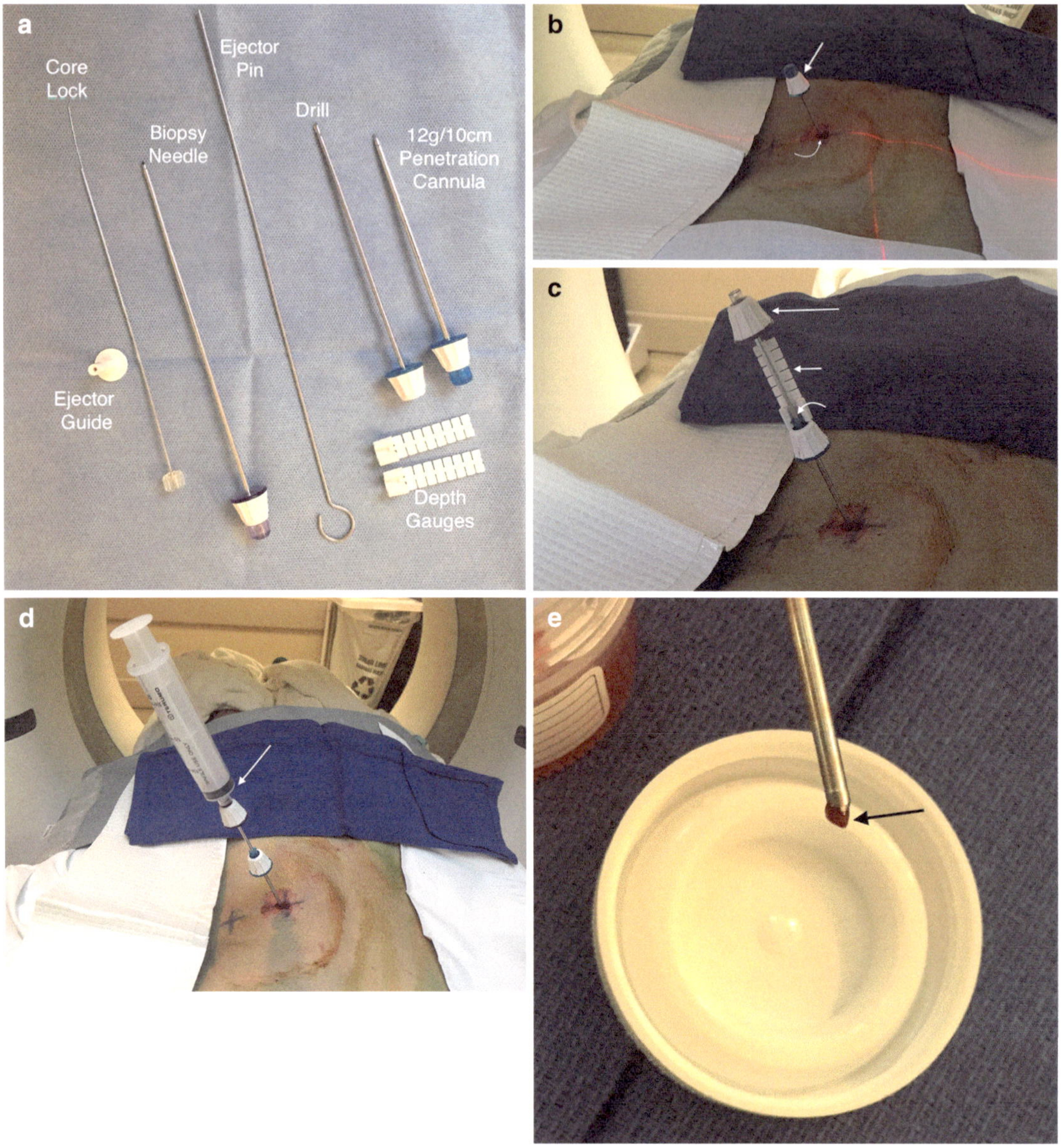

Fig. 3.21 Photograph of a bone biopsy system (**a**) that includes a trapping mechanism or core lock for the biopsy core within the bone cannula. Actual case demonstration (**b**) of inserted penetration cannula (*arrow*) using CT guidance; note the skin mark and laser line (*curved arrow*). Use of depth gauge (*small arrow*) attached to the penetration cannula (*curved arrow*) and coaxial placement (**c**) of a biopsy needle (*long arrow*). The operator elected to use an aspiration technique (**d**) with a 20 mL syringe (*arrow*). Photograph (**e**) of small bone core (*arrow*)

properly preparing and orienting the patient and their healthcare representatives. Hopefully, the operator has already seen the patient in consultation and can share this important information with the nurse. The more thoroughly debriefed that the nurse is regarding the intended procedure, the more efficiently the nurse is able to assist in it. This contributes significantly toward key procedure steps such as placement of the intravenous catheter, location of monitoring equipment, procedure verification, patient positioning, and intravenous sedation and analgesia. All of these

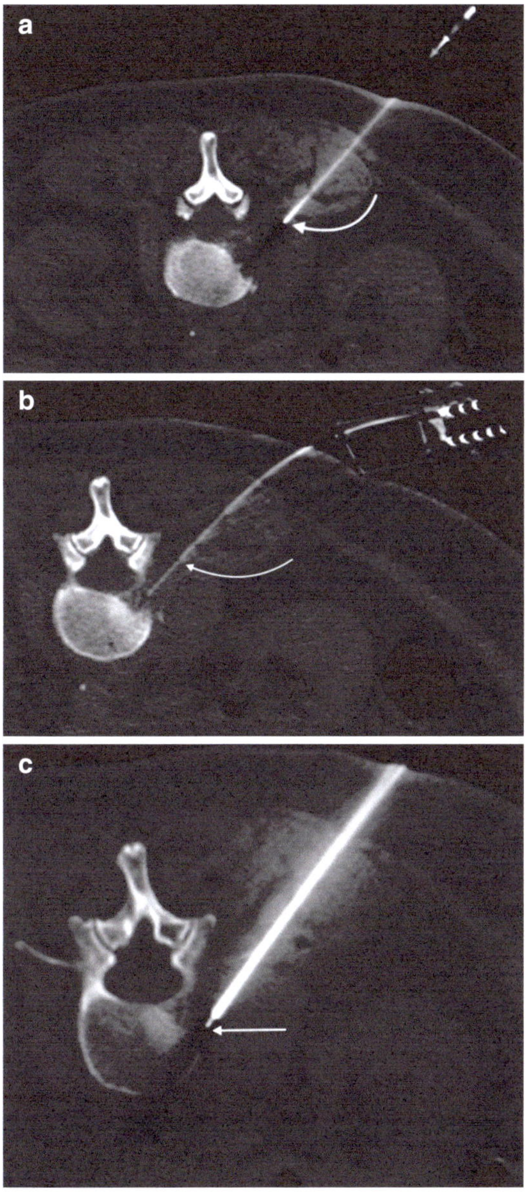

Fig. 3.22 A 63-year-old female with low back pain and abnormal MRI and CT examinations showing an L2 lesion. Axial CT image (**a**) showing FNA of paraspinal soft tissue mass (*arrow*). Axial CT image (**b**) shows soft tissue core needle biopsy (*arrow*) (note the top-heavy bulky handle). Axial CT image (**c**) shows bone biopsy of the L2 vertebra (*arrow*)

factors, when executed properly, result in a smooth, safe procedure. The patient's comfort and recovery are therefore favorably impacted.

The CT technologist plays an important role as part of the team when performing a CT-guided spine or rib biopsy procedure. He or she is not present just to "take pictures." The technologist must completely understand the full functionality of their CT scanner and the logistics of the CT scan suite in order to optimize the biopsy procedure. An excellent technologist will understand how to set or override protocols. The technologist should be able to effectively and quickly program the scanner to generate good quality images for any biopsy procedure. They should also know how to use special features such as CT fluoroscopy and be able to generate quick multi-planar reformations when necessary (Figs. 3.23 and 3.24). The technologist is responsible for maximizing radiation safety during the procedure. A review of the pre-procedure studies with the technologist prior to the biopsy procedure helps to increase the chances of a correct level, correct side biopsy. The technologist performs multiple tasks before, during, and after the procedure. Once the patient is brought into the CT scan suite, the technologist introduces themselves to the patient, explains their important role in the procedure, and performs patient verification (Table 3.6). The technologist is a valuable assistant to the operator through all phases of the biopsy procedure and should be a major contributor to an efficient and safe biopsy.

References

Adapon BD, Legada Jr BD, Lim EV, Silao Jr JV, Dalmacio-Cruz A. CT-guided closed biopsy of the spine. J Comput Assist Tomogr. 1981;5:73–8.

CT technique directly impacts upon biopsy technique. Therefore, the operator and the CT technologist should work cohesively in order to optimize the spine or rib biopsy procedure.

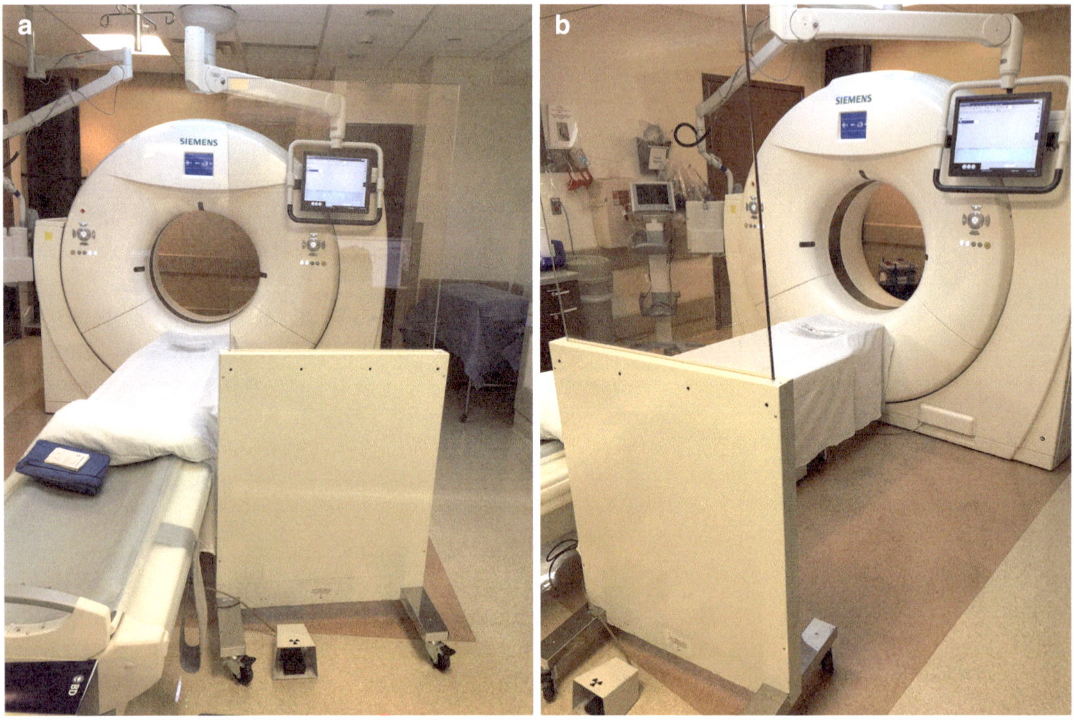

Fig. 3.23 Photographs of CT scan suite just prior to a procedure. The scanner gantry, fluoroscopy monitor, CT fluoroscopy pedal, and lead shield are in position (**a**). The procedure table is in the background and is covered with a sterile sheet. A slightly different angle of the room (**b**) shows the patient monitoring equipment in the background

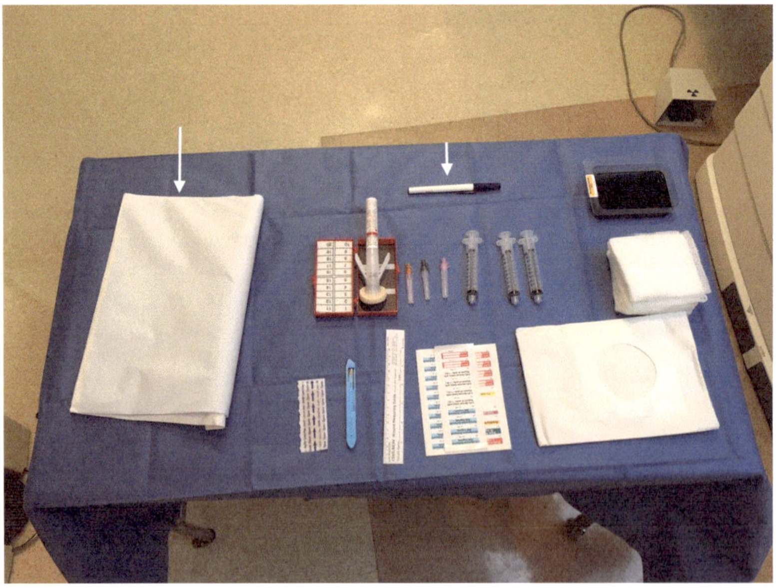

Fig. 3.24 Photograph of basic procedure table setup for a CT-guided procedure. The large arrow indicates a sterile pad for radiation protection (for the operator). The small arrow indicates a sterile marker pen. 10 mL syringes for local anesthetic and small needles, to draw up the local anesthetic and infiltrate the skin and subcutaneous tissues, are necessary as is the scalpel blade for making a crosshair skin incision. Betadine and ChloraPrep sterile scrubs are available as is a mini-procedure drape and plenty of sterile gauze. A ruler can assist with simple measurements, and pre-printed labels are used for identifying anesthetic agents such as lidocaine

Table 3.6 Role of the CT technologist in the CT-guided spine or rib biopsy procedure

1. Prepare the procedure room and assist in assembling the sterile table including biopsy tray and biopsy needles (infection prevention).
2. Set up the CT fluoroscopy equipment in the procedure room including monitor, floor pedal, and a lead shield.
3. Preprogram the CT scanner with patient information, position, and technique.
4. After the room has been prepped, the patient is brought into the room. Greet and double identify the patient (patient verification). The process is explained to the patient. The region of interest is confirmed with the patient, and they are placed on the scanner table and positioned accordingly (procedure verification). Assure that all lines and leads are in safe and appropriate locations. Place security strap on the patient (fall prevention).
5. Place a radiopaque skin grid on the patient.
6. Obtain topograms or scout images in the frontal and lateral projection.
7. Review the topograms with the operator in order to identify the area of interest and decide upon the area of coverage and the field of view. Perform scan using a spiral technique in a bone or soft tissue algorithm, as instructed by the operator.
8. Allow the operator to review the images in order to determine biopsy target(s) and the skin entry site using the skin grid as a reference. Activate laser line to determine the correct axial section at the level of interest. The skin entry site is marked with a surgical pen by the operator. The patient is prepped and draped.
9. Participate in a "time-out" with all members of the biopsy team and the patient (patient safety).
10. Switch scanner to CT fluoroscopy mode and adjust technique (MAS and kV) to accommodate patient's size and stature. Assure that only individuals with protective lead garments are in the procedure suite during CT fluoroscopy (radiation safety).
11. The patient is positioned at the level of the marked skin entry site, and the operator can now proceed with the biopsy procedure.
12. The technologist is vigilant with respect to monitoring the progress of device insertion and visualization with CT fluoroscopy. Slight adjustments in table position due to patient motion or based upon needle device location may have to be made.
13. It is the responsibility of the technologist to continuously review images making sure that they are centered appropriately and are of diagnostic quality.
14. The technologist also assists in maintaining patient comfort and cooperation throughout and immediately after the procedure.
15. Case completion and documentation.

Key Review Points

1. The tools that can be used for image-guided spine or rib biopsy procedures include fine needles, soft tissue core biopsy needles, and bone biopsy needles.
2. FNA procedures are optimally performed with CT -guidance using coaxial technique in order to facilitate multiple needle passes.
3. Soft tissue core biopsies can be performed in the spine and ribs in the setting of destructive osseous lesions.
4. Spine biopsies are optimally performed with coaxial technique and can also be performed with tandem- needle or single -needle biopsy techniques.
5. Rib biopsies are best performed with coaxial technique.
6. Intervertebral disk biopsy may require a percutaneous diskectomy device in order to obtain actual disk tissue.
7. Another approach that is used to assess for spine infection is to simultaneously perform a disk end plate biopsy with a bone biopsy needle.
8. Fluoroscopic guidance is ideal for lumbar or thoracic transpedicular approaches to large or diffuse vertebral body lesions and for intervertebral disk biopsy procedures.
9. CT guidance is optimal for small spine lesions, posterior element lesions, epi-

dural or paraspinal soft tissue masses, and rib lesions.

10. The CT biopsy team includes the operator, the nurse, and the CT technologist. Working proactively and together, these individuals can improve the likelihood of a favorable patient experience and a successful biopsy procedure.

Fenton DS, Czervionke LF. Percutaneous spine biopsy. In: Image-guided spine intervention. Philadelphia: Saunders; 2003. p. 141–86.

Geremia GK, Charletta DA, Granato DB, Raju S. Biopsy of vertebral and paravertebral structures with a new coaxial needle system. AJNR Am J Neuroradiol. 1992;13:169–71.

Gupta RK, Cheung YK, Al Ansari AG, Naran S, Lallu S, Fauck R. Diagnostic value of image-guided needle aspiration cytology in the assessment of vertebral and intervertebral lesions. Diagn Cytopathol. 2002;27:191–6.

Hardy DC, Totty WG, Funk KC. CT-directed rib biopsy. J Comput Assist Tomogr. 1987;11:994–7.

Hewes RC, Vigorita VJ, Freiberger RH. Percutaneous bone biopsy: the importance of aspirated osseous blood. Radiology. 1983;148:69–72.

Jakanani GC, Saifuddin A. Percutaneous image-guided needle biopsy of rib lesions: a retrospective study of diagnostic outcome in 51 cases. Skeletal Radiol. 2013;42:85–90.

Jelinek JS, Murphey MD, Welker JA, Henshaw RM, Kransdorf MJ, Shmookler BM, Malawer MM. Diagnosis of primary bone tumors with image-guided percutaneous biopsy: experience with 110 tumors. Radiology. 2002;223:731–7.

Omura MC, Motamedi K, Uybico S, Nelson SD, Seeger LL. Revisiting CT-guided percutaneous core needle biopsy of musculoskeletal lesions: contributors of biopsy success. AJR Am J Roentgenol. 2011;197:457–61.

Puri A, Shingade VU, Agarwal MG, Anchan C, Juvekar S, Desai S, Jambhekar NA. CT-guided percutaneous core needle biopsy in deep seated musculoskeletal lesions: a prospective study of 128 cases. Skeletal Radiol. 2006;35:138–43.

Ray-Coquard I, Ranchère-Vince D, Thiesse P. Evaluation of core needle biopsy as a substitute to open biopsy in the diagnosis of soft-tissue masses. Eur J Cancer. 2003;39:2021–5.

Robertson RC, Ball RP. Destructive spine lesions: Diagnosis by needle biopsy. J Bone Joint Surg Am. 1935;37:443–64.

Shpilberg KA, Delman BN, Tanenbaum LN, Esses SJ, Subramaniam R, Doshi AH. Radiation dose reduction in CT-guided spine biopsies does not reduce diagnostic yield. AJNR Am J Neuroradiol. 2014;35:2243–7.

Wattamwar AS, Ortiz AO. Use of a percutaneous diskectomy device to facilitate the diagnosis of infectious spondylitis. ANJR Am J Neuroradiol. 2010;31:1157–8.

Wu JS, Goldsmith JD, Horwich PJ, Shetty SK, Hochman MG. Bone and soft-tissue lesions: what factors affect diagnostic yield of image-guided core needle biopsy? Radiology. 2008;248:962–70.

Yaffe D, Greenberg G, Leitner J, Gipstein R, Shapiro M, Bachar GN. CT-guided percutaneous biopsy of thoracic and lumbar spine: a new coaxial technique. AJNR Am J Neuroradiol. 2003;24:2111–3.

Yu WY, Siu C, Wing PC, Schweigel JF, Jetha N. Percutaneous suction aspiration for osteomyelitis: report of two cases. Spine. 1991;16:198–202.

4 Cervical Spine Biopsy

A. Orlando Ortiz

Learning Objectives

1. To understand the value and importance of radiologic anatomy as it pertains to cervical spine biopsy
2. To review the indications and contraindications for cervical spine biopsy
3. To learn image-guided coaxial cervical spine biopsy approaches and techniques

4.1 Introduction

Of all the percutaneous image-guided biopsy procedures that can be performed along the spinal axis, cervical spine biopsy remains the most challenging of these procedures. Indeed, many operators are reluctant to perform cervical spine procedures due to the perceived risk of the procedure in an area where the anatomy may present barriers to safe lesion access. The relatively small size of the cervical vertebrae pedicles limits the traditional "shielded" transpedicular pathway to the vertebral body for tissue sampling. The critical vascular structures of the neck, the carotid and vertebral arteries and the internal and external jugular veins, surround the anterior and lateral aspects of the cervical spine. These vascular structures, at initial inspection, may appear to prevent direct access to a vertebrae or intervertebral disk. Close proximity to other critical structures such as the lung apices, trachea, esophagus, thyroid gland and submandibular glands raises appropriate concerns for injury to these structures. The aerodigestive tract and adjacent glandular structures may also limit the access to the target lesion(s) within the cervical spine. The prominent cervical spinal cord and exiting nerve roots may also discourage attempts at sampling nearby lesions. Some operators are more comfortable with single access bone biopsy needles which make repeat passes in the neck somewhat precarious. Other operators have tried to improve their targeting using tandem needle techniques in which the biopsy needle is passed alongside a previously placed smaller gauge guide needle, but this requires a minimum of two needle passes in an area that contains numerous critical structures and, therefore, is a rarely utilized technique in the cervical spine. Cervical spine biopsy is an infrequently performed procedure when compared to thoracic or lumbar spine biopsy, hence many operators lack experience with the tools and techniques that are required to make cervical spine biopsy an effective, efficient and low risk procedure. In a single institution experience 22 cervical spine biopsies out of 703 total spine biopsies (3.1%) were performed over a period of 18 years whereas at another institution 9 out of 410 (2.2%) spine biopsies performed to assess for neoplasm, over an 8-year period, were performed in the cervical spine (Rimondi et al. 2011; Lis et al. 2004) . When a procedure is performed infrequently, the comfort level with performing it decreases. The objective of this chapter is to introduce the reader

A.O. Ortiz, *Image-Guided Percutaneous Spine Biopsy*, DOI 10.1007/978-3-319-43326-4_4

to the approaches and techniques that will assist them in the performance of percutaneous image-guided cervical spine biopsy.

4.2 Anatomic Considerations

While the cervical spine consists of seven cervical vertebrae and the intervening intervertebral disks, the overall smaller size of these structures compared to the remainder of the spinal axis is associated with a relatively lower incidence of suspicious lesions in this location. The neck is bordered superiorly by the skull base and foramen magnum. Inferiorly, the neck is separated from the thoracic cavity by the thoracic inlet, including the lung apices, brachial plexus and brachiocephalic vasculature. From a biopsy perspective, with respect to approach, the neck can be divided into anterior and posterior compartments. Anterior compartment lesions will involve either the cervical vertebral bodies, intervertebral disks or the adjacent paraspinal soft tissues. Posterior compartment lesions will involve the articular masses or facet joints, the posterior elements (pedicle, laminae or spinous processes) or the adjacent paraspinal soft tissues within the perivertebral space – paraspinal component. The anterior compartment can be further subdivided into suprahyoid and infrahyoid compartments. The pertinent suprahyoid compartments include the masticator space, parapharyngeal space, perivertebral space – prevertebral component, submandibular space, retropharyngeal space and carotid space. The oropharynx and hypopharynx are located within the suprahyoid neck and are quite prominent; a breach of these structures could contaminate the spine and biopsy specimen with adverse consequences in either situation. The carotid space contains the carotid artery and the internal jugular vein, and these critical vascular structures determine the choice of approaches when considering an anterior compartment biopsy procedure (Fig. 4.1). The vertebral arteries, likewise critical vascular structures, influence the types of approaches that can be used to access the posterior compartment (Fig. 4.1). The proximity of visceral and carotid space in the infrahyoid neck will constrain the types of approaches that can be used to access the anterior cervical spine.

The carotid space is the key anatomic landmark for determining the majority of anterior-lateral or posterior-lateral approaches for image-guided percutaneous cervical spine biopsy.

Essentially, all needle passes within the anterior compartment will be made either anterior or posterior to the carotid space (Fig. 4.2). For fluoroscopy-guided procedures, the carotid space is a palpable structure – in other words, the operator can palpate the carotid pulse and use a manual displacement technique to move the carotid space out of the way prior to needle insertion. For computed tomography (CT) – guided procedures, the carotid space is readily identified, even on non-contrast CT studies of the neck. The primary objective is to determine a trajectory towards a lesion that avoids puncturing the carotid artery or jugular vein.

The posterior compartment of the neck includes the posterior cervical space. This includes the posterior neck muscles and the posterior elements of the cervical vertebrae. The critical anatomic structures to be aware of when attempting to biopsy lesions in this compartment are the vertebral arteries and the spinal cord. The vertebral arteries are particularly exposed in the upper cervical spine near the craniocervical junction; hence a detailed knowledge of the size and course of these vessels is mandatory when considering upper cervical spine biopsy (Fig. 4.1). The presence of a dominant vertebral artery or a hypoplastic or absent vertebral artery should be noted on the initial diagnostic studies as this will help to prevent a potential major complication. Given the small size and thickness of the posterior elements it is

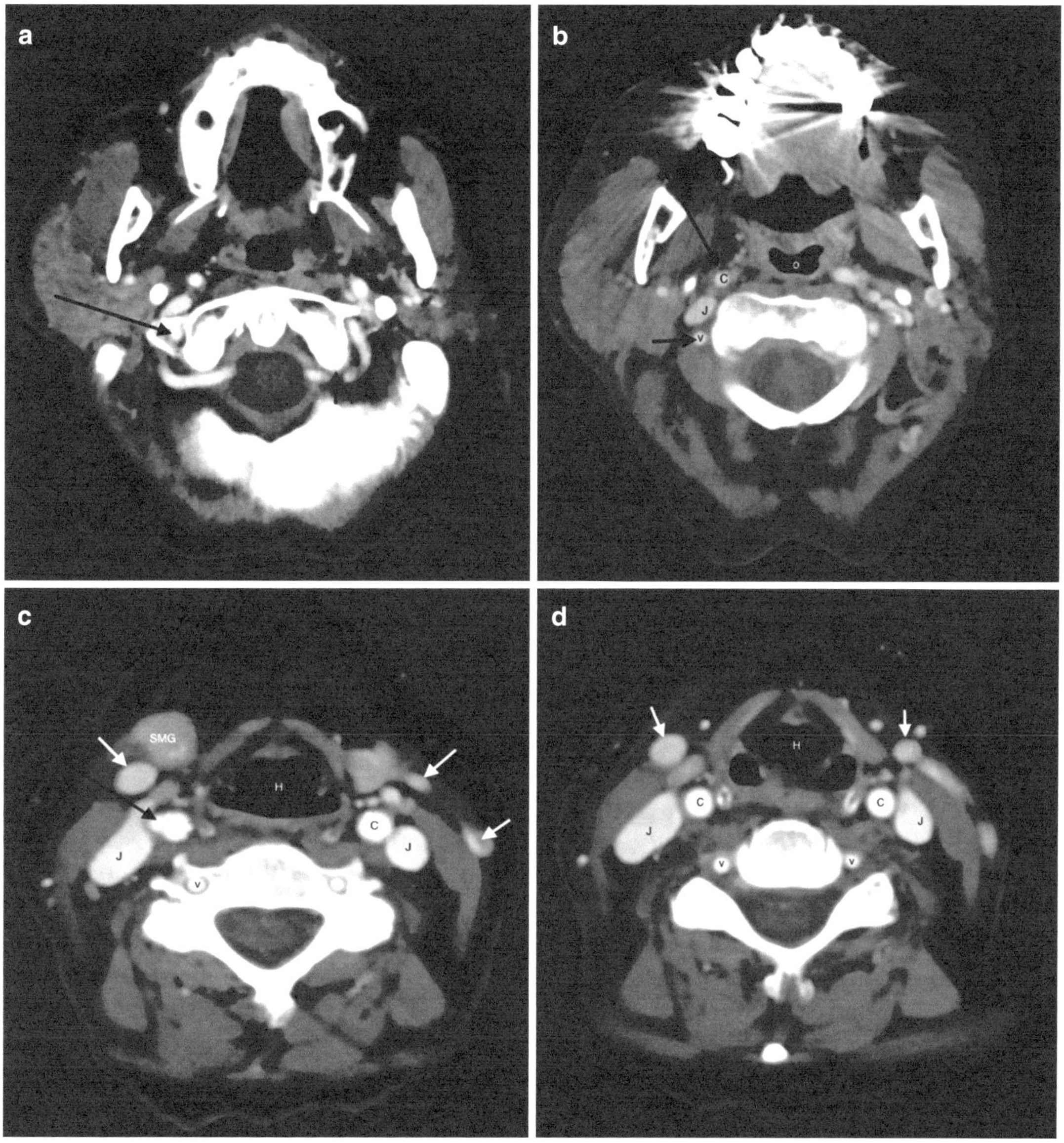

Fig. 4.1 Axial contrast-enhanced CT image (**a**) at C1 level shows course of vertebral arteries as they emerge from the C1 transverse foramen (*large arrow*) to course posterior to the lateral mass (*small arrow*), along a groove on the superior surface of the C1 neural arch, and then enter the spinal canal. Axial contrast-enhanced CT image (**b**) at C2 level shows enhancing vascular structures adjacent to lateral aspect of C2 (internal carotid artery (*c*; *large arrow*), internal jugular vein (*J*) and vertebral artery (*V*; *small arrow*)). If this were a biopsy case, this vascular anatomy effectively forms a barrier to biopsy needle access from these directions. The oropharynx (*O*) forms the anterior relation of the C2 vertebral body. Axial contrast-enhanced image (**c**) at C5 level shows external jugular vein branches (*small arrows*), internal jugular vein (*J*), carotid artery bifurcation on the right (*large arrow*) and common carotid artery (*c*). The vertebral artery (*V*) is located within the foramen transversarium. The submandibular gland (SMG) is seen anteriorly while the hypopharynx (*H*) forms the anterior relation at this level. Axial contrast-enhanced image (**d**) at the C5–6 disk space level shows external jugular vein branches (*small arrows*), internal jugular veins (*J*), common carotid arteries (*C*) and vertebral arteries (*v*). The hypopharynx (*H*) forms the anterior relation at this level

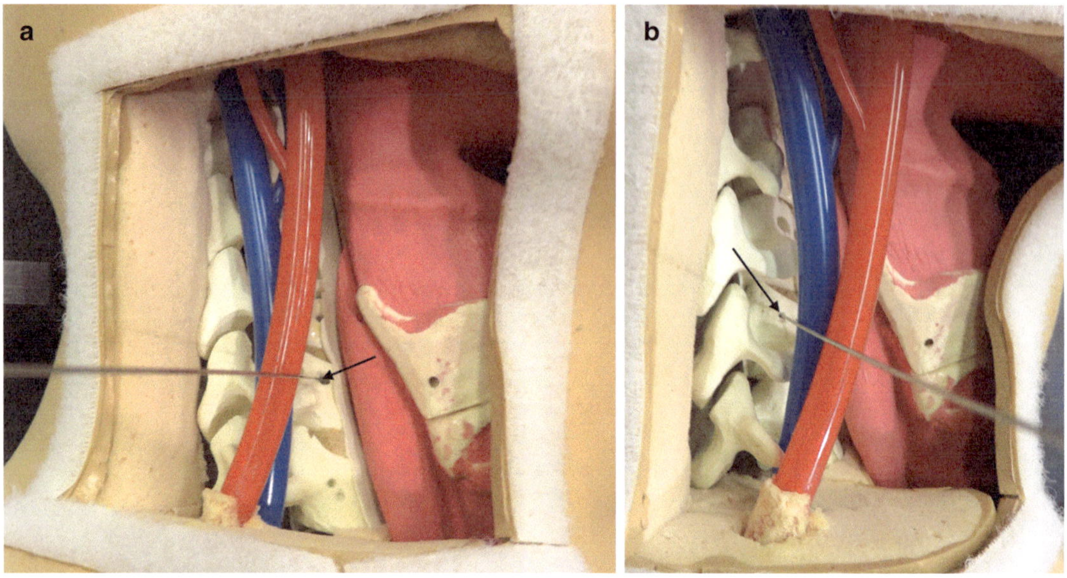

Fig. 4.2 Photographs of neck model showing a spinal needle inserted into a cervical vertebral body (**a**) anterior (*arrow*) and (**b**) posterior (*arrow*) to the carotid space

important to be aware of the location of the spinal cord and exiting nerve roots relative to the lesion.

> A constant awareness and vigilance of the important neck compartments and critical anatomic structures is required before, during and even after the cervical spine biopsy procedure.

This is an important principle that must be adhered to when performing image-guided percutaneous spine biopsies (Ortiz et al. 2010). A detailed review of pertinent imaging studies, such as magnetic resonance imaging (MRI) studies of the cervical spine or positron emission tomography (PET) – CT examinations, is therefore mandatory prior to considering and planning a biopsy procedure. The prior study or studies should be readily available for immediate consultation during the biopsy procedure.

4.3 Indications

Image-guided percutaneous cervical spine biopsy is performed to obtain tissue samples from the cervical vertebrae (including the vertebral bodies, articular masses and posterior elements) intervertebral disks and surrounding paraspinal soft tissues. The two most common indications for performing percutaneous image-guided cervical spine biopsy include the evaluation of a neoplastic process or the assessment for possible spine infection (Table 4.1). Secondary or primary neoplastic lesions of the spine may be considered for biopsy when their histopathologic identification impacts the subsequent management of the patient. Secondary neoplastic lesions of the cervical spine include metastases, myeloma, lymphoma and leukemia; these may occur in patients with a known primary malignancy, or be the first presentation of an unknown primary tumor. Alternatively, a patient may be afflicted with two or more neoplastic conditions, and further characterization

Table 4.1 Indications for image-guided percutaneous cervical spine biopsy

1. Secondary neoplastic involvement
   - Metastasis
     - Known primary neoplasm
     - Two or more known primary neoplasms
     - Unknown primary neoplasm
   - Extension from systemic neoplasm (myeloma, lymphoma, leukemia)
2. Primary neoplastic involvement
3. Spine infection
4. Spine infection mimics
   - Inflammatory spondyloarthropathy (chronic hemodialysis, gout)
5. Other
   - Pathologic vertebral compression fracture
   - Langerhans Cell Histiocytosis
   - Evaluate recurrence of neoplasm after surgical, medical and/or radiation treatment
   - Distinguishing radiation change from neoplasm

of a cervical spine mass will determine which of these processes is responsible. Primary spine tumors, though rare, do occur and may require a biopsy in order to optimize the subsequent management. Now that tailored immune-modulating therapies are available and that an analysis of cellular genomics is readily feasible, biopsies for tissue acquisition and detailed characterization are critical for both treatment planning and prognosis. A pathologic cervical vertebral compression fracture may also require a biopsy.

> It must be emphasized that when a neoplastic process is identified within the cervical spine, the remainder of the spinal axis and body should be evaluated for the possible presence of a more readily accessible lesion for biopsy sampling (Fig. 4.3)

In patients in whom there is an infectious or inflammatory process that involves the cervical disk space and adjacent vertebral endplate(s) a biopsy may be necessary in order to confirm the diagnosis and guide subsequent therapeutic interventions.

4.4 Contraindications

The major contraindication to performing percutaneous image-guided cervical spine biopsy is uncorrected coagulopathy (Table 4.2). Given the increased modern day use of anticoagulants and anti-platelet agents, it is imperative that the operator be aware of whether or not a patient is being treated with one or more of these medications (Refer to Chap. 2*)*. A discussion with the referring clinician and patient is often required in order to determine the necessary steps in either holding or reversing the effects of these medications in order to perform the biopsy procedure. The focus of the conversation should include a risk-benefit analysis in order to ascertain the absolute need for the cervical spine biopsy procedure. The rationale for the both the cervical spine biopsy procedure and the temporary management of the coagulation status should be documented by the operator. In specific situations the patient may need to be admitted for in-hospital management of their coagulation status prior to performance of the biopsy. It must be kept in mind that the majority of these cervical spine biopsy procedures are elective or semi-urgent procedures that by default provide sufficient opportunity for adequate evaluation and communication in order to maximize the chances for a safe and effective procedure. If patient, custodial agent or administrative consent cannot be obtained then the procedure should not be performed.

The other contraindications to image-guided percutaneous cervical spine biopsy are relative, that is, the procedure can be performed provided that the specific management steps are taken. For example, pre-procedure

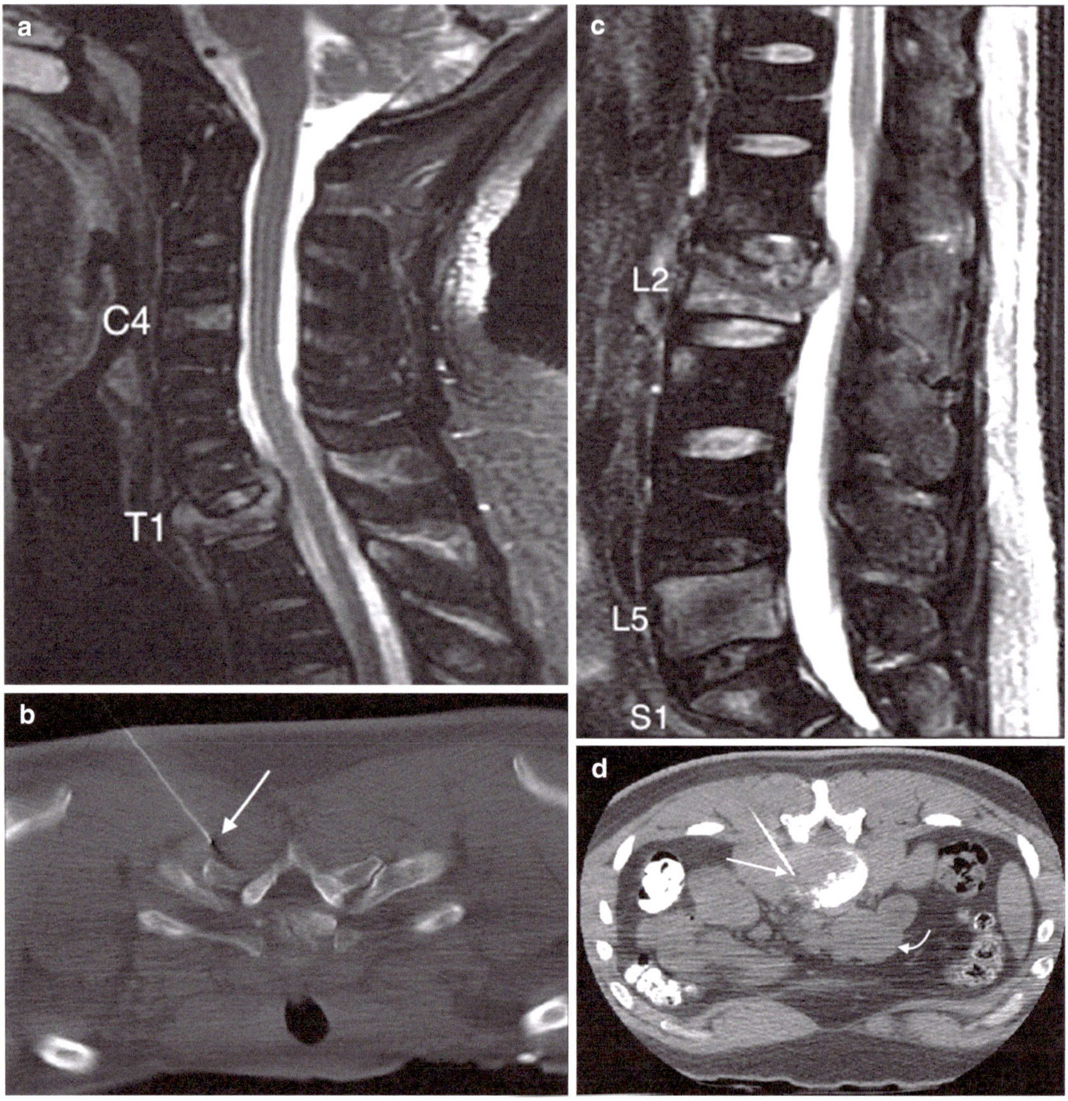

Fig. 4.3 30 year-old male with multiple spine lesions. Fat-suppressedT2 sagittal MR image of cervical spine (**a**) shows a C4 and T1 vertebral body lesions. The operator attempted to biopsy T1 via a posterior approach (*arrow*) without success (**b**). STIR sagittal MRI image of lumbar spine (**c**) shows L2 and L5 and S1 lesions. CT-guided biopsy (**d**) of the L2 lesion via a posterior approach (*arrow*) confirmed the presence of lymphoma; note the extensive retroperitoneal adenopathy (*curved arrow*)

Table 4.2 Contraindications to image-guided percutaneous cervical spine biopsy

Absolute
Uncorrected coagulopathy
Unable to obtain consent for the procedure
Relative
Uncooperative patient
Unstable patient
Suspected vascular lesion
Small (<5 mm diameter) lesion located adjacent to critical structure

catheter angiography with our without embolization may be required prior to performing a biopsy of a suspected vascular tumor such as a renal or thyroid metastasis, aneurysmal bone cyst, or aggressive hemangioma. Alternatively, a very small (<5 mm diameter) if not tiny lesion may just not be amenable to tissue sampling, especially if it is located in close proximity to the spinal cord or a vascular structure.

4.5 Risks and Complications Associated with Cervical Spine Biopsy and How to Minimize Them

The risks and complications that occur as a result of image-guided percutaneous cervical spine biopsy are uncommon and can be kept to a minimum (Wu et al. 2014). Complications that occur as a result of cervical spine biopsy include hemorrhage. As previously stated, this risk can be reduced by temporarily correcting a pre-existing coagulopathy. Identifying critical vascular structures when planning an approach to the lesion and determining an optimal trajectory will also reduce the likelihood of a hemorrhagic complication. Use of coaxial biopsy needle technology, with one needle pass and placement of a guiding cannula through the biopsy trajectory, also reduces the chances of hemorrhage. The occasional, but necessary use of intravenous contrast enhancement with CT guidance may identify subtle vascular structures that can subsequently be avoided. Pre- and peri-procedure management of suspected vascular lesions will also help to reduce the possibility of hematoma formation. Some vascular lesions may require an embolization procedure (pre-procedure endovascular embolization or post-procedure biopsy tract embolization with a small amount of surgifoam), while others can be safely sampled with fine needle aspiration techniques. Adequate blood pressure management and control during and after the biopsy procedure will also help to reduce the likelihood of hemorrhage (Fig. 4.4). There is no substitute for appropriate hand compression techniques following removal of the biopsy needle system at the puncture site, as this will help to stop bleeding at the puncture site. A few minutes (2–5 min) of manual compression will help to stabilize the biopsy tract. Bleeding into one of the neck spaces can lead to hematoma formation and possible airway compromise. Therefore, it is important to monitor the patient during and after the procedure (Fig. 4.4). Patients with hematoma formation can be imaged with CT in order to assess for stability of the hematoma and the airway.

Other procedural risks are related to needle puncture and include vascular injury, spinal cord puncture and, with lower cervical spine biopsy, lung perforation with pneumothorax formation. Fortunately with careful planning and meticulous technique, injury to these critical structures can usually be prevented. Spine infection is a potential complication of any biopsy procedure. This applies to situations where the cervical

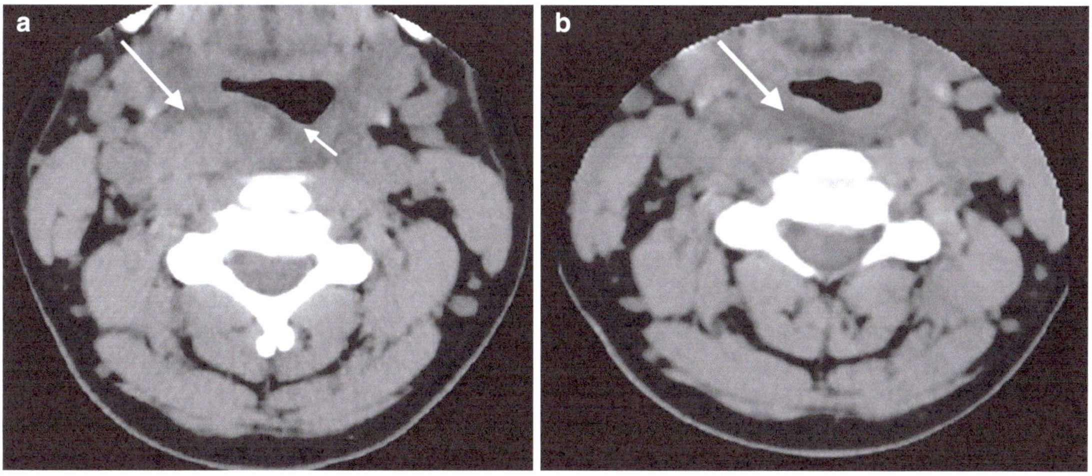

Fig. 4.4 48F for fluoroscopy guided disk aspiration at C4–5 (**a**). The patient's blood pressure increased significantly during the procedure (240/120 mmHg) and she complained of difficulty swallowing. Axial CT image (**a**) shows acute soft swelling with hematoma formation (*large arrow*) and mass effect on oropharynx (*small arrow*). This responded to conservative management including blood pressure control. A follow-up limited CT (**b**) at 1 week shows partial resolution of the swelling and residual retropharyngeal fluid (*arrow*)

spine biopsy is being performed to evaluate for non-infectious conditions, such as neoplastic lesions of the cervical spine. The use of strict aseptic technique including shaving and hair removal at the biopsy puncture site will help to reduce the chance of infection. The use of coaxial technique, by reducing the number of times that the skin is breached, will also help to reduce the inadvertent introduction of cutaneous microbes into the deep tissues of the cervical spine. The routine use of pre-procedure intravenous antibiotic prophylaxis for the performance of cervical spine biopsy is not required unless there is a specific clinical concern that might warrant their use such as a patient that is immunocompromised. Seeding of tumor along a biopsy tract is an extremely rare complication of biopsy procedures and theoretically is even less likely to occur with coaxial biopsy techniques (Saghieh et al. 2010).

The types of complications that can occur or have been reported with cervical spine biopsy are listed in Table 4.3. It must be kept in mind that these are potential complications, many of which can be avoided if careful steps are taken to minimize the chances of their occurrence. The overall incidence of complications that can occur with skeletal biopsy is less than 0.2% (Murphy et al. 1981). The overall complication rate for percutaneous spine biopsy ranges from less than 1% to 3% (Tehranzadeh et al. 2007). A review of the literature shows that the overall incidence of complications that can occur with image-guided percutaneous cervical spine biopsy is rare (Brugieres et al. 1992; Kattapuram and Rosenthal 1987; Rimondi et al. 2008; Wu et al. 2014). The other important risk that can occur with cervical spine biopsy procedures is the possibility of a "non-diagnostic" biopsy. In this situation, tissue is obtained from the sampled lesion; nevertheless the histopathologic analysis is not able to arrive at a conclusive diagnosis. This potential outcome should always be discussed with the patient at the time of the informed consent process in order to clarify expectations and to make them aware that another biopsy procedure, percutaneous or open, might be required.

Table 4.3 Cervical spine biopsy procedure risks and complications

Hemorrhage
Superficial – at puncture site
Deep – potential hematoma formation – airway compromise
Needle injury
Artery or vein puncture
Spinal cord puncture
Cervical nerve root puncture
Lung puncture – pneumothorax
Glandular injury: thyroid gland, parathyroid gland, submandibular gland, parotid gland
Aerodigestive tract perforation
Other
Non-diagnostic biopsy
Wrong level or wrong side biopsied
Infection (cellulitis, infectious spondylitis)
Tumor seeding along the biopsy tract
Transient paresis of lower extremities
Transient recurrent laryngeal nerve palsy
Systemic – anesthesia complication, contrast agent reaction
Increased pain
Radiation exposure
Death
Equipment failure – broken needle

4.6 Imaging Guidance

While there are a few sporadic case reports of image-guided percutaneous spine biopsy performed with ultrasound or magnetic resonance imaging guidance the principal imaging modalities that are used for cervical spine biopsy include CT and fluoroscopy (Ortiz et al. 2010). Each of these modalities possesses advantages and disadvantages. Both modalities allow for ease of access to the cervical spine, variable patient positioning and ready access to the patient for continuous monitoring and management, and the ability to use any number of tools or instruments for the biopsy procedure. CT provides good axial spatial resolution and a thorough view of all anatomic and critical structures within the cervical spine as well as localizing the target lesion. The major vascular structures within the neck can usually be visualized on unenhanced axial images and intravenous contrast agents are not routinely required. The axial CT images can be compared to the pre-biopsy studies in order to plan the optimal approach and trajectory for the biopsy procedure. The precise location of the biopsy needle tip relative to the lesion and adjacent critical structures can readily be monitored with CT. CT-guided cervical spine biopsies were first performed with conventional stepwise advancement of needles with intermittent acquisitions of a small number of images through the area of interest between needle advancements or repositioning (Brugieres et al. 1992; Kattapuram and Rosenthal 1987). This technique facilitated procedure safety, but was associated with a longer procedure time. CT fluoroscopy improves the efficiency of the procedure by keeping the operator in the procedure room and allowing for immediate image acquisition through the area of interest. CT does have limited longitudinal or Z-axis visualization, which can be a challenge if the patient moves during the procedure or if needle angulation is required. These challenges are partially mitigated by using CT fluoroscopy with the trade-off being a slight increase in radiation dose. Nevertheless, the use of CT fluoroscopy increases the efficiency and safety of the procedure as it combines the real time benefits of fluoroscopy with the axial resolution of CT (Wu et al. 2014).

Fluoroscopy can be used to perform anterior cervical spine biopsy. The advantages of this modality include real time, instantaneous feedback on needle trajectory and depth of the needle tip. The operator's hands, however, are often within the fluoroscopy field during the procedure and this increases radiation exposure to the operator. The absence of soft tissue contrast limits the anatomic detail and subtle or small lesions may not be visualized with fluoroscopy. Fluoroscopic guidance is helpful in performing intervertebral disk biopsies using an anterolateral approach with manual displacement of the carotid space by the operator (the operator uses his/her hand to pull the carotid out of the way) and efficient prompt insertion of the biopsy needle into the abnormal disk.

4.7 Approaches

The objective of any biopsy is to obtain as much tissue as possible to improve the chances of obtaining an accurate diagnosis and to perform this safely without injuring critical structures. The choice of a percutaneous approach to a lesion is paramount to determining the optimal biopsy needle trajectory or trajectories (Table 4.4) (Gupta et al. 2007). The approach for cervical spine biopsy is determined by several factors (Ortiz et al. 2010). First, the location of the lesion – is it within the anterior compartment or the posterior compartment? Second, the level of the lesion – is the lesion at the level of the suprahyoid neck or the infrahyoid neck? Is the lesion located within the upper cervical spine at C1 or C2 or is it located in the mid to lower cervical spine (C3-C7) (Sun et al. 2009)?

Table 4.4 Approaches used to perform cervical spine biopsy

Lesion	Level	Location	Approach
Osseous	C1	Lateral mass	Posterior or lateral
		Posterior arch	Posterior or lateral
Osseous	C2	Dens/body	Infra-maxillary, transoral, transpedicular
		Posterior arch	Posterior or lateral
Osseous	C3 – C7	Vertebral body	Anterolateral
		Facet joint	Posterior or lateral
		Posterior arch	Posterior or lateral
		Spinous process	Posterior or lateral
Intervertebral disk			Anterolateral
Prevertebral soft tissues			Anterolateral
Paraspinal soft tissues			Posterior or lateral

Third, what is the specific anatomic location of the lesion – vertebral body, intervertebral disk, articular mass or facet joint, laminae, spinous process or paravertebral soft tissues? Lesion size will also influence the approach. In general, when sampling a lesion it is desirable to have the needle pass through the greatest diameter of the lesion. This allows for both more sampling and for a margin of safety in that the needle stays within the lesion and does not extend beyond into a possible critical structure. Larger lesions provide a large diameter for sampling whereas smaller lesions may have limited areas for needle excursion thereby resulting in fewer and/or smaller samples. Larger lesions, especially those that involve the paraspinal soft tissues, may displace critical structures out of the path of the intended needle trajectory. Of equal importance is the identification of all critical structures, from skin surface to spinal cord, along all possible trajectories to the lesion. These factors will not only contribute towards determining the approach to lesion, but will also influence the patient's position within the operative field. In addition to supine and prone patient positions for standard anterior and posterior approaches, respectively, it may be necessary to place a patient in oblique or decubitus positions to facilitate access to specific lesions or cause slight displacement of critical structures such that the intended trajectory becomes more feasible.

4.8 The Cervical Spine Biopsy Procedure

4.8.1 General Considerations

4.8.1.1 Patient Factors

Cervical spine biopsy procedures can be performed on inpatients or outpatients and should only be performed on cooperative patients. Therefore, whenever and as much as possible it is important to evaluate and examine the patient. This objective can be accomplished at the time of the informed consent process. This consultation serves several purposes as it allows the operator to assess the patient's mental status and to establish a doctor – patient relationship with the patient and the patient's family and healthcare proxies. It also enables the operator to examine the neck for any possible wounds, scars, tattoos and hair, to assess the patient's ability to flex, extend or rotate the head and neck, to assess shoulder mobility and to determine ahead of time, which positions the patient can or cannot tolerate. These factors along with the intended approach will influence the patient position. The patient should be as comfortable as possible just before and throughout the procedure as this will improve their ability to cooperate during the biopsy procedure. An informed and comfortable patient will tend to be a cooperative and less anxious patient. The upfront opportunity to clarify expectations with the patient and the patient's representatives cannot be understated. Patients should also be informed that the other diagnostic alternative to a percutaneous biopsy procedure is an open biopsy procedure. Open biopsy procedures are performed in the operating room under general anesthesia, require a somewhat longer recovery period and carry the risks (bleeding, infection, tissue damage) associated with open surgical procedures (Mankin et al. 1996).

In addition to obtaining a thorough medical and surgical history, the operator should also be aware of the patient's medications, especially antiplatelet and anticoagulant medications, any concurrent antibiotic therapy and any herbal or vitamin supplements. Patient allergies should be documented and recent laboratory parameters for hematologic status (serum hematocrit, hemoglobin, platelet count), coagulation status (serum Prothrombin Time, Partial Thromboplastin Time, International Normalized Ratio), and renal function (serum Blood Urea Nitrogen, Creatinine, Glomerular Filtration Rate) should be available. In those patients with a suspected spine infection, consideration ought to be given to obtaining a white blood cell count with differential, an erythrocyte sedimentation rate and a C-reactive protein. Patients should be instructed to not eat or drink, in other words, remain in NPO status after midnight on the day of the procedure.

4.8.1.2 Staff Factors

It is helpful to discuss the procedure ahead of time with the procedural staff, including the radiology technologist, nurse(s), anesthesiologist (if consulted), pathologist and/or microbiologist. These communications maximize the chances for a smoother, more successful procedure. They facilitate specimen collection, handling and analysis. For example, if a fine needle aspiration procedure is performed, then a cytopathologist or cytotechnologist may be present on site to evaluate the tissue samples and determine if there is adequate diagnostic tissue.

4.8.1.3 Anesthesia

The choice of anesthesia is influenced by the type of biopsy, the patient's preference, the patient's medical condition, the patient's position and the operator's discretion. If an anesthesiologist is assisting in the case, then they will help to decide the preferred method of anesthesia. The options for anesthesia range from the use of local anesthetics, to intravenous sedation and analgesia to the use of intravenous anesthesia. It is strongly advised to avoid the antecubital fossa for securing intravenous access as the arms are often flexed during the procedure, impeding the efficacy of intravenous medications.

4.8.1.4 Patient Preparation

The patient is placed on the procedure table in the desired position and monitoring equipment (pulse oximeter, electrocardiogram and blood pressure monitor) is placed on the patient. Cervical spine biopsy is performed with strict aseptic technique. The skin should be shaved in order to remove hair from the sterile field. It is important to discuss the need for hair removal at the craniocervical junction ahead of time with patients. Once the patient is positioned, the skin is shaved and the patient is on the procedure table, then a time-out protocol is exercised in order to confirm patient, procedure, site and side.

4.8.2 Technique

4.8.2.1 CT Guidance

Scout images are obtained in both the frontal and lateral projections with a radiopaque skin grid in place covering the side and area of the intended approach (Fig. 4.5). The intended skin puncture site is marked with a skin marker. The skin is then prepped with a sterile solution and draped. In patient's that are receiving intravenous sedation/analgesia or anesthesia, this can be initiated at this time or just after the time out process. The skin is anesthetized with a local anesthetic agent (such as 1 or 2% lidocaine or 0.25% bupivacaine) using a 25 gauge needle. A small cross hair incision is made at the skin insertion site using a #11 scalpel blade.

Cervical spine biopsies were first performed with tandem needle techniques; a biopsy needle was maneuvered alongside and parallel to an initially placed small gauge (20 gauge) spinal needle, but these entailed a minimum of 2 skin punctures (Kattapuram and Rosenthal 1987). Coaxial needle technique is well suited for performing cervical spine biopsy (Geremia et al. 1992; Wu et al. 2014;). With a coaxial needle technique, a 15 cm long, 20 gauge guide needle with a removable hub is slowly advanced under CT fluoroscopic guidance towards the target lesion, carefully avoiding critical structures. When the needle tip approaches the margin of the lesion or an osseous surface, additional local anesthetic (approximately 1 mL volume) can be administered in order to minimize patient discomfort. Once the optimal trajectory and needle position are established with imaging guidance and the periosteal or lesion surface have been anesthetized, then the needle hub is removed (Fig. 4.5). The needle then serves as a guidewire or guidepin for subsequent coaxial insertion of a guiding cannula. The guiding cannula provides a safe access port to the target lesion, reducing if not obviating the requirement for repeat needle passes in the vicinity of critical structures (Figs. 4.6 and 4.7). For bone biopsy, a removable blunt dissector is inserted into the guiding cannula; this facilitates safe passage of the guiding cannula through the deep soft tissues over the hub-less guide needle. For any type of soft tissue biopsy (disk or paraspinal) a guiding cannula and blunt dissector can be advanced over the guide needle or, alternatively, a soft guide needle can be advanced using its own stylet (Fig. 4.8). In the anterior neck, the platysma can present as a stubborn barrier to advancement of the blunt dissec-

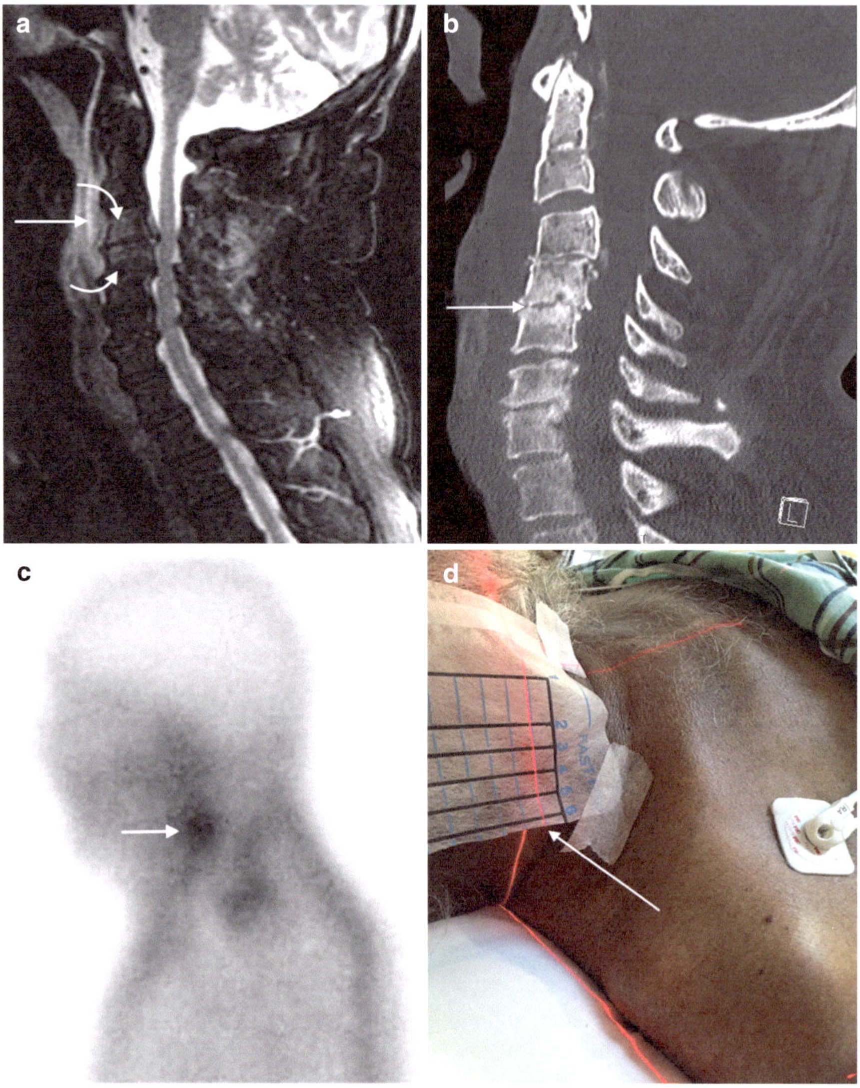

Fig. 4.5 83 M with neck pain. Fat suppressed T2 sagittal MR image (**a**) shows a small prevertebral fluid collection (*arrow*) with subtle increased signal within the adjacent vertebral bodies at C3 and C4 (*curved arrows*). A sagittal reconstructed CT image (**b**) shows multi-level disk space height loss with endplate irregularity (*arrow*) at C4–5. Lateral static image from a gallium scan (**c**) shows intense uptake within the cervical spine (*arrow*). An erythrocyte sedimentation level and C reactive protein level were noted to be elevated and the patient was referred for an image-guided biopsy. A grid line sheet (*arrow*) was placed on the right side of the patient's neck (**d**). A CT scout frontal radiograph (**e**) shows the radiopaque lines (*arrows*) which aid in marking the skin entry site with an indelible ink marker pen. An axial CT image in bone algorithm (**f**) shows the grid points (*arrows*) relative to the C4–5 disk space. The skin was then prepped and draped with strict aseptic technique, the skin anesthetized with 0.5 mL 2% lidocaine, and a 20 gauge guide needle (*arrow*) was advanced into the skin (**g**) and passed along the lateral margin of the thyroid ala (*arrow*) as shown on the axial image (**h**). Photograph of guide needle (**i**) after removal of the hub (*arrow*). An 18 gauge spinal needle (*large arrow*) was subsequently passed over what is now essentially a firm guidewire (*medium arrow*) in order to adequately penetrate the platysma (*small arrow*) as shown on the axial image (**j**). Axial CT (K) shows advancement of the spinal needle over the hub-less guide needle to the anterior aspect of the C4–5 disk (*arrow*). The 18 gauge spinal needle is removed, but the 22 gauge hub-less guide needle (guidewire) is kept in place in order to maintain safe access for subsequent placement of the blunt dissector. Axial CT image (**l**) shows advancement of the blunt dissector over the guide needle (*arrow*). The blunt dissector was removed and then inserted into the guide cannula such that this coaxial system was subsequently advanced over the guide needle to the anterior aspect of the C4–5 disk (*arrow*) as shown in the axial CT image (**m**). The blunt dissector was exchanged for a trephine bone biopsy needle (*arrow*) which was advanced through the guide cannula and into the disk and endplate as shown on the axial CT image (**n**). The microbiology specimens were positive for enterococcus species and the pathology specimens showed inflammatory changes consistent with osteomyelitis

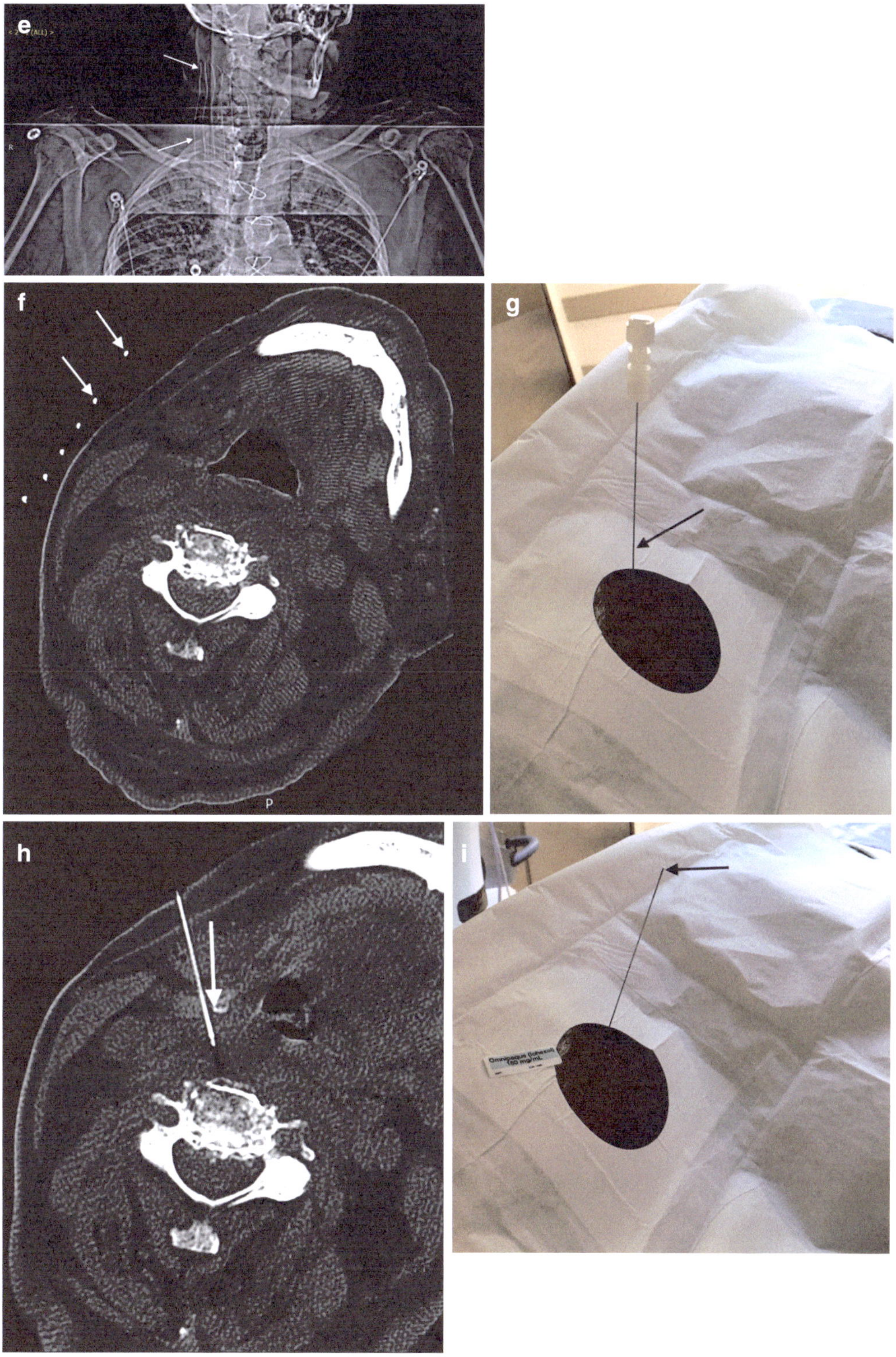

Fig. 4.5 (continued)

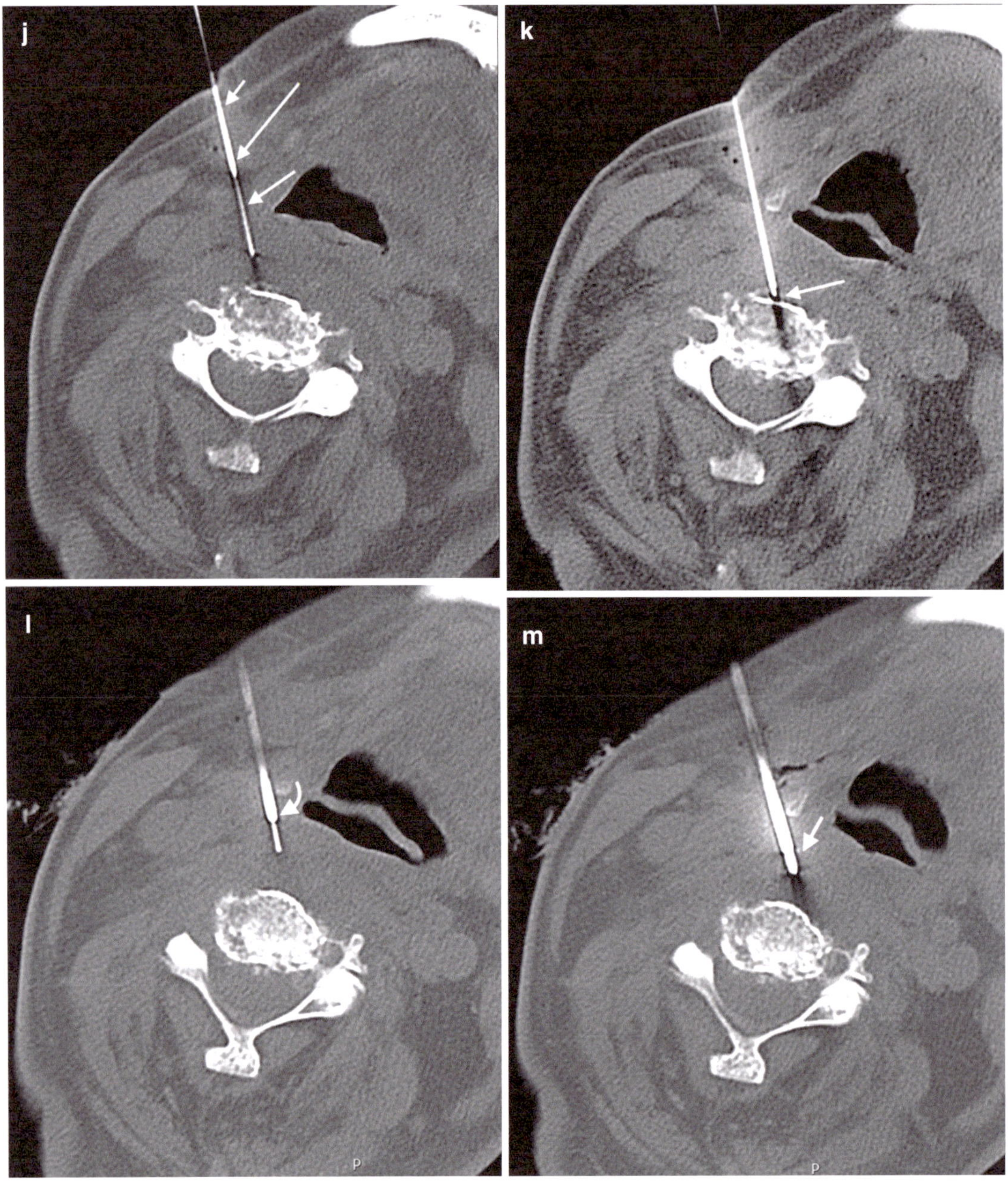

Fig. 4.5 (continued)

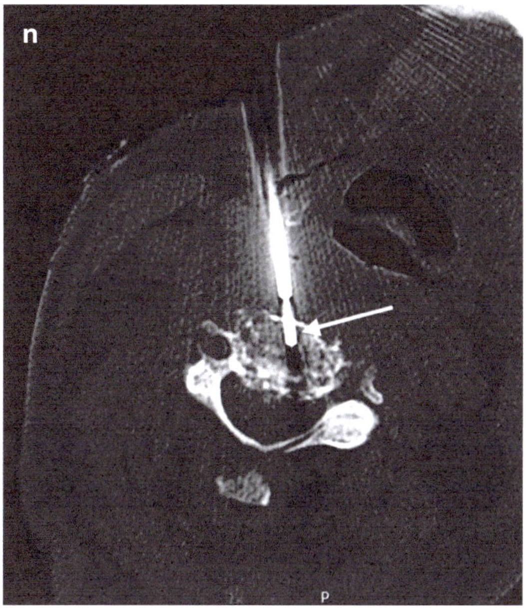

Fig. 4.5 (continued)

tor and/or guiding cannula. If this occurs, then the operator should first advance an 18 gauge spinal needle over the guide needle in order to make a small perforation in the platysma (Fig. 4.5). This maneuver will allow the blunt dissector, initially without, and then with the guiding cannula to readily pass through the platysma.

Once the guiding cannula reaches the margin of the bone or the lesion then the guide needle and blunt dissector are removed after satisfactory positioning is confirmed with CT. Other needles can now be safely inserted through this working cannula. The biopsy sample can be obtained using fine needle (1 mm diameter or less) aspiration or core needle (diameter greater 1.5 mm) biopsy via this coaxial technique. In some situations, the guiding cannula is not supported by the soft tissues of the neck and tends to move. When this occurs it is helpful to hold the guiding cannula and insert the biopsy needle in order to gain purchase within the structure to be sampled. A trephine needle, which has a serrated cutting edge, or other bone cutting needle can be inserted into osseous structures while a soft tissue cutting needle or a fine needle can be inserted into a soft tissue lesion. The guiding cannula can also be stabilized at the skin surface with either sterile towels or a small stack of sterile gauze. The position of the guiding cannula and biopsy needle, relative to the lesion and other critical structures, can be confirmed with the acquisition of sequential CT images (Figs. 4.6 and 4.7).

For soft tissue masses, fine needle aspiration should be performed prior to core biopsy in order to minimize hemorrhage into the needle tract (Fig. 4.8) (Ayala et al. 1995). The latter adversely impacts on the utility of the fine needle aspiration procedure by contaminating the biopsy specimen with blood. Sequential needle passes can be made into the soft tissue mass with slight angulations in order to sample areas of "fresh" tissue. CT image acquisition should be used to monitor the direction and depth of the biopsy needle and assess its proximity to other critical structures. Fine needle aspiration and soft tissue biopsy needles can be used to obtain tissue samples from osteolytic lesions provided that the peripheral cortex, if very thin, can be penetrated by these needles or a bone needle is used to create a tract for subsequent soft tissue needle use. Many soft tissue biopsy needle systems possess a sampling chamber that must be exposed within the substance of the lesion; the needle tip therefore must travel a short distance further (often 1 or 2 cm) in order for the cutting mechanism to work within the lesion matrix. It is important to account for the excursion distance of the soft tissue cutting needle when deploying this instrument in order to avoid injury to a critical structure. The number of passes that can be made will be determined by the size of the lesion and its location relative to critical structures; small, less than 1 cm diameter, lesions will yield only a small sample volume. If the fine needle aspiration shows diagnostic tissue then, at the operator's discretion, the procedure can be stopped. If the situation permits an attempt should be made to obtain at least 3 soft tissue cores (Ortiz et al. 2010).

Bone biopsy needles are used to obtain osseous matrix from bone lesions. Trephine needles are manually rotated with alternating short clockwise and counterclockwise motions, with slight downward pressure, in order to be advanced into the bone. A similar maneuver can be used with other bone cutting needles. The gradual advance-

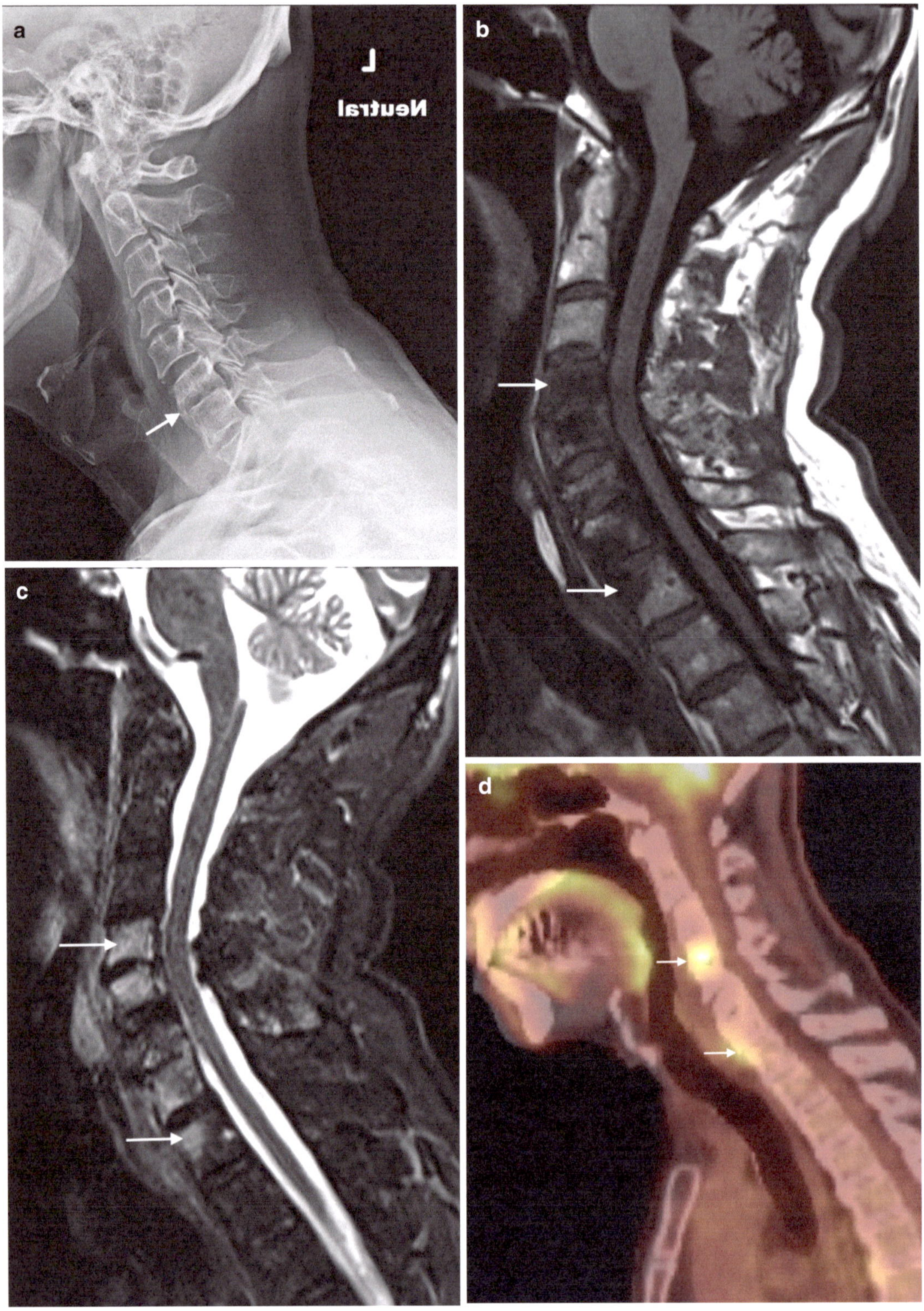
a
L
Neutral
b
c
d

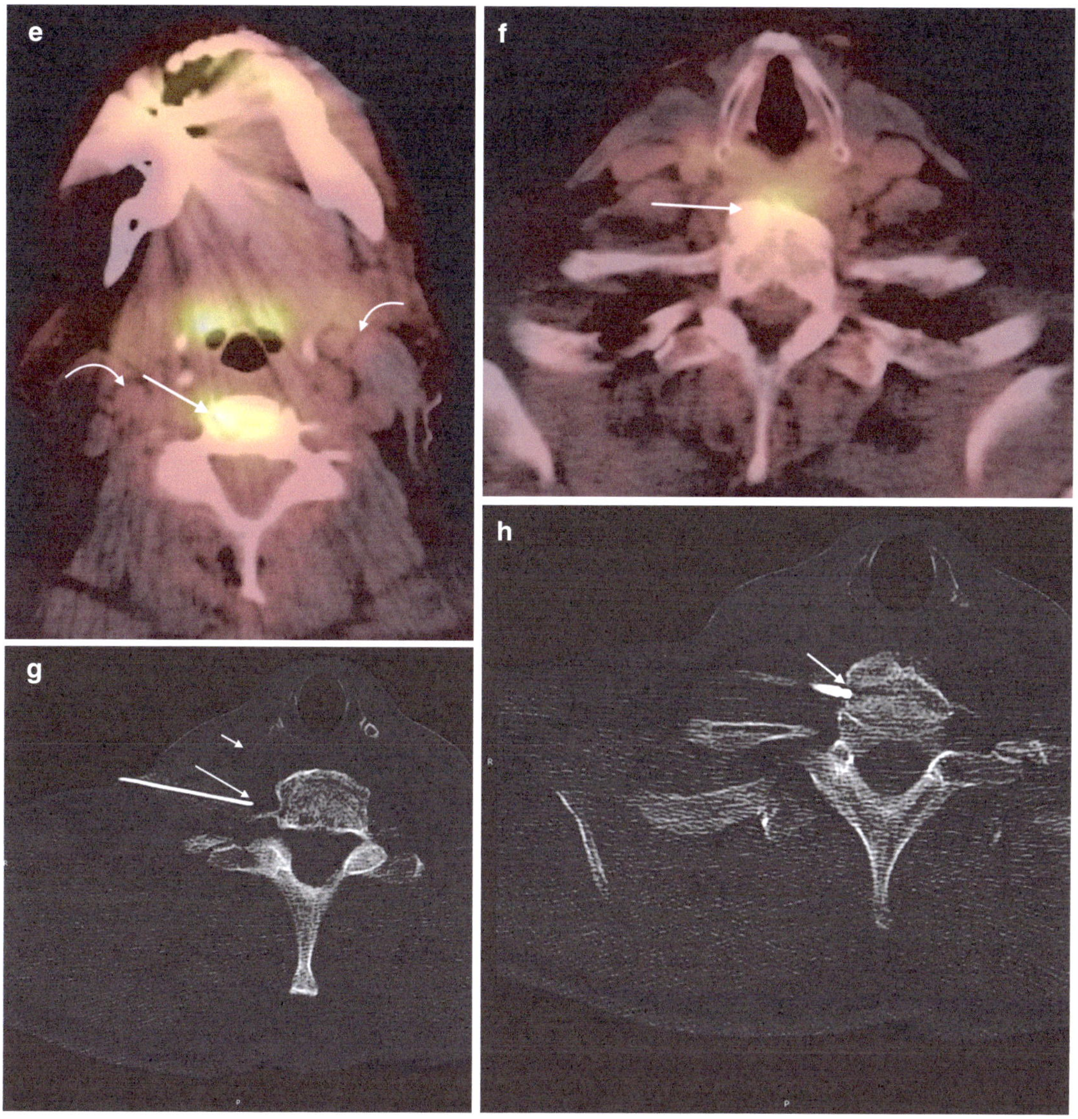

Fig. 4.6 (continued)

Fig. 4.6 73M with history of prostate cancer complains of neck pain. Lateral radiograph of the cervical spine (**a**) shows endplate irregularity and a bridging osteophyte at C6–7 (*arrow*) and no gross lytic or blastic bone lesions. T1 (**b**) and T2 (**c**) weighted sagittal MR images show a diffuse marrow replacement process that extends from C4 to T1 (*arrows*). Sagittal fused PET-CT image (**d**) shows hypermetabolic activity at the C4–5 level and the C7 level (*arrows*). Fused axial PET-CT images at C4–5 (**e**) and C7-T1 (**f**) levels confirm the areas of hypermetabolism (*arrow* in **e**), but also show multiple vascular structures preventing access to the C4–5 level (*curved arrows* in **e**). A more feasible approach posterior to the carotid space (*large arrow* in **f**) is possible at C7-T1. A lateral approach commencing with an 18 gauge spinal needle (*large arrow*) posterior to the carotid space (*small arrow*) was used (**g**). This enabled the bone needle (*arrow*) to be advanced across the C7 vertebra (**h**, **i**). Photograph of specimen container (**j**) shows multiple bone cores (*arrows*)

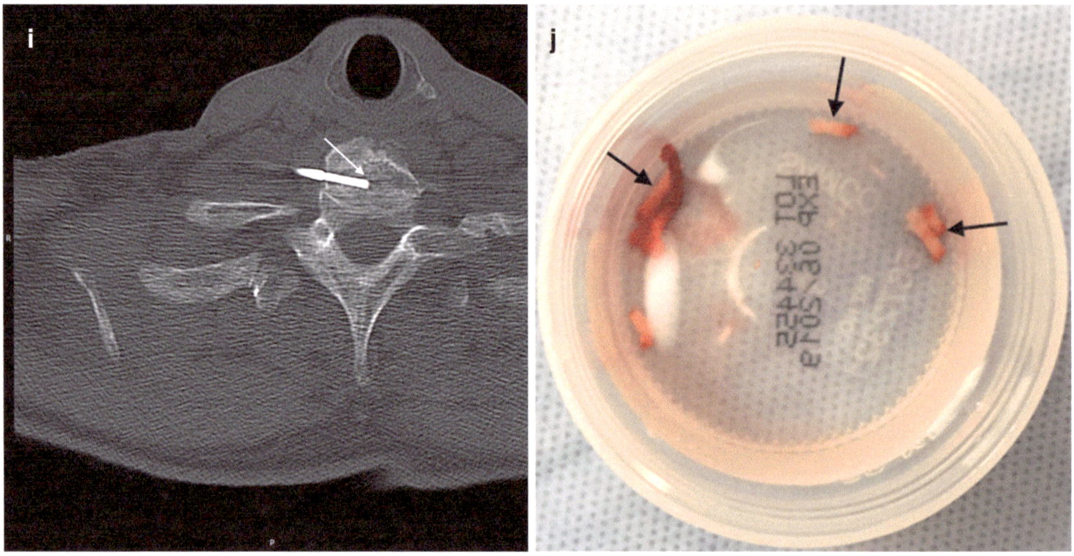

Fig. 4.6 (continued)

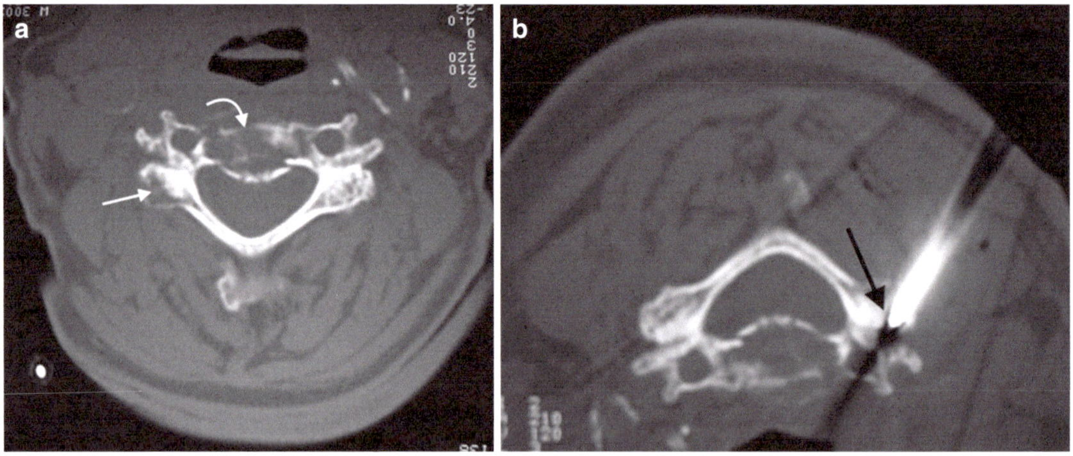

Fig. 4.7 Axial CT image in bone window algorithm (**a**) shows lytic lesions within the vertebral body (*curved arrow*) and the right articular pillar (*arrow*). Axial CT image with patient prone (**b**) shows that the articular pillar was biopsied (*arrow*) with a posterior approach in this patient with biopsy proven multiple myeloma

ment of the needle should be monitored with serial CT scans. Extreme caution should be observed in elderly patients with osteoporosis, or patients with very osteolytic lesions as the bone needle may advance briskly in these situations. It is helpful to sample as much tissue as safely as possible, scanning and checking needle position, between and during biopsy attempts. Since the bone tissue will require de-calcification prior to histopathologic analysis, whenever possible the operator should attempt obtain at least three bone cores (Fig. 4.6).

4.8.2.2 Fluoroscopic Guidance

Fluoroscopic guidance can be used to biopsy large or diffuse osseous lesions when CT is not available. This modality is particularly useful in providing prompt access to the intervertebral disk

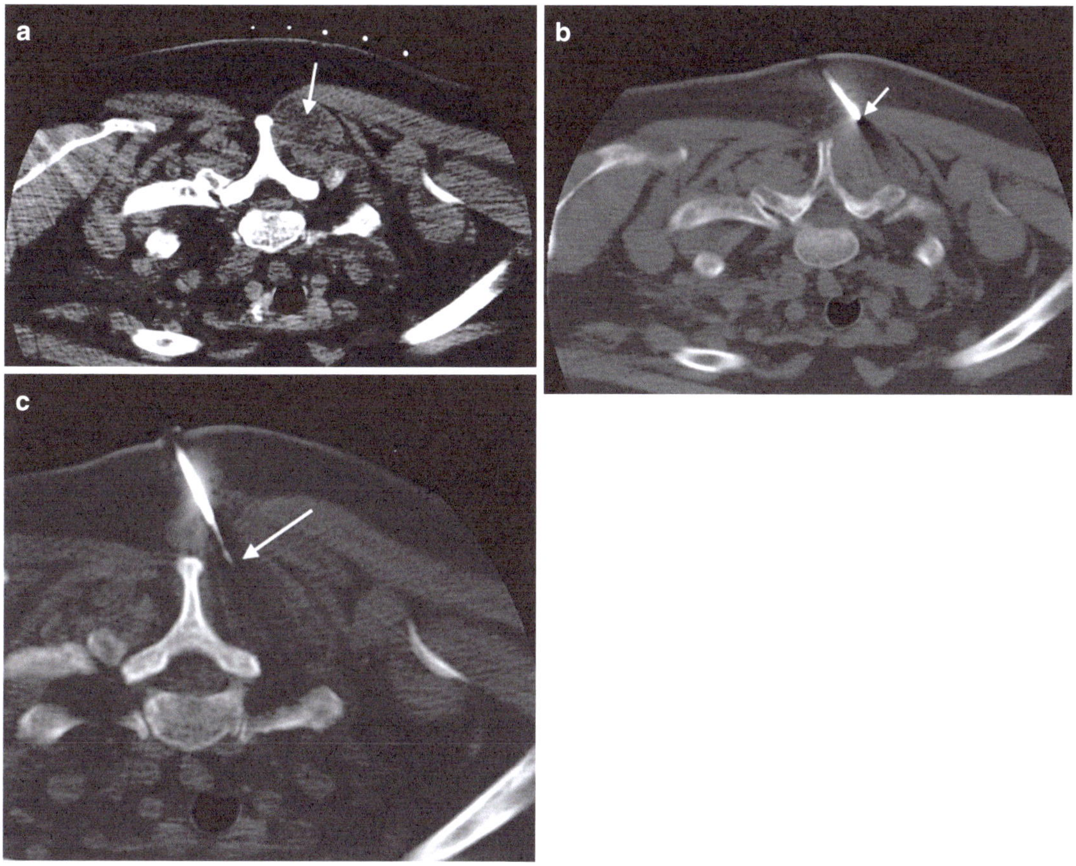

Fig. 4.8 63F with palpable posterior neck mass. Axial CT image in soft tissue algorithm (**a**) shows skin markers placed above a slightly hypodense mass that is located beneath the trapezius muscle (*arrow*). Axial CT image in bone window algorithm (**b**) shows guide needle placement just superficial to the lesion (*arrow*). Note that the guide needle is obliquely angled away from the spinal canal in order to (1) prevent spinal canal access and spinal cord injury and, (2) to maximize biopsy needle excursion through the greatest diameter of the lesion. Axial CT image in bone window algorithm (**c**) shows deployment of a cutting needle within the matrix of this biopsy proven schwannoma

space using an anterolateral approach with manual posterior displacement, by the operator, of the carotid artery and jugular vein. With the patient supine and the neck extended, an oblique approach with the cervical vertebral endplates aligned at the level of interest, the intervertebral disk is accessed at a minimum of a few millimeters anterior to the uncovertebral joint (Fig. 4.9). The extent and depth of needle insertion is monitored with frontal, lateral and contralateral oblique projections. Coaxial approaches with a guide needle/cannula and smaller gauge aspiration needles can be used to attempt to obtain tissue from the disk. Alternatively, automated percutaneous aspiration systems are available and can be used to obtain disk material for microbiologic and pathologic analysis (Ortiz et al. 2010; Wattamwar and Ortiz 2010). As the majority of these disk biopsy procedures are being performed to evaluate for infection, additional coaxial passes with bone biopsy needles, angling them toward the endplate, may help to yield more tissue (Michel et al. 2006). The number of passes that can be made with these approaches will be limited by the final location of the biopsy needle tip, which should be maintained within the confines of the disk space throughout the procedure. Performing disk biopsies prior to the initiation of

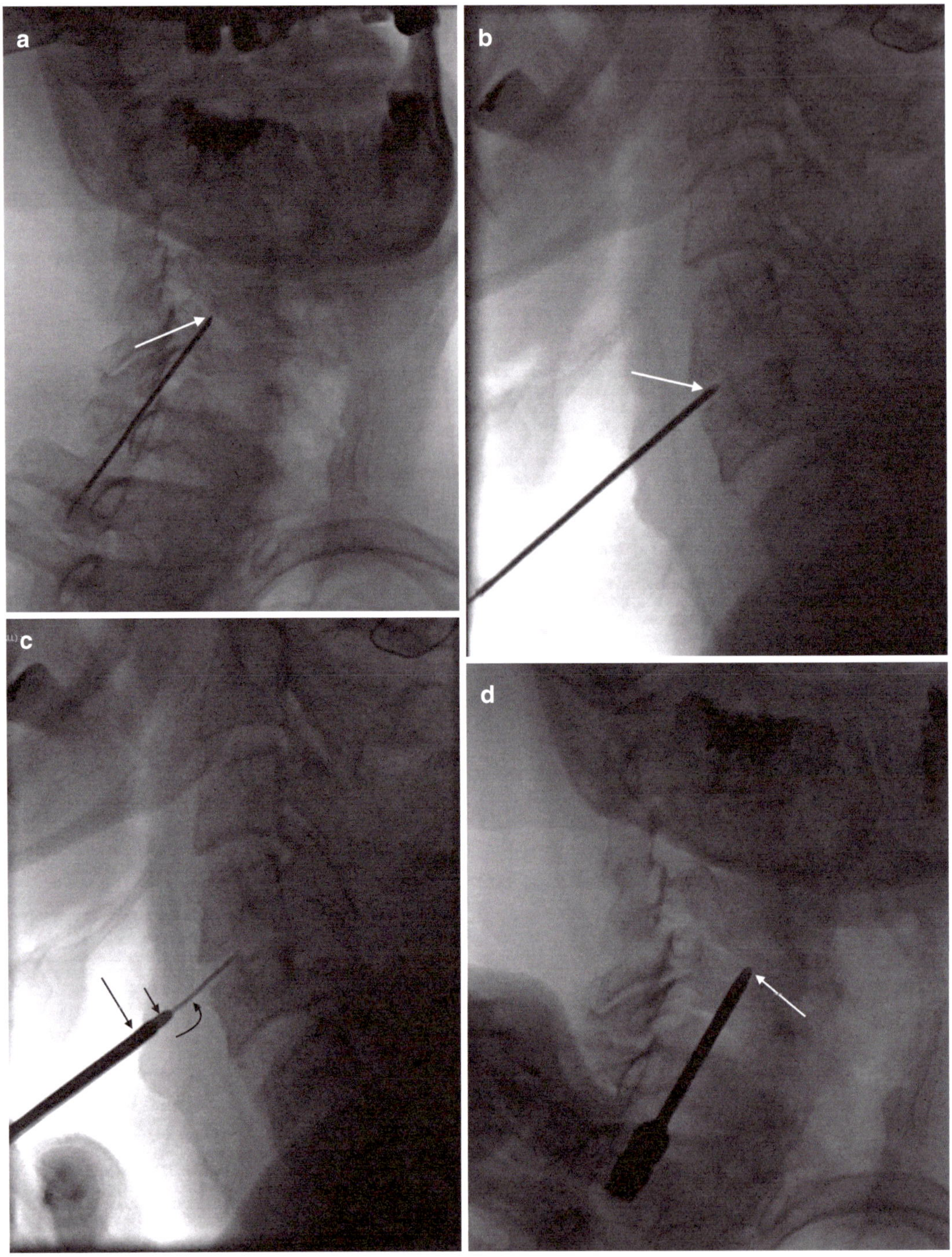

Fig. 4.9 Fluoroscopic images showing oblique approach (**a**) to disk space with an 18 gauge spinal needle; note the position of the spinal needle anterior to the uncovertebral joint adjacent to the lateral margin of the disk space (*arrow*). A lateral projection (**b**) shows the tip of the needle within the disk space (*arrow*). After disk aspiration is performed through the spinal needle, a hub-less long 22 gauge exchange (*insert*) needle is inserted into the spinal needle using coaxial technique and the spinal needle is exchanged for a12 gauge bone biopsy guide cannula (*large arrow*) and introducer (*small arrow*) which are then advanced over the guide needle (*curved arrow*) as shown on the lateral projection (**c**). The insert needle is removed and the guide cannula is stabilized and slightly re-positioned within the disk (*arrow*) as shown of the oblique projection (**d**). Frontal projection (**e**) shows replacement of the introducer with a bone biopsy needle (*arrow*) as the guide cannula is held firmly in place. The bone biopsy needle is carefully advanced with to and fro clockwise/counterclockwise rotations; the position of the biopsy needle tip is monitored with frontal, oblique and lateral (**f**) fluoroscopic images

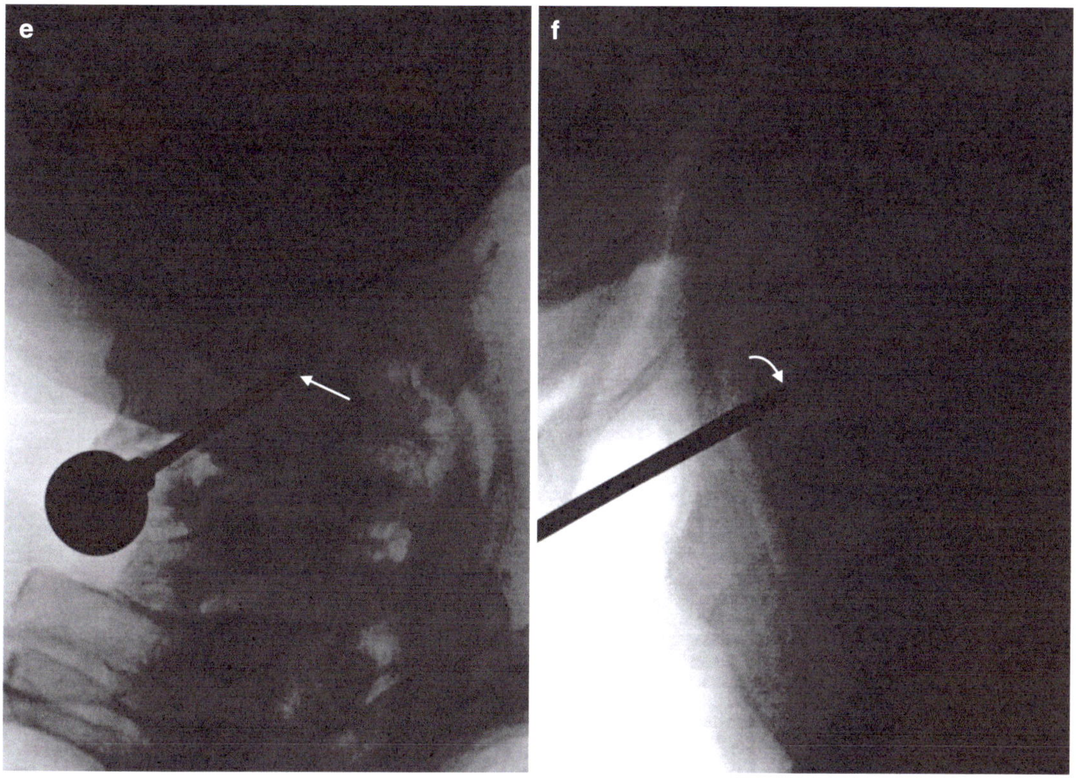

Fig. 4.9 (continued)

antibiotic therapy will help to increase the likelihood of a positive diagnostic yield (Howard et al. 1994; Rankine et al. 2004).

Once biopsy specimens are obtained, they should be labeled and processed immediately. Microbiology specimens should be placed in sterile containers and immediately transported to the microbiology laboratory with the appropriately completed requisition. Pathology specimens should be placed in 10% formalin (bone and soft tissue cores) or a cytology compatible ethanol mixture for fine needle aspirates, labeled, and brought to the pathology laboratory with the appropriately completed requisitions. If there is a clinical concern for specific clinical conditions, such as lymphoma or leukemia, special measures for specimen handling will be necessary, and this should be discussed with a pathologist as flow cytometry and/or other special stains will be performed. Specimen transport should be performed by responsible personnel as part of an organized process; unfortunately, not a year goes by when at some institution or facility, that after a biopsy procedure is performed, the specimen is lost. It is highly recommended that the operator provide as much detailed information about the case and the imaging findings along with their specific clinical concerns in order to improve the chances of obtaining an accurate diagnosis.

The diagnostic accuracy of image-guided percutaneous cervical spine biopsy has improved with the use of CT fluoroscopy and coaxial needle techniques (Wu et al. 2014). Factors that impact on the diagnostic accuracy of the spine biopsy procedure include the lesion location, lesion type, size and matrix, needle size (gauge) and type, sample volume and the experience of the operator and pathologist (Kreula 1990; Ortiz et al. 2010; Rimondi et al. 2011). Small and difficult to access lesions will yield less volume of tissue as compared to other lesions; this is not an infrequent scenario in the cervical spine. Malignant neoplastic lesions are more readily detected as compared to some benign tumors or other benign, non-neoplastic processes (Rimondi et al. 2011). The diagnostic accuracy is lower for sclerotic lesions (76%), which are technically more difficult to sample, as compared to lytic lesions (93%) (Lis et al. 2004). A review of the literature shows that the accuracy of image-guided percutaneous spine biopsy with core sampling ranges from 70 to 97% (Hau et al. 2002; Issakov et al. 2003; Madhavan et al. 2002; Schweitzer et al. 1996). A few reports have shown 100% accuracy, but these are small case series (Wu et al. 2014). With CT-guidance the diagnostic accuracy of coaxial core biopsy techniques is in the range of 90%, especially when sampling a neoplastic process (Lis et al. 2004). The diagnostic accuracy of fine needle aspiration is 60% (Rimondi et al. 2008; Gupta et al. 2002; Yang and Damron 2004). This lower accuracy rate reflects the smaller sampling volume that is obtained with smaller gauge needles as well as sample contamination by hemorrhage. When performing an image-guided percutaneous spine biopsy for infection the diagnostic accuracy is lower, in the range of 50–60% (Rimondi et al. 2008). Antibiotic therapy decreases the diagnostic yield for spine biopsies intended to assess for the presence of infection and antibiotics either should ideally not be administered until the biopsy is performed or should be held for 48 h prior to the performance of the procedure.

4.9 Post-procedure Care

Following cervical spine biopsy, the patient should be monitored and recovered for at least 2 h. The biopsy skin puncture site should be immediately covered with a sterile bandage and monitored for signs of bleeding or expanding hematoma. Pain medication can be given if necessary. An ice-pack can be placed over the area of the puncture site in order to reduce swelling and irritation. Once stable the patient can be discharged home or transported back to their hospital room. The patient should be reminded that the biopsy specimen(s) may take several days to process prior to analysis and that the biopsy results, especially with bone biopsies, will not be immediately available. The patient is instructed to follow up with the referring clinician for the biopsy results. Outpatients are also instructed to call the operator's office and/or staff if they notice any increased swelling, irritation, or increased difficulties with breathing or swallowing. After the procedure, the operator can contact the referring clinician and update them on the procedure and the patient's status. A day after the procedure, a courtesy follow-up telephone call to the patient (for outpatients) or a direct visit with an inpatient is very helpful in terms of clarifying any post-procedure concerns, identifying delayed complications and reassuring the patient. The operator and/or a staff designee should follow up with the appropriate laboratories in order to obtain the biopsy results and ascertain that the referring clinician also has the biopsy results.

Key Review Points

1. A primary objective of image-guided percutaneous cervical spine biopsy is to determine a trajectory towards a lesion that avoids injury to a critical structure while at the same time yielding access to the target lesion.
2. A constant awareness and vigilance of the important neck compartments and critical structures is required before, during and even after the cervical spine biopsy procedure.
3. When a cervical spine neoplasm is detected, always evaluate the remainder of the axial skeleton and body for the possibility of a more accessible lesion.
4. An absolute contraindication to cervical spine biopsy is uncorrected coagulopathy.
5. The risks and complications that can occur as a result of image-guided percutaneous cervical spine biopsy are uncommon and can be kept to a minimum.
6. CT fluoroscopy is a useful modality for performing cervical spine biopsy.
7. Coaxial techniques improve the sampling rate and safety margin of the cervical spine biopsy procedure.
8. Another important objective of cervical spine biopsy is to obtain as much tissue as possible in order to improve the chances of obtaining an accurate diagnosis and to perform the procedure safely without injuring the patient.

References

Ayala AG, Ro JY, Fanning CV, Flores JP, Yasko AW. Core needle biopsy and fine needle aspiration in the diagnosis of bone and soft tissue lesions. Hematol Oncol Clin North Am. 1995;9:633–51.

Brugieres P, Gaston A, Voisin MC, Ricolfi F, Chakir N. CT-guided percutaneous biopsy of the cervical spine: a series of 12 cases. Neuroradiology. 1992;34:358–60.

Geremia GK, Charletta DA, Granato DB, Raju S. Biopsy of vertebral and paravertebral structures with a new coaxial needle system. AJNR Am J Neuroradiol. 1992;12:169–71.

Gupta RK, Cheung YK, Al Ansari AG, Naran S, Lallu S, Fauck R. Diagnostic value of image-guided needle aspiration cytology in the assessment of vertebral and intervertebral lesions. Diagn Cytopathol. 2002;27:191–6.

Gupta S, Henningsen JA, Wallace MJ, Madoff DC, Morello FA, Ahrar K, Murthy R, Hicks E. Percutaneous biopsy of head and neck lesions with CT guidance: various approaches and relevant anatomic and technical considerations. RadioGraphics. 2007;27:371–90.

Hau MA, Kim JI, Kattapuram S, Hornicek FJ, Rosenberg AE, Gebhardt MC, Mankin HJ. Accuracy of CT-guided biopsies in 359 patients with musculoskeletal lesions. Skelet Radiol. 2002;31:349–53.

Howard CB, Einhorn M, Dagan R, Yagupski P, Porat S. Fine-needle bone biopsy to diagnose osteomyelitis. J Bone Joint Surg Br. 1994;76:311–4.

Issakov J, Flusser G, Kollender Y, Merimsky O, Lifschitz-Mercer B, Meller I. Computed tomography-guided core needle biopsy for bone and soft tissue tumors. Isr Med Assoc J. 2003;5:28–30.

Kattapuram SV, Rosenthal SI. Percutaneous biopsy of the cervical spine using CT guidance. AJR Am J Roentgenol. 1987;149:539–41.

Kreula J. Effect of sampling technique on specimen size in fine needle aspiration biopsy. Investig Radiol. 1990;25:1294–9.

Lis E, Bilsky MH, Pisinski L, Boland P, Healey JH, O'Malley B, Krol G. Percutaneous CT-guided biopsy of osseous lesion of the spine in patients with known or suspected malignancy. AJNR Am J Neuroradiol. 2004;25:1583–8.

Madhavan VP, Smile SR, Chandra SS, Ratnakar C. Value of core needle biopsy in the diagnosis of soft tissue tumours. Indian J Pathol Microbiol. 2002;45:165–8.

Mankin HJ, Mankin CJ, Simon MA. The hazards of biopsy, revisited. J Bone Joint Surg Am. 1996;78:656–63.

Michel SC, Pfirrmann CW, Boos N, Hodler J. CT-guided core biopsy of subchondral bone and intervertebral space in suspected spondylodiskitis. AJR Am J Roentgenol. 2006;186:977–80.

Murphy WA, Destouet JM, Gilula LA. Percutaneous skeletal biopsy1981: a procedure for radiologists – results, review, and recommendations. Radiology. 1981;139:545–9.

Ortiz AO, Zoarski G, Brook A. Image-guided percutaneous spine biopsy. In: Mathis JM, Golovac S, editors. Image-guided spine interventions. 2nd ed. New York: Springer; 2010. p. 75–106.

Rankine JJ, Barron DA, Robinson P, et al. Therapeutic impact of percutaneous spinal biopsy in spinal infection. Postgrad Med J. 2004;80:607–9.

Rimondi E, Staals EL, Errani C, Bianchi G, Casadei R, Alberghini M, Malaguti MC, Rossi G, Durante S, Mercuri M. Percutaneous CT-guided biopsy of the spine: results of 430 biopsies. Eur Spine J. 2008;17:975–81.

Rimondi E, Rossi G, Bartalena T, Ciminari R, Alberghini M, Ruggieri P, Errani C, Angelini A, Calabro T, Abati CN, Balladelli A, Tranfaglia C, Mavrogenis AF, Vanel D, Mercuri M. Percutaneous CT-guided biopsy of the musculoskeletal system: results of 2027 cases. Eur J Radiol. 2011;77:34–42.

Saghieh S, Masrouha KZ, Musallam KM, Mahfouz R, Abboud M, Khoury NJ, Haidar R. The risk of local recurrence along the core-needle biopsy tract in patients with bone sarcomas. Iowa Orthop J. 2010;30:80–3.

Schweitzer ME, Gannon FH, Deely DM, O'Hara BJ, Junega V. Percutaneous skeletal aspiration and core biopsy: complementary techniques. AJR Am J Roentgenol. 1996;166:415–8.

Sun HY, Lee JW, Kim KJ, Yeom JS, Kang HS. Percutaneous intervention of the C2 vertebral body using a CT-guided posterolateral approach. AJR Am J Roentgenol. 2009;193:1703–5.

Tehranzadeh J, Tao C, Browning CA. Percutaneous needle biopsy of the spine. Acta Radiol. 2007;48:860–8.

Wattamwar AS, Ortiz AO. Use of a percutaneous discectomy device to facilitate the diagnosis of infectious spondylitis. ANJR Am J Neuroradiol. 2010;31:1157–8.

Wu R, Tseng YA, Drexler S, Ortiz O. Image-guided percutaneous cervical spine biopsies: A review of techniques, results, and complication avoidance. Neurographics. 2014;4:78–85.

Yang YJ, Damron TA. Comparison of needle core biopsy and fine needle aspiration for diagnostic accuracy in musculoskeletal lesions. Arch Pathol Lab Med. 2004;128(7):759–64.

Thoracic Spine Biopsy

5

A. Orlando Ortiz

Learning Objectives

1. To review the radiologic anatomy that is pertinent toward the safe performance of thoracic spine biopsy
2. To review the indications and contraindications for thoracic spine biopsy
3. To learn image-guided percutaneous thoracic spine biopsy approaches and techniques

5.1 Introduction

Image-guided percutaneous thoracic spine biopsies are the second most commonly performed biopsy procedure of the spinal axis, second to lumbar spine biopsies (Rimondi et al. 2008; Heyer et al. 2008). The proximity to the lungs can be a source of major concern for operators who perform this procedure. Fortunately, the presence of consistent osseous landmarks, including the posterior ribs and their articulation with the vertebral body, can be used to avoid injuring the lung. A sound understanding of the radiologic anatomy of the thoracic spine can assist in enhancing the safety margin of this procedure. In general, posterior approaches are required to access the thoracic vertebrae, as the overwhelming majority of lesions are usually located within the vertebral body and/or pedicle, with a lesser proportion of lesions seen within the intervertebral disk and even fewer lesions in a paraspinal soft tissue location. The biopsy needle size and number of passes may be limited depending on the lesion size, extent, and location within the thoracic spine. While this may increase the challenge of the image-guided percutaneous spine biopsy procedure, thoracic spine biopsy is a procedure that is associated with a high diagnostic yield, 92% in one large series (Rimondi et al. 2008). Most thoracic spine biopsies are performed at the mid or lower thoracic spine levels. The majority of thoracic spine biopsies are requested to assess for the possibility of a neoplastic process. The suspected thoracic spine abnormality is often identified on an MRI examination. The increased use of post-treatment imaging surveillance with PET-CT has also resulted in the identification of spine lesions that may require additional evaluation. Whenever possible, these prior studies should be carefully scrutinized to determine if alternative, and possibly safer, biopsy sites within the lumbar spine, sacrum, or pelvis are present. When thoracic spine biopsy is indicated, an understanding of the pertinent radiologic anatomy, the possible approaches to the target lesion, and the available biopsy devices and techniques will increase the efficiency, safety, and success of the image-guided percutaneous thoracic spine biopsy procedure.

A.O. Ortiz, *Image-Guided Percutaneous Spine Biopsy*, DOI 10.1007/978-3-319-43326-4_5

5.2 Anatomic Considerations

There are usually 12 rib-bearing thoracic vertebrae. In the presence of a transitional vertebral anatomy at the thoracolumbar junction, 11 or 13 thoracic vertebrae may occasionally be encountered. It is critical that the operator and the diagnostic radiologist be vigilant to the occurrence of these findings when present, in order to prevent the possibility of a wrong-level biopsy. Counting the vertebral bodies starting from the cervical spine can be helpful as there are seven cervical segments (Carrino et al. 2011). Alternatively, the counting scheme for the biopsy procedure should match the numbering scheme on the pre-procedure studies that identify the site and vertebral level of the lesion in question (Fig. 5.1). As occurs in the lumbar spine, the thoracic vertebrae share morphologic features in common from the first thoracic vertebra to the twelfth thoracic vertebra (Fig. 5.2). The major change that occurs within the thoracic spine as the vertebrae are studied from cranial to caudal is that the vertebral bodies get slightly larger within the lower thoracic spine. This also includes the size of the thoracic pedicles; for example, the T12 pedicles are larger than the T1 pedicles. This observation likely reflects the increased biomechanical load that the lower thoracic vertebrae are exposed to. Unlike the lumbar spine, where the pedicles are obliquely

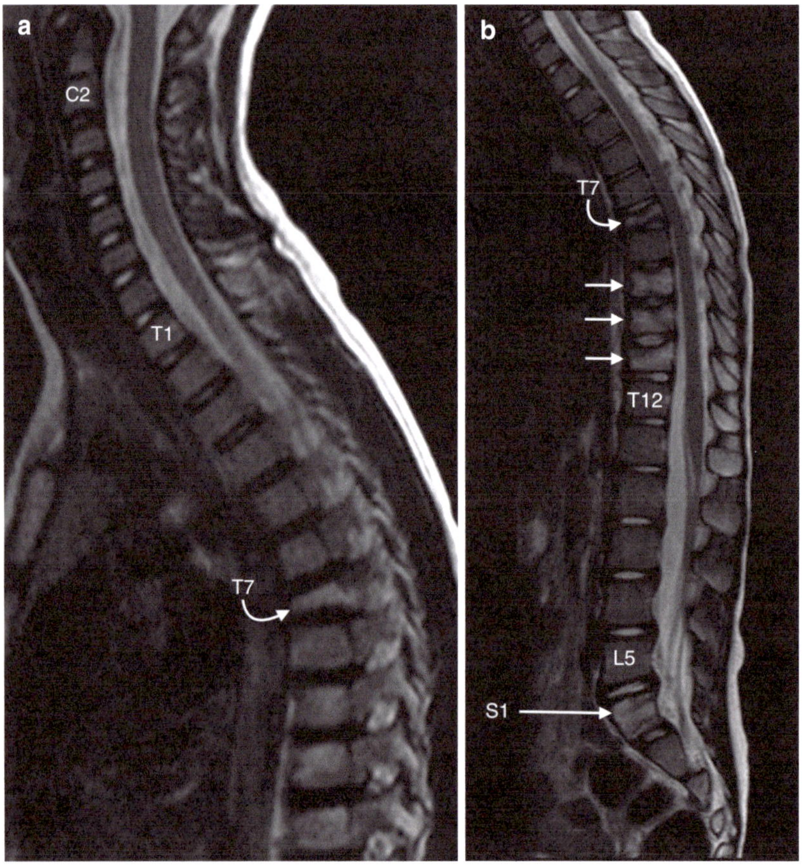

Fig. 5.1 Counting and labeling thoracic vertebral levels can be performed with scout MR or CT images or with fluoroscopy. This becomes particularly important when dealing with subtle thoracic lesions or when sampling thoracic disks. T2-weighted sagittal scout image (**a**) of the cervical and upper thoracic spine; C2 and T1 are labeled and a partial vertebral compression deformity is present at T7 (*arrow*). T2-weighted sagittal scout image (**b**) of thoracic and lumbar spine shows the T7 vertebral compression deformity (*curved arrow*) with marrow edema and three additional mild vertebral compression deformities (*arrows*) with marrow edema; T12, L5, and S1 (with marrow edema) are labeled

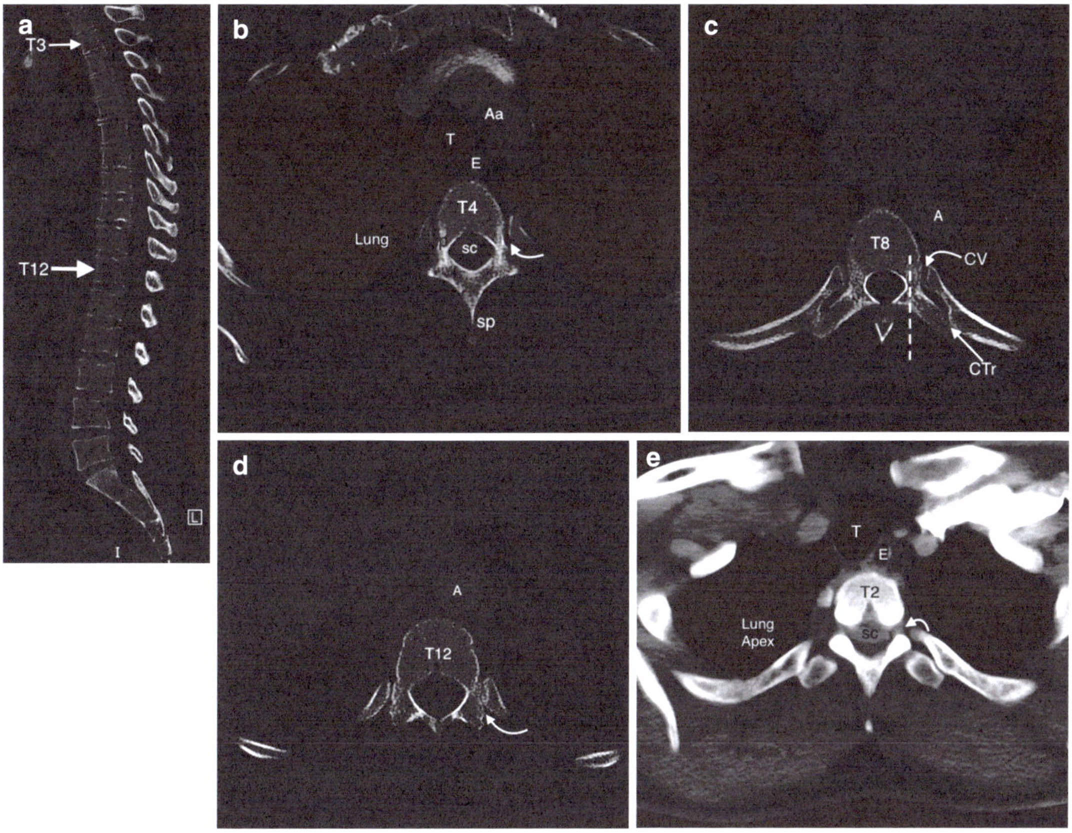

Fig. 5.2 CT anatomy of the thoracic spine. Reformatted midline sagittal CT image (**a**) shows progressive enlargement of thoracic vertebrae moving in a caudal direction; compare T3 to T12. Axial CT image (**b**) from contrast enhanced CT study at the T4 level shows the vertebral body (*T4*), pedicle (*p*), lamina (*L*), spinous process (*sp*) and costovertebral junction (*curved arrow*). Key anterior structures include the lung, esophagus (*E*), trachea (*T*) and aortic arch (*Aa*). Axial CT image (**c**) from contrast-enhanced CT study at the T8 level shows the costotransverse (*CTr*) and costovertebral (*CV*) articulations. The aorta (*A*) is well visualized even on bone window algorithm. Note the tangential orientation (*dashed line*) of the pedicle relative to the vertebral body. Axial CT image (**d**) from contrast-enhanced CT study at the T12 level shows a more prominent pedicle and a larger vertebral body; the costovertebral articulation is noted (*arrow*); the transverse process is rudimentary; the aorta (*A*) is well visualized. Axial CT image (**e**) from same study in soft tissue algorithm at the T2 level shows the spinal cord (*sc*) within the spinal canal and the exiting nerve root (*curved arrow*) within the neural foramen; critical structures at the level of the cervicothoracic junction include the lung apex, the esophagus (*E*), and the trachea (*T*); the great vessels lie anterior and lateral to the latter structures

angled toward the vertebral body, the thoracic pedicles maintain a relatively tangential orientation toward the vertebral body. This orientation of the thoracic pedicles, as well as their size, must always be taken into account when considering a transpedicular approach for thoracic spine biopsy. Some thoracic spine lesions, therefore, especially lesions within the posterior median aspect of the vertebral body, may not be accessible with a transpedicular approach. The rib articulates with a vertebra at two junctures, posterior at the transverse process or costotransverse articulation and, more anteriorly, at the posterior aspect of the lateral vertebral body or costovertebral junction. Each vertebra consists of the posterior elements which form the neural arch and include the spinous process, lamina, articular facets, transverse process, and pedicles. The pedicles connect the posterior elements to the vertebral body.

> When counting the vertebrae within the spinal axis, the possible presence of a transitional vertebra at the thoracolumbar junction should be considered in order to prevent a wrong-level thoracic spine biopsy procedure.

The critical structures that partially surround the thoracic spine are best understood in the context of their anatomic relations. The posterior elements of the thoracic vertebra are surrounded by the posterior paraspinal musculature which includes the erector spinae muscles. The neural arch, medial pedicle cortex, and posterior vertebral body cortex form the margins of the spinal canal. The spinal canal includes the epidural space, which contains fat and a venous plexus, and the meningeal lined spinal cord which is surrounded by cerebrospinal fluid. Spinal nerves and vascular structures pass through the neural foramina that are located between the pedicles of adjacent vertebral bodies. These vascular structures include branches of the intercostal arteries, some of which provide blood supply to the spinal cord. The lateral relations of the thoracic spinal column include the lungs and pleura. The anterior relations of the spinal column include the posterior mediastinum and mediastinum. The aorta is located anterior and to the left with respect to the vertebral column. The sympathetic plexus lies anteriorly and laterally along the vertebral column. When deciding upon the feasibility of an image-guided percutaneous thoracic spine biopsy procedure, the operator must always factor these critical structures into their approach.

Critical structures at the thoracic spine level
Spinal cord
Lung
Aorta
Intercostal vessels

5.3 Indications

Image-guided percutaneous thoracic spine biopsy is indicated for the evaluation of pathologic lesions that are located within the thoracic vertebrae, intervertebral disks, and/or adjacent paraspinal soft tissues (Table 5.1). The two most common indications for performing thoracic spine biopsy are evaluation of a neoplastic process and spine infection. Neoplastic processes within the thoracic spine are usually secondary lesions associated with metastatic disease, multiple myeloma, or lymphoma. Primary tumors within the thoracic spine, though uncommon, may also require a biopsy procedure. A biopsy may also be required in order to distinguish between a pathologic and an osteoporotic vertebral compression fracture (Figs. 5.3 and 5.4). As with all clinically indicated invasive interventions, the biopsy result should clearly influence the clinical management of the patient. This is the primary benefit of the biopsy procedure. If this benefit will not be achieved with the requested procedure, then it might not be necessary to subject the patient to an invasive procedure. The importance of reviewing all imaging studies prior

Table 5.1 Indications for image-guided percutaneous thoracic spine biopsy

1. Infection
Spondylitis-diskitis
Paraspinal abscess
2. Neoplastic
Primary osseous neoplasm
Evaluation of solitary bone lesion
Secondary osseous neoplasm
Osseous metastatic disease or involvement by systemic malignancy
Diffuse marrow replacement process
Evaluation of neoplastic lesions with diffusion restriction or FDG-PET avidity post-treatment to assess for treatment response
Paraspinal soft tissue mass
Pathologic vertebral body compression fracture
3. Pretreatment (including the above categories)
Tissue characterization prior to treatment initiation

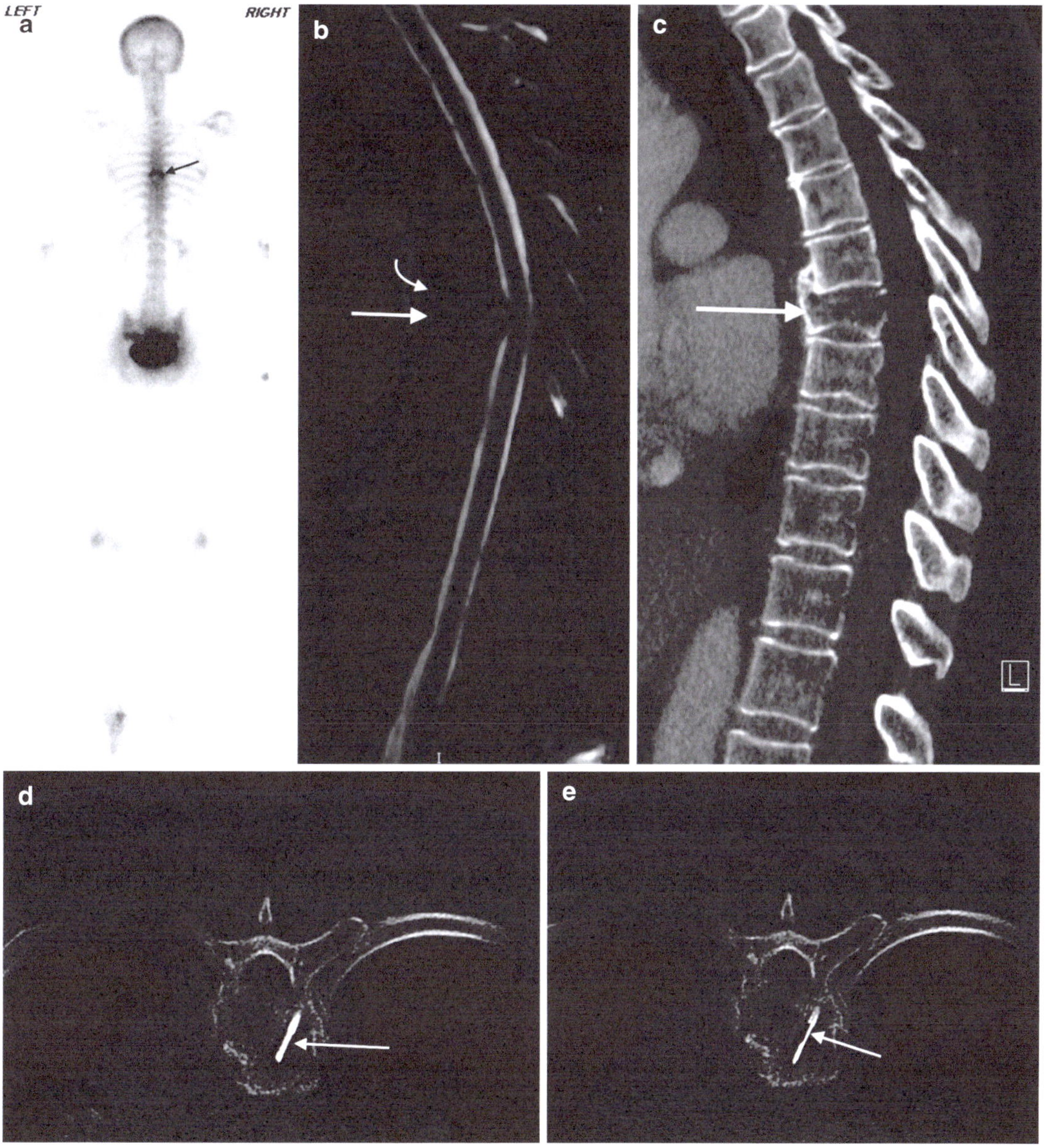

Fig. 5.3 A 65-year-old female with history of breast cancer and back pain. Single posterior projection from a whole body bone scan (**a**) shows focal radionuclide uptake (*arrow*) within the mid-thoracic spine. T2-weighted sagittal image (**b**) shows a partial vertebral compression deformity with marrow edema (*arrow*) and bone retropulsion into the spinal canal. Focal inferior vertebral endplate edema and disk edema (*curved arrow*) are seen above the vertebral compression deformity. Reformatted sagittal CT image (**c**) in bone window algorithm shows a partial vertebral compression deformity (*arrow*) with loss of the trabecular striations and anterior bone formation. Axial CT image (**d**) from the bone biopsy procedure shows the tip of a bone needle (*arrow*) within the predominantly lytic vertebral body lesion; scant tissue was obtained with this needle. Axial CT image (**e**) shows a soft tissue cutting needle within the lesion. Multiple soft tissue cores confirmed the presence of metastatic breast cancer in this patient with a pathologic vertebral compression fracture

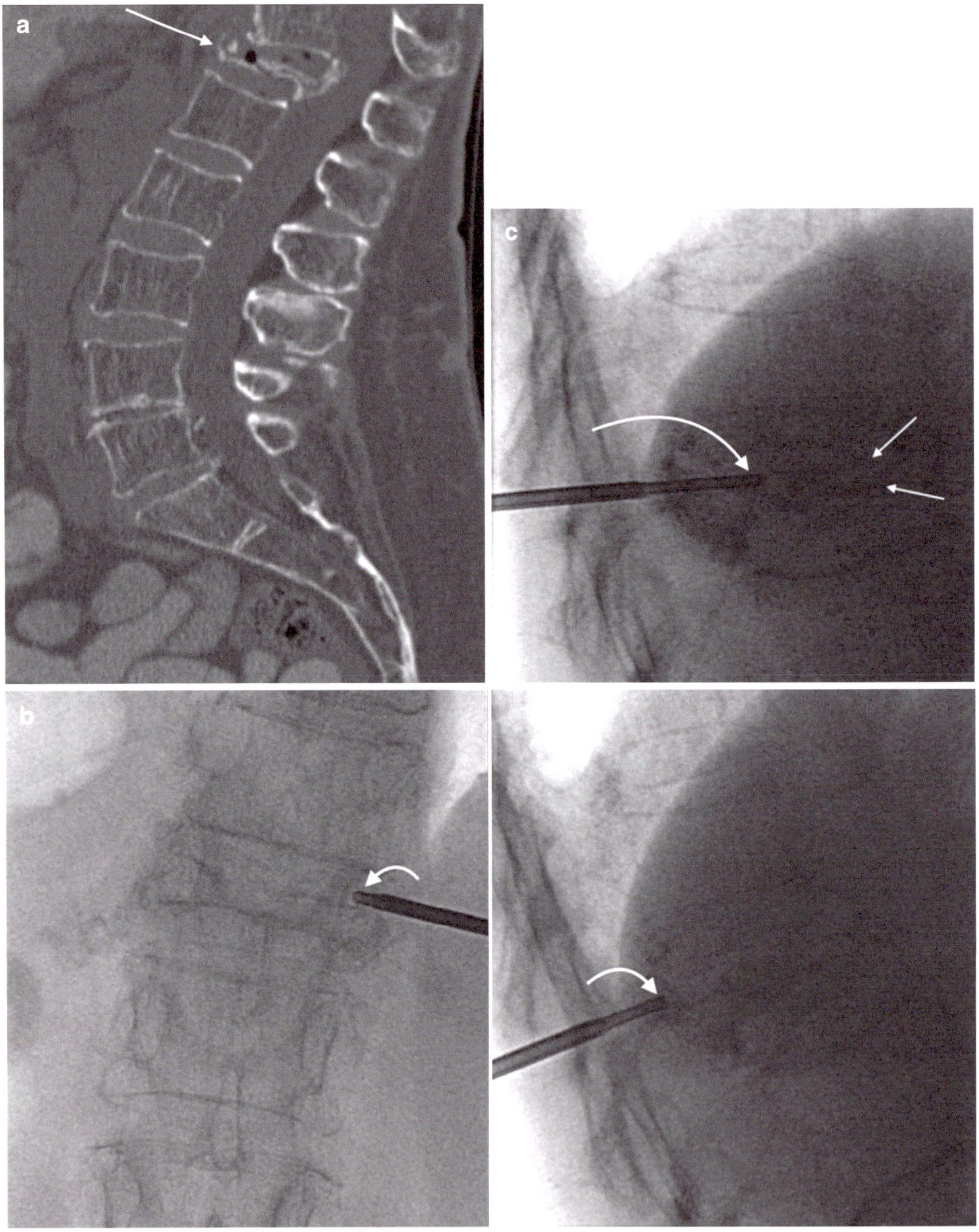

Fig. 5.4 A 77-year-old female with chronic, severe low back pain. Reformatted sagittal CT image (**a**) in bone window algorithm shows a vertebra plana deformity of the T12 vertebral body (*arrow*) with small amounts of gas with the anterior vertebral body and adjacent disk space; mild bone retropulsion into the spinal canal is noted as is focal kyphosis. Marked osteopenia is seen. Biplane fluoroscopic images (**b**) in the frontal and lateral projection show coaxial advancement of a bone biopsy needle into the pedicle (*arrow*). Lateral fluoroscopic image (**c**) shows further advancement of the bone needle into the posterior vertebral body (*curved arrow*); the vertebral endplates (*arrows*) show the severity of this collapse, which limits advancement of the bone needle. The biopsy samples showed no evidence of malignant cells in this patient with an osteoporotic vertebral compression fracture

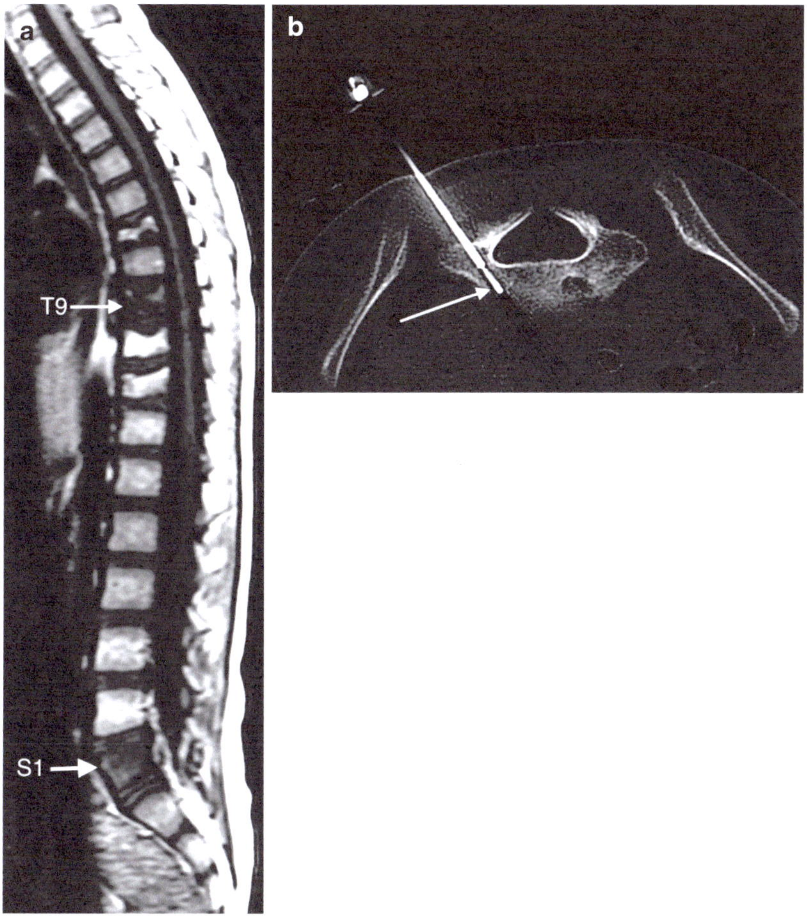

Fig. 5.5 A 7-year-old female with back pain (same patient as in Fig. 5.1). T1-weighted sagittal scout image (**a**) of the thoracic and lumbar spine shows multiple thoracic vertebral compression deformities and hypointense vertebral body marrow signal within the T9 and S1 vertebra (*arrows*). Axial CT image (**b**) shows biopsy of the S1 vertebra (*arrow*); 5 bone cores were submitted to pathology. The biopsy was nondiagnostic

to considering a thoracic spine biopsy is again emphasized. The remainder of the spinal axis and body should be studied in order to identify other possible sites, for example, within the lumbar spine, sacrum, or pelvis, which can be more safely sampled (Fig. 5.5).

5.4 Contraindications

The major contraindication to performing a thoracic spine biopsy is uncorrected coagulopathy (Table 5.2). Special consideration is also given to patients with neurologic compromise and in whom the imaging findings are consistent with acute spinal cord compression. These patients will require immediate surgical decompression of the spine, and this important intervention should not be delayed by a spine biopsy procedure. As with image-guided percutaneous spine biopsy procedures in the other segments of the spinal axis, thoracic spine biopsy procedures should not be performed on unstable patients. Given the risk of spinal cord or lung injury, the procedure should be avoided in uncooperative patients. As there are 12 thoracic vertebrae, the possibility of occurrence of benign lesions with certain pathognomonic imaging features is not uncommon in the thoracic spine. Bone islands and Schmorl's nodes may not require a biopsy

Table 5.2 Contraindications to image-guided percutaneous thoracic spine biopsy

Absolute
Uncorrected coagulopathy
Acute spinal cord compression
Untreated infection in patient with suspicious mass lesion
Relative
Patient factors
Combative or uncooperative patient
Clinically unstable patient
Lesion type
Vascular lesion
Probable benign lesion
Lesion size
Discretion must be exercised with smaller lesions (<5 mm in diameter)
Limited or no specimen yield may result in a false-negative biopsy
Lesion location
Defer biopsy for lesions located adjacent to critical structures or inaccessible locations

Table 5.3 Percutaneous thoracic spine biopsy – potential risks and complications

Tissue injury
Pneumothorax
Spinal cord injury
Vascular injury
Hemorrhage
Superficial or subcutaneous
Deep – hemorrhage into tumor and/or spinal canal can result in acute neurologic changes or retroperitoneal hemorrhage can result in hypotension or severe pain
Infection (superficial or deep) in those cases being performed to assess for neoplasm
Inappropriate needle placement
Breach of the anterior vertebral body or medial pedicle cortex
Needle placement within the spinal canal
Wrong level
Inadequate tissue sampling
Technical failure – biopsy system failure, lost specimen
Tumor seeding along the biopsy tract
Radiation exposure
Anesthesia complications
Aspiration, airway compromise, respiratory depression

procedure. For probably benign lesions, it may also be helpful to obtain and review the patient's prior studies, if available, or clinically correlate the finding and perform follow-up imaging surveillance only if deemed clinically necessary.

5.5 Risks and Complications Associated with Thoracic Spine Biopsy and How to Minimize Them

The risks and complications that are associated with image-guided percutaneous thoracic spine biopsy are similar to those observed with lumbar spine biopsy (Olscamp et al. 1997; Tehranzadeh et al. 2007) (Table 5.3). There are, however, two major differences between thoracic spine biopsy and biopsy in other segments of the spinal axis. First, the risk of pneumothorax takes on a greater priority when performing a thoracic spine biopsy. There is much greater surface area of lung parenchyma at risk in thoracic spine biopsy as compared to cervical or lumbar spine biopsies where the lung apices and bases, respectively, are at risk. Second, the thoracic spinal cord is a structure at risk when performing a thoracic spine biopsy. Careful attention to technique and utilization of the appropriate osseous landmarks whether using CT or fluoroscopic guidance will help to reduce the likelihood of a lung or spinal cord injury. Similarly, the use of coaxial technique, by incurring only one single pass with a guide cannula, will decrease the likelihood of injuring normal anatomic structures. All biopsy instruments can then be passed through the guide cannula multiple times without disturbing the surrounding soft tissue structures. Active monitoring of the location and excursion of these biopsy instruments will also enhance the margin of safety for any biopsy procedure (Fig. 5.6). Procedure-related hemorrhage can be mitigated by adhering to appropriate coagulation status protocols, holding anticoagulant or antiplatelet medications for an appropriate period of time, and using coaxial technique. In the thoracic spine, it is important to be extremely careful navigating needles adjacent to the ante-

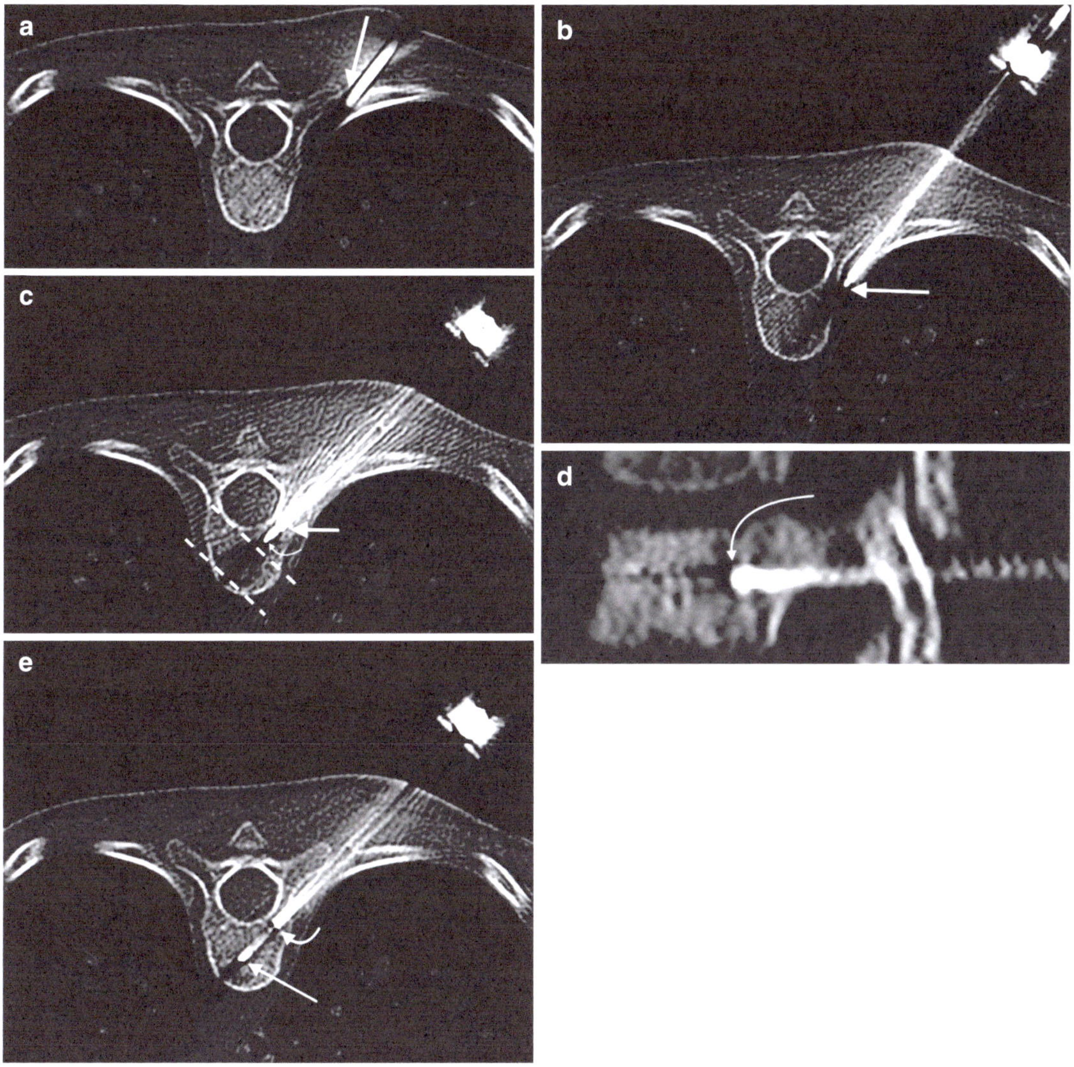

Fig. 5.6 A 7-year-old female with back pain, 1 month later. Axial CT image (**a**) from a T9 biopsy procedure shows advancement of a bone needle via a costotransverse approach (*arrow*). Axial CT image (**b**) shows needle tip at lateral margin of vertebral body (*arrow*); because of the steep nature of this approach, the needle tip points at the vertebral body, not the lung. Axial CT image (**c**) shows entry of the bone needle (*curved arrow*) into the posterior vertebral body. The beam hardening artifact distal to the needle provides a good estimate of the needle trajectory within the remainder of the vertebral body (*dashed lines*); the needle trajectory was adjusted at the point of insertion within the lateral vertebral cortex (compare to image **b**). A reformatted sagittal image obtained with CT fluoroscopy (**d**) shows the needle tip's (*curved arrow*) relationship to the vertebral endplates and anterior vertebral cortex. Axial CT image (**e**) shows coaxial advancement of the bone needle (*arrow*) through the guide cannula (*curved arrow*) in order to obtain additional bone cores (a total of 6 bone cores). Compare this final trajectory with that estimated in Figure **c**. Subsequent histopathologic analysis showed Langerhans cell histiocytosis

rior neural foramina and near the inferior margins of the posterior ribs as these are anatomic locations where normal vascular structures are located. Utilization of standard thoracic biopsy techniques such as the transpedicular, costotransverse, and costovertebral approaches help to reduce the likelihood of injury to these vascular structures.

5.6 Imaging Guidance

CT and fluoroscopy are the two modalities that are used to perform image-guided percutaneous thoracic spine biopsy (Lis et al. 2004; Ortiz et al. 2010). The key osseous landmarks for imaging guidance are visualized with both modalities. CT does provide additional soft tissue resolution to identify, with better detail, the critical structures in the thoracic spine. In general, many operators tend to use fluoroscopic guidance for transpedicular approaches in the thoracic spine, especially when attempting to sample large or diffuse lesions within the thoracic vertebral body (Fig. 5.7) (Pierot and Boulin 1999). More experienced operators will also use fluoroscopy to perform percutaneous disk biopsies utilizing a posterior oblique approach that keeps the needle between the medial aspect of the rib and the lateral aspect of the pedicle. The ability of CT to visualize the lesion and its relation to the vertebra and to nearby critical structures tends to make CT the preferred modality for image-guided percutaneous thoracic spine biopsy. It is particularly helpful in sampling the posterior elements and the paraspinal soft tissues (Fig. 5.8). CT fluoroscopy increases the efficiency of the procedure by allowing faster monitoring of needle advancement and position. Since both CT and fluoroscopic guidance entail radiation exposure, adherence to sound radiologic imaging and shielding principles will assist in limiting radiation exposure not only to the patient but also to the operator and the operator's staff.

5.7 Approaches

Posterior approaches are required to access the thoracic vertebrae, intervertebral disks, and paraspinal soft tissues. These posterior approaches are performed with the patient in the prone, prone oblique, or lateral decubitus position. The most optimal position, barring specific patient factors, is the prone position; however, some patients are unable to maintain this position due to pain or breathing issues. The prone position is the most common position with which spine interventions are performed at the thoracic spine level; hence, operators tend to have a comfort level with the imaging landmarks and with the angulations of their biopsy devices with the patient in this position. Each of the approaches to the thoracic spine is determined by the lesion location and size and by the local anatomic constraints that are seen with imaging guidance (Table 5.4) (also refer to Chap. 9). The two major approaches are either transpedicular or extrapedicular (Figs. 5.9 and 5.10) (Renfrew et al. 1991). Commonly used extrapedicular approaches within the thoracic spine include the costotransverse and costovertebral approaches. Intercostal approaches are occasionally required for posterior paraspinal soft tissue masses (Fig. 5.11). A major anatomic constraint within the upper thoracic spine tends to be the smaller size of the thoracic pedicle (Fig. 5.2). This may either limit the size of the instruments that can be used in the biopsy procedure or restrict the procedure to an extrapedicular approach, or both. It is imperative for the operator to review all pertinent pre-procedure imaging

Fig. 5.7 An 80-year-old male with history of prostate, colon, and lung cancer. Fat-suppressed contrast-enhanced T1-weighted sagittal image (**a**) shows multiple hypointense foci (*curved arrows*) with mild peripheral enhancement; the largest lesion (*arrow*) is located within the T10 vertebral body. Axial CT image (**b**) from a T10 biopsy procedure shows the use of coaxial technique and a costovertebral approach (*curved arrow*) with subsequent placement of a bone needle (*arrow*) into a large sclerotic lesion. Five bone cores were obtained with this 12 gauge system; the biopsy showed no evidence of malignant cells. T1weighted sagittal image (**c**) performed 3 months later shows progression of a vertebral marrow replacement process, particularly at T10 (*arrow*). Frontal fluoroscopic projection (**d**) shows transpedicular coaxial placement (*arrow*) of a trephine bone needle into the sclerotic T10 vertebral body. Lateral fluoroscopic image (**e**) shows a guide cannula (*arrow*) within the distal pedicle and a biopsy needle (*curved arrow*) within the anterior vertebral body. Nine small bone cores were obtained in this procedure, and pathology revealed metastatic prostate cancer

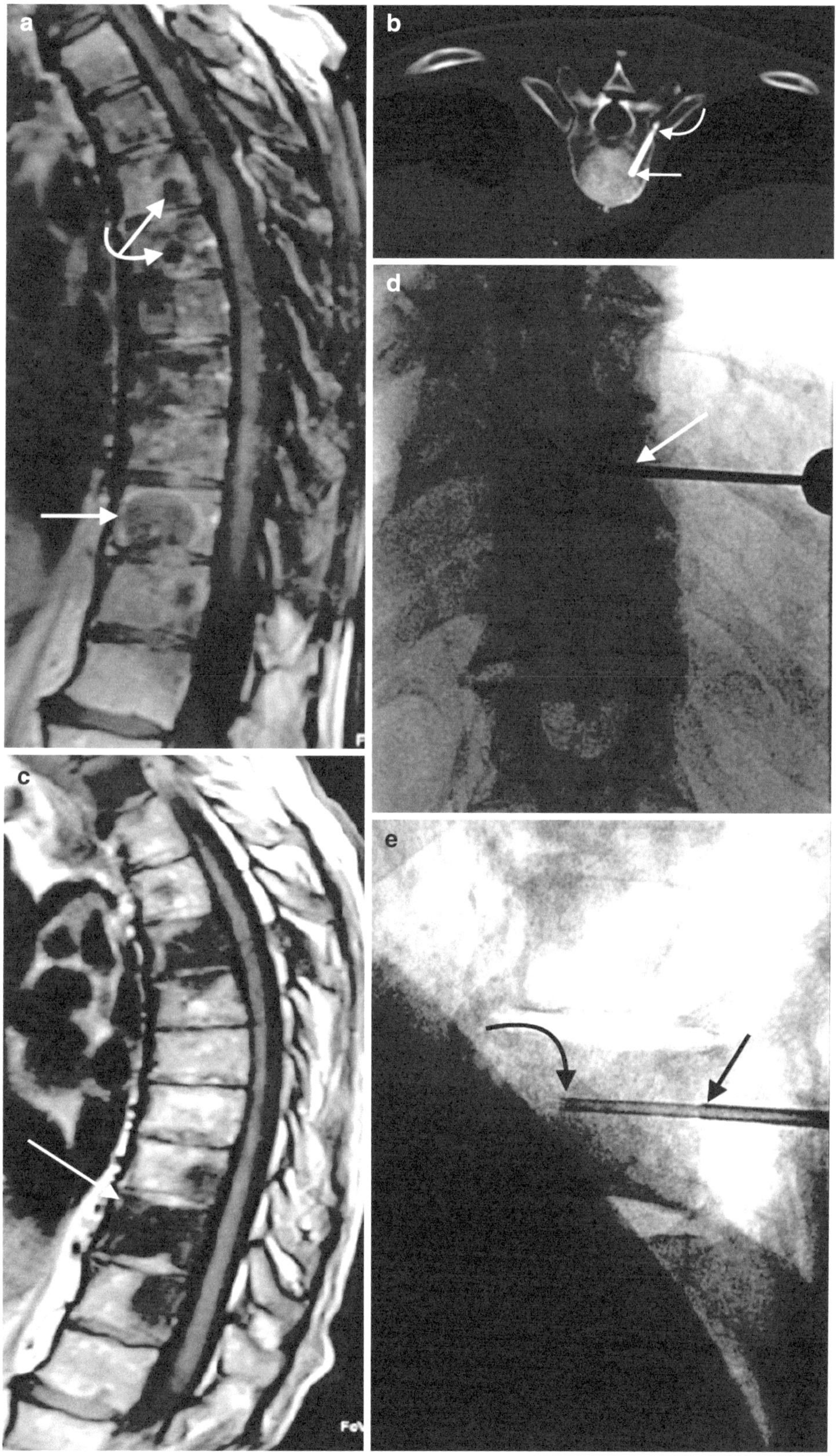
a
b
c
d
e

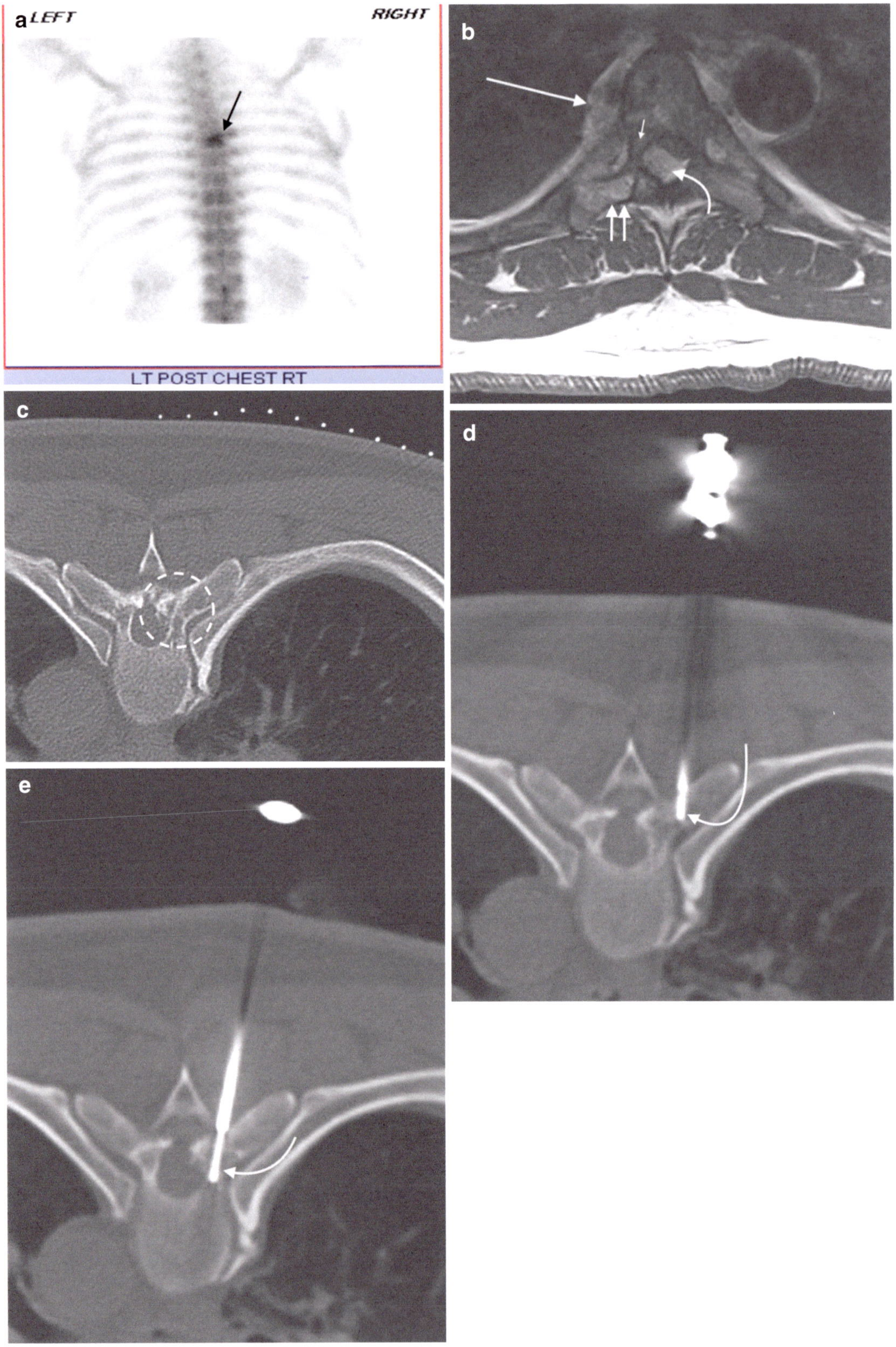
a
LEFT
RIGHT
LT POST CHEST RT
b
c
d
e

Table 5.4 Approaches for thoracic spine biopsy

Transpedicular
Needle tip advanced through the center of the pedicle into the vertebral body
Advantages: (1) Avoids spinal canal and contents; (2) does not disturb adjacent paraspinal soft tissues including blood vessels and lungs; (3) can apply more local anesthetic to posterior pedicle cortex, so often well tolerated by patient; (4) can be performed with either fluoroscopic or CT guidance
Disadvantages: (1) May be difficult to visualize pedicle (fluoroscopy) or pedicle may be too small to accommodate biopsy device; (2) may not be able to sample lesions within the posterior and median aspect of the vertebral body; (3) difficult access for disk space
Extrapedicular
Needle tip advanced outside of the pedicle toward the lesion in the vertebral body, intervertebral disk, or adjacent paraspinal soft tissue
Costotransverse
Needle tip passes between vertebral transverse process and posterior cortex of adjacent rib
Advantages: (1) Avoids spinal canal and contents; (2) avoids the lung; (3) allows access to lesions within the superior aspect of the vertebral body
Disadvantages: (1) Only performed under CT guidance; (2) cannot sample pedicle
Costovertebral
Needle tip passes between the dorsal aspect of the posterior rib and the pedicle
Advantages: (1) Avoids the lung and the spinal canal; (2) rib helps to guide the needle into the vertebral body or the intervertebral disk; (3) can be performed with CT or fluoroscopic guidance
Disadvantages: (1) Cannot sample pedicle
Intercostal
Needle placement is within the posteromedial intercostal space, anterior to the head of the rib and the costovertebral joint
Direct (paraspinal soft tissue lesion)
Needle tip advanced directly into lesion; a variant of intercostal approach
Advantages: (1) Directly sample the lesion
Disadvantages: (1) Risk of lung or vascular injury; (2) performed with CT guidance only

examinations in order to plan the most optimal approach to a thoracic spine lesion. Another decision to be made in thoracic spine biopsy is whether to approach the lesion from the right side or the left side of the thoracic spine. Certainly, if the lesion is located unilaterally, then this is the side that the posterior approach is initiated from. But, if the lesion is diffuse or large, and when anatomic structures permit, then a right-sided approach might be used in order to reduce the chance of injury to the aorta (Fig. 5.7).

> It is imperative for the operator to review all pertinent pre-procedure imaging examinations in order to plan the most optimal approach to a thoracic spine lesion.

Fig. 5.8 A 56-year-old male with thoracic back pain. Single posterior projection (**a**) from a bone scan shows focal radionuclide uptake within a single thoracic vertebra (*arrow*), T6. Contrast-enhanced T1-weighted axial image (**b**) shows mild focal enhancement within the right T6 transverse process (*double arrow*) and pedicle (*small arrow*). Epidural (*curved arrow*) and paraspinal (*large arrow*) soft tissue enhancement is also seen. Axial CT image (**c**) from the biopsy procedure with skin grid in place shows a subtle mixed lytic and sclerotic pattern with the T6 posterior elements (*dashed circle*). Axial CT image (**d**) shows coaxial insertion of a bone needle (*arrow*) into the right transverse process. Axial CT image (**e**) shows repositioning of the guide cannula, avoiding another skin puncture, and transpedicular placement of the bone needle. The histopathology confirmed the presence of a hemangioma

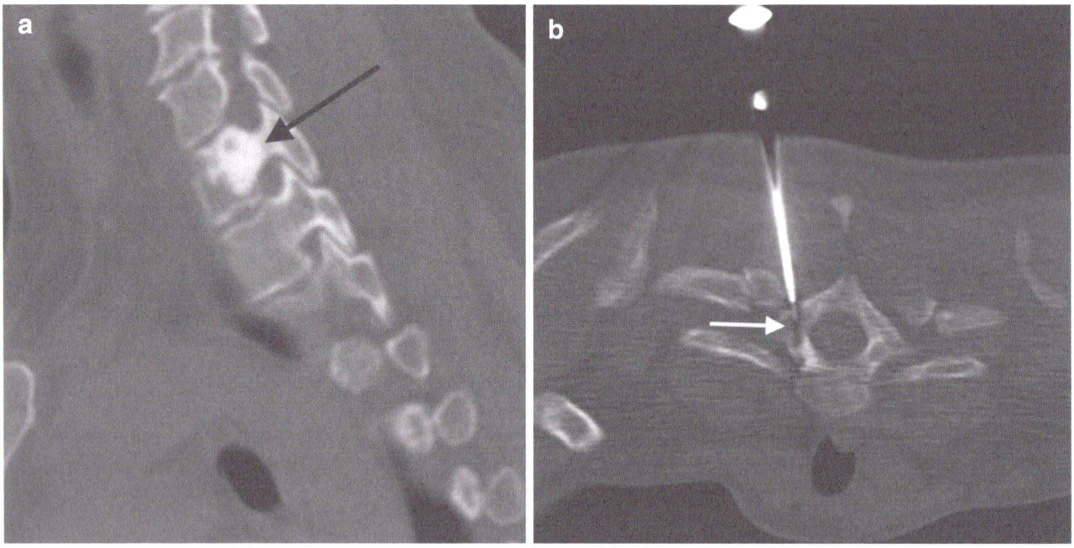

Fig. 5.9 A 50-year-old female. Reformatted parasagittal CT image (**a**) shows well-defined sclerotic lesion within the posterior T1 vertebral body and pedicle (*arrow*). Axial CT image (**b**) shows a transpedicular approach (*arrow*) to the sclerotic lesion. The biopsy showed normal bone formation and no evidence of malignant cells

5.8 The Thoracic Spine Biopsy Procedure

5.8.1 General Considerations

5.8.1.1 Patient Factors

Image-guided percutaneous thoracic spine biopsy procedures should only be performed on cooperative patients. The patient should be evaluated to ascertain whether or not they can lie in the prone position. In rare instances, it is sometimes necessary to use the prone oblique position. The patient's back should be examined in order to make sure that the skin is intact and that there are no pressure ulcers at the level of the intended biopsy procedure. Skin tattoos may also pose a barrier to biopsy, and these are often located in the upper back, near the cervicothoracic junction or the interscapular area. The patient's medical history, pertinent laboratory values, allergies, imaging studies, and NPO status should be reviewed (Talac and McLain 2009). If certain medications, such as anticoagulants, antiplatelets, or antibiotics, require discontinuation prior to the procedure, then the details of these actions are confirmed. Informed consent is obtained from the patient or their designated representative. The risks and benefits of the biopsy procedure, and alternatives to this procedure including open biopsy and continued medical surveillance, should be discussed with the patient. The post-procedure recovery and any wound care instructions are briefly discussed and reinforced after the procedure.

5.8.1.2 Staff Factors

When needed, anesthesiology and pathology consultations should be obtained on a timely basis such that if the services of these medical consultants are required, then they will be able to assist with the performance of the procedure. The staff should be well trained and able to exercise the appropriate patient and procedure verification protocols. The staff is made aware that a thoracic spine biopsy will be performed. A procedure table has been prepared and sterilely draped prior to the procedure and can be positioned based upon the procedure logistics. The staff is instructed to place the patient in the prone position and to make sure that the patient is as comfortable as reasonably possible. The application of security straps around the lower body of the patient will help to prevent falls off of the procedure table. The patient is

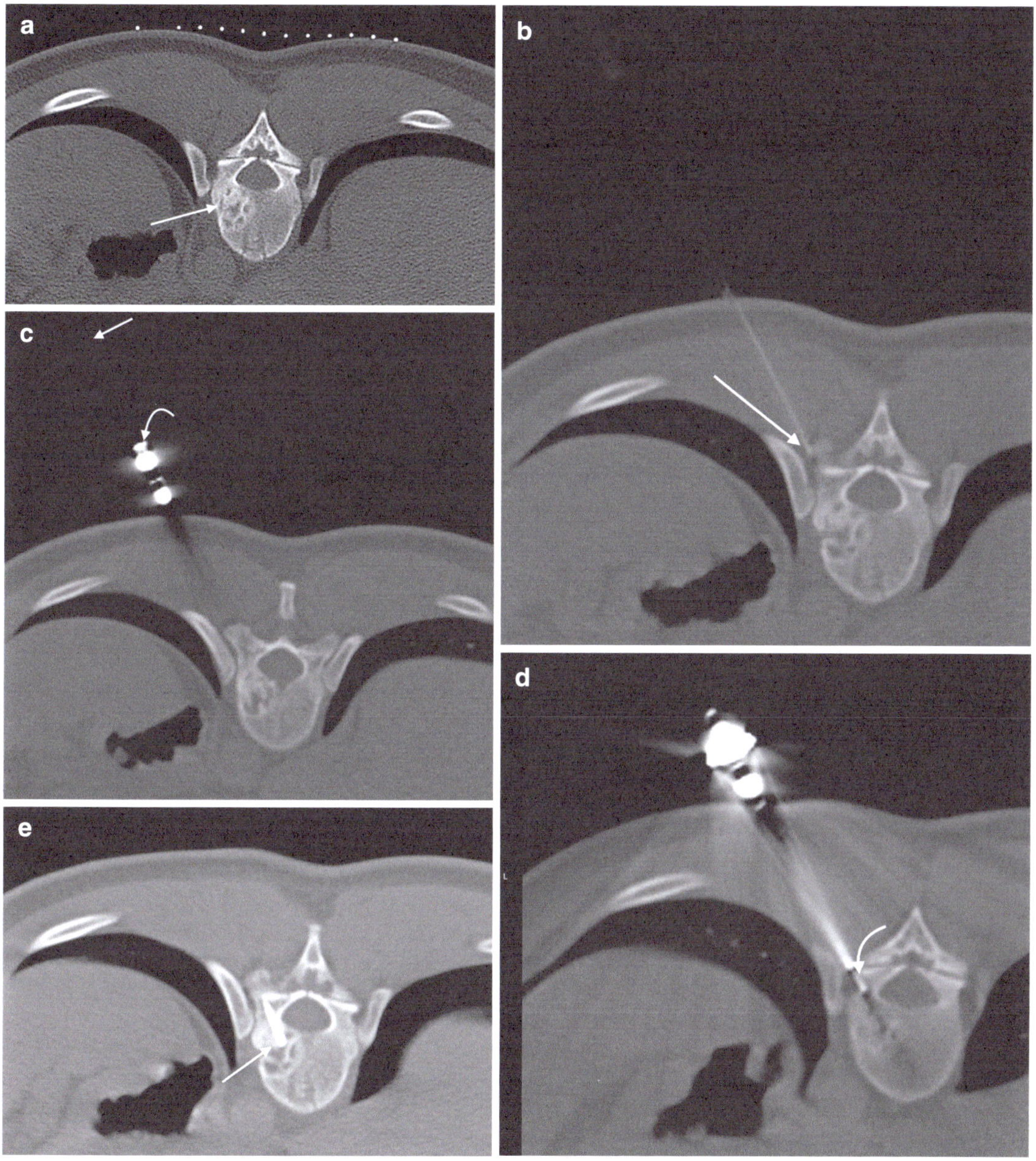

Fig. 5.10 A 29-year-old male with incidental lesion detected on outside study. Axial CT image (**a**) from the biopsy procedure with a skin grid in place shows a mixed sclerotic lesion within the posterior vertebral body (*arrow*). Axial CT image (**b**) shows tip of 20 gauge insert needle (*arrow*) adjacent to the transverse process. This needle was used to administer 2% lidocaine; the hub of the needle is removable so that it becomes a guidewire. Axial CT image (**c**) shows the hubless (*arrow*) 20 gauge needle and coaxial insertion of a 12 gauge introducer (*curved arrow*) and guide cannula (not seen on this image due to angled introduction of the coaxial system). Axial CT image (**d**) shows coaxial insertion of a trephine bone needle via a parapedicular approach (*curved arrow*). Axial CT image (**e**) shows the bone needle tip (*arrow*) within the lesion – a hemangioma

asked to place their arms up, whenever possible, with intravenous access in the forearm, wrist, or dorsum of the hand. Remember, antecubital intravenous catheters are problematic in these procedures as they tend to get occluded by a bent arm position. Monitoring equipment is placed on the

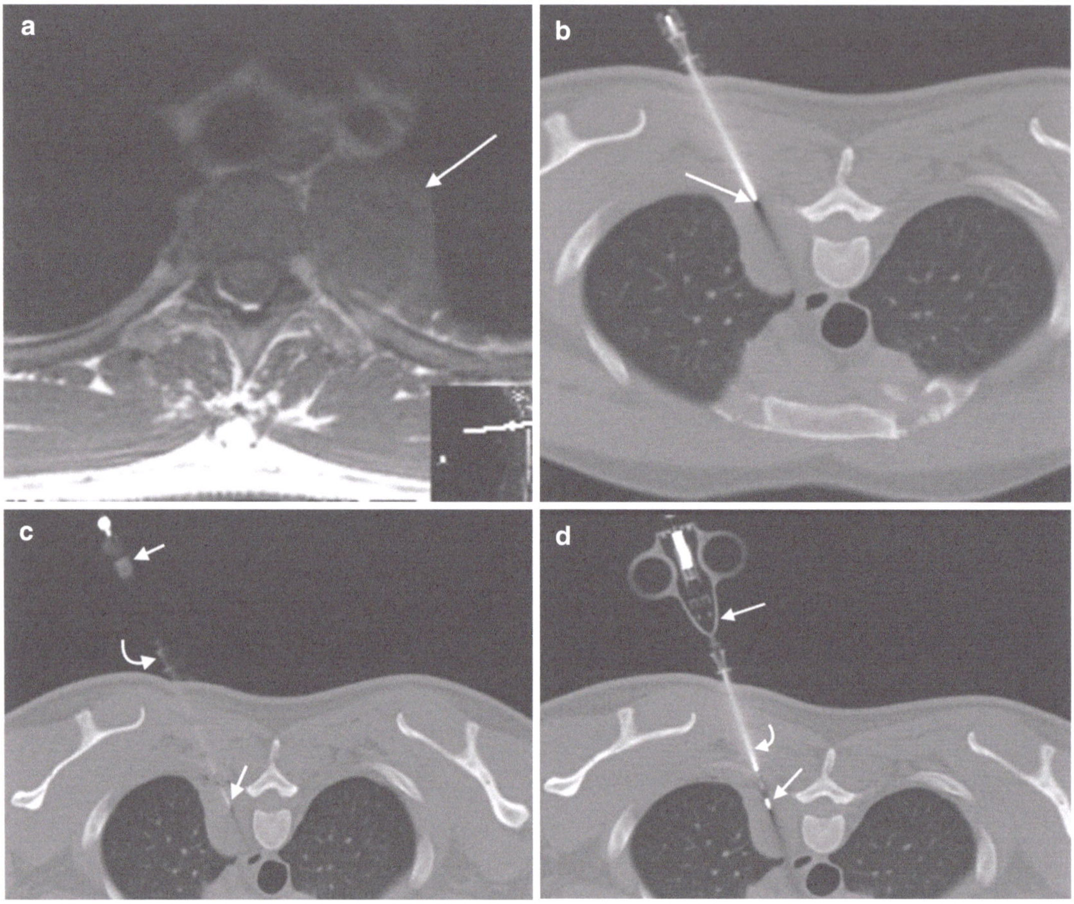

Fig. 5.11 A 30-year-old male with incidental mass seen on chest radiograph. T1-weighted axial image (**a**) shows solid intermediate signal intensity soft tissue mass (*arrow*) adjacent to the upper thoracic spine. Axial CT image (**b**) shows placement of a guide needle with advancement of the needle tip to the margin of the lesion (*arrow*); the needle is purposely angled away from the lung. Axial CT image (**c**) shows coaxial insertion of a 22 gauge Chiba needle (*small arrows*) via the guide cannula (*curved arrow*) for the purposes of fine needle aspiration. Several FNA passes were performed and submitted for cytologic evaluation. Axial CT image (**d**) shows the subsequent placement of a 16 gauge cutting needle (*arrows*) via the same guide cannula (*curved arrow*). The cytopathologic evaluation showed that this was a schwannoma

patient, and the staff is reminded to keep leads, lines, and wires away from the intended sterile field and area of the biopsy. These wires can obscure the area of interest, especially with fluoroscopic procedures. The back is shaved, when necessary, with electric clippers.

5.8.1.3 Anesthesia

As with other percutaneous spine biopsy procedures, thoracic spine biopsy is performed with local anesthesia and either with intravenous sedation and analgesia or with intravenous anesthesia provided by an anesthesiologist or anesthetist. The level of anesthesia will be determined by the patient, the patient's medical condition, the operator, and, when involved, the anesthesiologist. The patient is actively monitored, with respect to vital signs, oxygen saturation, and comfort level, by properly trained and qualified staff.

5.8.2 Patient Preparation

After the patient is positioned on the procedure table and the monitoring equipment placed, a time-out with the staff and patient is initiated so that the correct patient has the correct procedure at the correct level and, when applicable, on the correct side. For CT procedures a skin grid is placed on the back, and the intended level of skin entry is identified with CT imaging such that the skin can be marked with an indelible ink marker prior to prepping the skin. The skin is prepped and draped using strict aseptic technique. For fluoroscopy procedures, a clamp can be used to localize the level and side of interest in order to make a skin mark with a sterile marker pen. Once the monitoring equipment is recording the patient's vital signs, oxygen saturation, and a continuous electrocardiogram, the patient can start to receive their sedation and analgesia or their intravenous anesthesia. In rare instances, for example, in patients who are immunocompromised, it may be necessary to provide intravenous antibiotic prophylaxis within one hour of starting the procedure (Santiago et al. 2014).

5.8.3 Technique

5.8.3.1 CT Guidance

After the operator reviews the pertinent prior examinations and decides upon the thoracic level of interest, a skin grid is placed upon the patient's back. Scout frontal and lateral images of the thoracic spine are obtained; these may include the cervical spine for upper thoracic biopsies or the lumbar spine for lower thoracic biopsies in order to facilitate counting the vertebral body levels. This step takes on great importance in patients with transitional vertebrae or in patients in whom the pathology is difficult to visualize with CT (as compared to their initial MRI or nuclear medicine test). Having the prior examination available at the time of the biopsy procedure for additional review is also very helpful. After skin grid placement and scout CT images are obtained, the thoracic level of interest is scanned using serial axial sections. The preliminary axial CT study will often include the vertebral level above and below the level of interest. Additionally, the field of view should permit the visualization of the skin surface in order to identify the reference grid and the eventual skin entry site. These initial axial CT images are obtained with thin section technique (1–3 mm thick axial sections), often with bone algorithm when a vertebral biopsy is planned and occasionally with soft tissue algorithm when sampling large paraspinal soft tissue masses or fluid collections. The skin entry site is identified, and the skin is marked with an indelible ink marker prior to prepping with sterilizing solutions. The choice of trajectory and approach are at the operator's discretion and will generally include a path that safely accesses the lesion and avoids normal structures using standard thoracic spine approaches. In general, a transpedicular approach can be used to access the pedicle and anterior and/or lateral vertebral body lesions. An extrapedicular approach tends to be used for some posterior and median vertebral body lesions and for sampling intervertebral disk or paraspinal soft tissue pathology (Fig. 5.12).

A small amount of anesthetic agent, such as 1 or 2% lidocaine is used to anesthetize the skin entry site as well as the deep soft tissues of the needle tract down to the level of the vertebral periosteum. The application of the deep tissue anesthetic is performed with imaging guidance in order to prevent injury to critical structures. This maneuver also will confirm that the chosen biopsy needle trajectory, with respect to safety, will be feasible (Fig. 5.10). A dermatotomy is performed with a #11 scalpel blade at the anesthetized skin entry site.

A coaxial biopsy system is often used for thoracic spine biopsies (Yaffe et al. 2003). This maintains access to the biopsy site via a guide cannula and allows the operator to use bone needles, soft tissue needles, or both. A bone needle can be advanced into the vertebra, and the bone needle stylet is then removed such that the bone needle cannula serves as a guide cannula for the coaxial

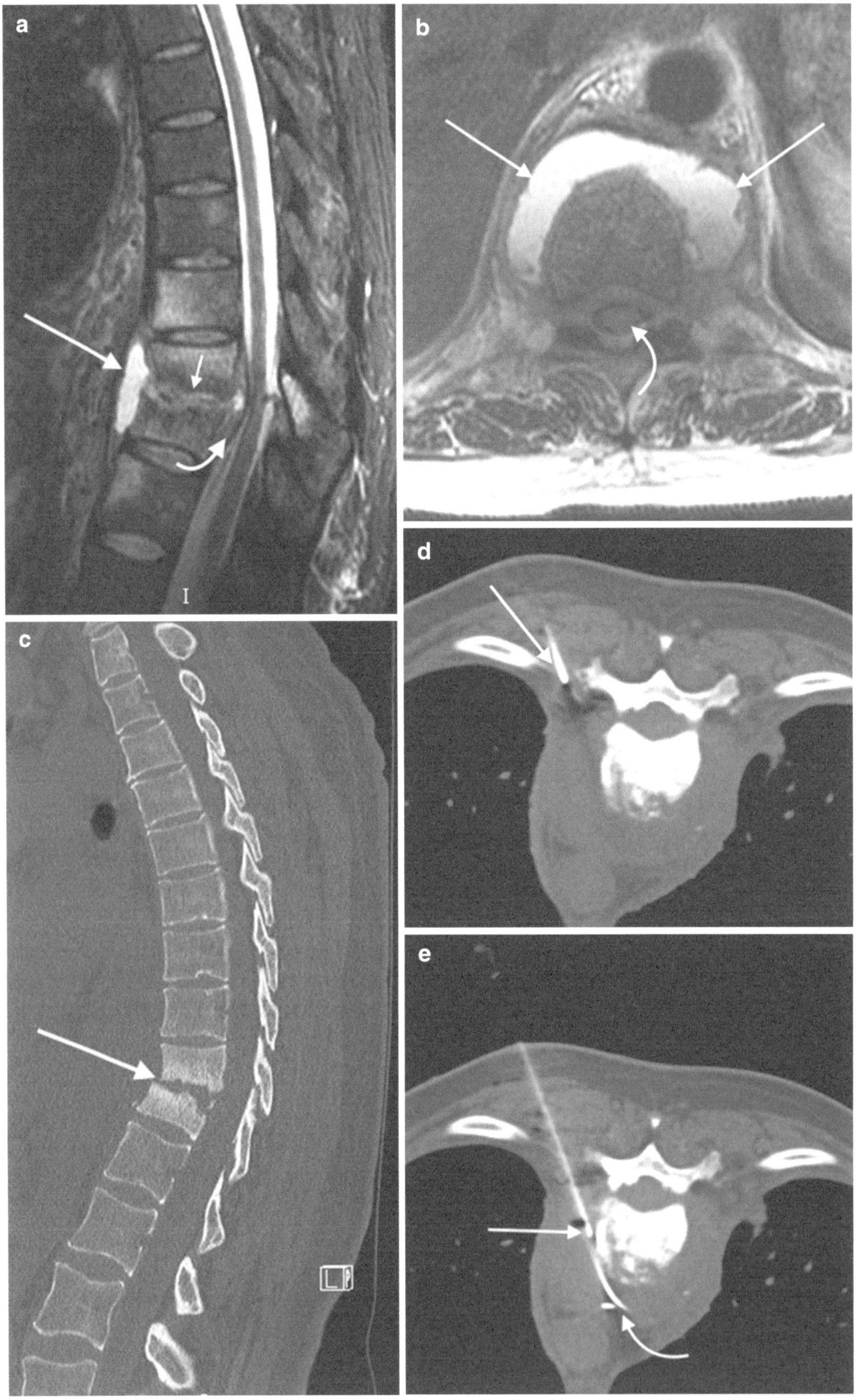
a
b
c
d
e

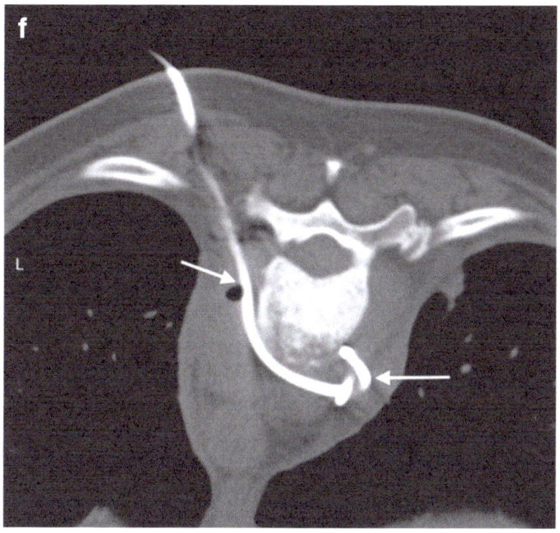

Fig. 5.12 (continued)

insertion of other biopsy needles (Geremia et al. 1992). Bone needles tend to be used for vertebral lesions, if at a minimum, to penetrate the vertebral cortex and gain access to the lesion margin (Fig. 5.3). Another type of guide cannula system entails the advancement of a guided cannula over an introducer or blunt dissector. The introducer fits inside the guide cannula such that the guide cannula–introducer unit can be advanced over a guidewire. When the guide cannula reaches the margin of the vertebra, disk, or paraspinal soft tissue lesion, the introducer and guidewire are removed and the guide cannula is left in place. The guide cannula acts a safe conduit for sharp instruments and guards against soft tissue injury (Fig. 5.10). The guide cannula also facilitates patient comfort by minimizing trauma to the skin entry site. Once the guide needle is advanced to the cortical entry site, it may have to be held in place with one hand, while the insert needle and introducer/blunt dissector cannula are removed with the other hand. A trephine bone needle is then inserted through the guide cannula with the other hand and then rotated clockwise and counterclockwise with gentle forward pressure to dock the system into the vertebral cortex. The bone needle entry site is quickly scanned, this is optimized with CT fluoroscopy, and the trajectory and position of the needle is monitored during subsequent advancements (Fig. 5.6).

One difference between thoracic spine biopsy as compared to lumbar spine or sacral biopsy procedures is that bone needle excursions are shorter with thoracic spine biopsies due to the inherent relatively smaller size of the thoracic vertebrae and their proximity to the lungs and the aorta. Another difference in these types of procedures is that with thoracic spine biopsy the overall sample size may be limited depending on the lesion size and extent. It must be kept in mind that there are two key locations for optimizing the biopsy needle trajectory: first, at the skin insertion site and, second, at the vertebral cortex insertion site. This is based upon the fact that biopsy needles are metallic constructs that tend to move in a straight direction. The bone needle is usually advanced about 5 mm. Bone material accumulates within the bone needle lumen as the needle is advanced. The bone needle can be removed and replaced with a second or "fresh" bone needle. This will allow for the bone sample within the first bone needle to be expressed, with a metal pusher, into the appropriate biopsy container. This bone needle swapping maneuver will require stabilization of the guide cannula at the vertebral entry site with one hand, while the bone

Fig. 5.12 A 43-year-old female with history of intravenous drug abuse and back pain. T2-weighted sagittal image (**a**) shows a prevertebral fluid collection (*large arrow*) that communicates with an abnormal disk (*small arrow*) and a posterior epidural phlegmon (*curved arrow*). The adjacent vertebral bodies show marrow edema. T2-weighted axial image (**b**) shows large paravertebral fluid collection (*large arrows*) and spinal cord edema (*curved arrow*). Reformatted sagittal CT image (**c**) shows disk and vertebral endplate destruction (*arrow*) with sclerotic reaction and focal kyphosis. Axial CT image (**d**) shows insertion of a guide needle via a costotransverse approach (*arrow*). Axial CT image (**e**) shows placement of a guidewire (*curved arrow*) into the paraspinal fluid collection via the guide needle (*arrow*). Axial CT image (**f**) shows over the wire placement of a drainage catheter (*arrows*) into the collection. Abundant purulent material was drained via this catheter, and the specimens were positive for *Streptococcus viridans*

needle exchanges are performed with the operator's other hand. Coaxial placement of the second bone needle will again require rotational movements with gentle forward pressure on this needle and with monitoring of needle progression with CT images. These procedural steps can be repeated as long as the biopsy needle tip is within the lesion and safely distant from critical structures. The operator should attempt to obtain at least three bone cores whenever possible. Another technique that can be used to obtain more tissue, after the initial traverse through the lesion, is to try to create a fresh biopsy tract by angling the bone needle slightly at the vertebral insertion site (Fig. 5.6). This latter maneuver also works very well with transpedicular technique using fluoroscopic guidance. Ultimately, however, the number of biopsy needle passes and trajectories are determined by the lesion location, size, and morphology.

For soft tissue masses, intraosseous lytic lesions, or disk space biopsies, the coaxial approach at the thoracic level may first include an attempt at FNA using small gauge needles that can be coaxially passed through a guide cannula (Fig. 5.13). FNA should be considered by the operator as an initial biopsy technique when the lesion to be sampled is potentially hypervascular (such as a renal or thyroid metastasis). Once the FNA passes are complete, whether or not abnormal cells have been detected, then a core soft tissue biopsy should be performed with a soft tissue cutting needle. The cutting needle is advanced coaxially to the margin of the lesion under CT guidance. The cutting compartment of the needle is exposed within the matrix of the lesion and this is confirmed with CT; the tip of the needle is monitored at all times with CT images, especially after any adjustments in needle position, and should not threaten critical structures (Fig. 5.14). Again the optimal goal is to obtain at least three soft tissue cores if possible. Another possible technique that can be used to sample lytic lesions is to sample the lesion margin with a trephine bone biopsy needle; this maneuver is sometimes able to sequester a small amount of cortical bone and the adjacent soft tissue abnormality (Figs. 5.15, 5.16, and 5.17). When sampling the disk or adjacent paraspinal soft tissues for possible infection, try to aspirate infected fluid first. If there is a definite fluid collection, but the viscosity of the collection is too thick, then try to use a larger gauge needle such as a 20 or an18 gauge needle and then aspirate with a 10 or 20 mL syringe. Alternatively, a small drainage catheter can be placed for larger collections (Fig. 5.12). If there is no fluid collection, then the disk-endplate complex can be biopsied with a trephine bone needle (Fig. 5.18). This latter maneuver usually yields tissue samples that can be submitted in their respective transport containers to microbiology and pathology. The other option is to use a percutaneous diskectomy device with coaxial technique and imaging guidance (Onik 1996; Chew and Kline 2001). Care should be taken in only advancing the diskectomy device slightly and with imaging guidance. Often after these types of deep tissue manipulation, there is a small amount of hemorrhage into the biopsy tract that can also be aspirated and submitted in a sterile container for microbiologic analysis.

5.8.4 Fluoroscopic Guidance

Thoracic spine biopsies can also be performed with fluoroscopic guidance. In the case of vertebral body lesions, these biopsy procedures tend to be performed in cases where there are either large lesions or the vertebral body is diffusely infiltrated by tumor. Suspected pathologic vertebral compression fractures are often biopsied

Fig. 5.13 A 67-year-old female with leukemia and fever; elevated CRP 76 and ESR 84. T2-weighted sagittal image (**a**) shows small anterior fluid collection (*curved arrow*) within the disk and superior endplate as well as prevertebral soft tissue swelling. Reformatted sagittal CT image (**b**) in bone window algorithm shows widening of the disk space (*arrow*) with endplate sclerosis and destruction. Axial CT image (**c**) shows coaxial placement of a 22 gauge needle (*arrow*) that was used to aspirate purulent material from the anterior disk; the microbiology was positive for coagulase-negative *Staphylococcus*

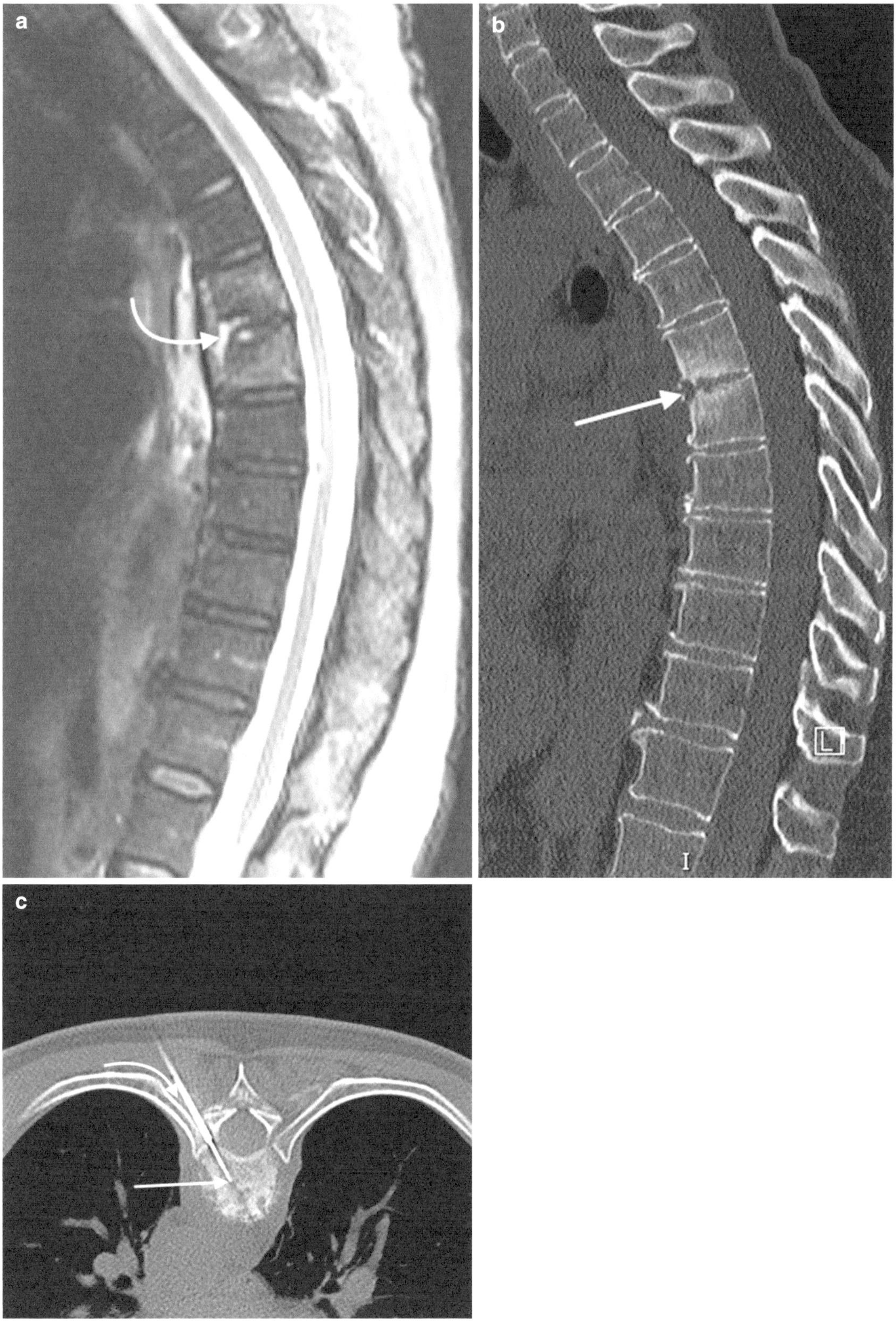
a
b
c

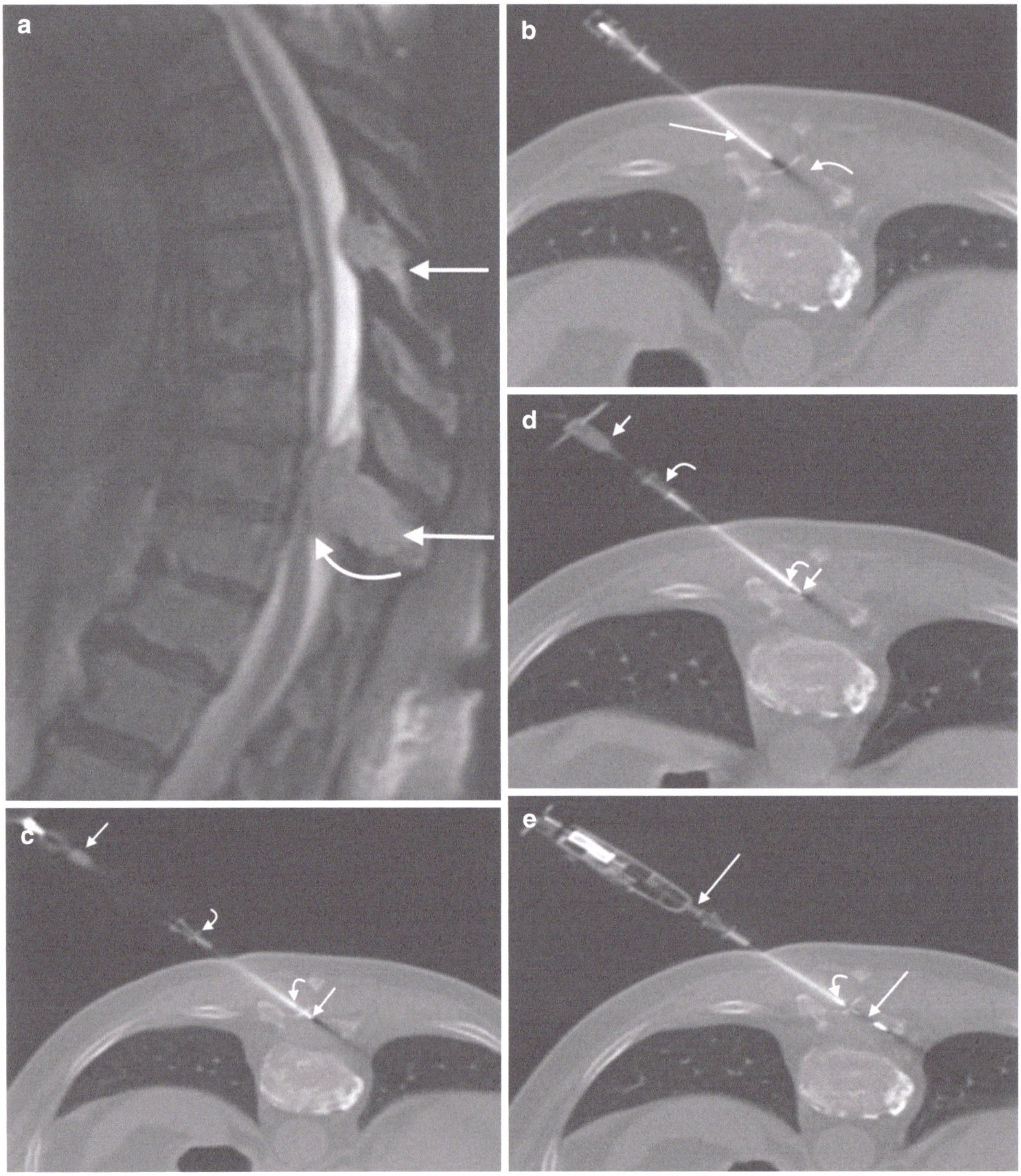

Fig. 5.14 An 82-year-old female with back pain. T2-weighted sagittal image (**a**) shows two spinous process lesions (*arrows*); the large lesion impinges upon the spinal cord (*curved arrow*). Axial CT image (**b**) shows placement of a guide cannula (*arrow*); note the orientation of the guide cannula relative to the expansile lesion within the laminae and base of the spinous process (*curved arrow*). Axial CT image (**c**) shows coaxial placement, via the guide cannula (*curved arrows*), of a 22 gauge needle (*arrows*) into the lesion. Axial CT image (**d**) shows placement of a 16 gauge self-aspirating biopsy needle (*arrows*) via the guide cannula (*curved arrows*). Axial CT image (**e**) shows the coaxial (*curved arrow*) use of a 16 gauge cutting needle. The biopsy was positive for carcinoma cells; unknown primary

under fluoroscopic guidance (Fig. 5.4). In general, these biopsies tend to be performed with a transpedicular approach, but they can also be performed with an extrapedicular approach. With transpedicular technique, the operator aligns the pedicle in the superior third of the vertebral body of interest. This often entails aligning the vertebral endplates. Then the fluoroscopic is rotated in

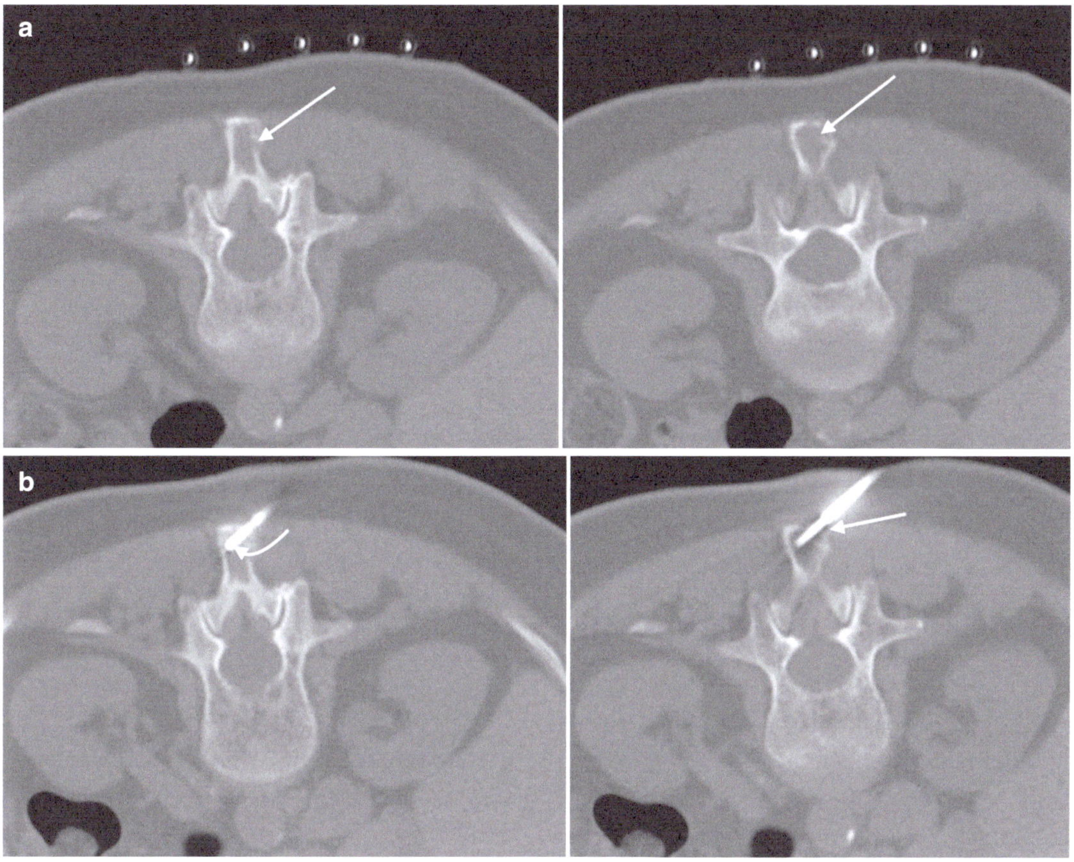

Fig. 5.15 A 74-year-old female with incidental spinous process lesion. Axial CT image (**a**) in bone window algorithm with a skin grid in place shows trajectory (*arrows*) for lytic lesion within the spinous process. Axial CT image (**b**) shows use of coaxial technique with a guide cannula (*arrow*) and trephine bone needle (*curved arrow*); the trephine needle is carefully rotated with gentle forward pressure to avoid fracturing the spinous process. Pathologic analysis of the biopsy specimens showed metastatic papillary thyroid carcinoma

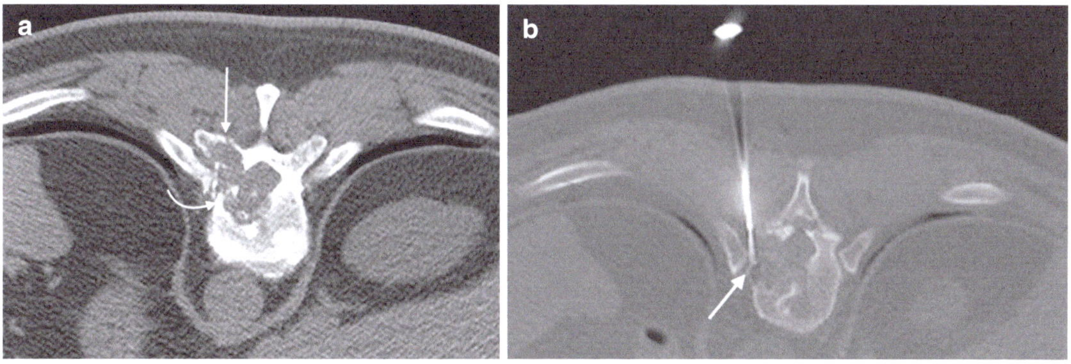

Fig. 5.16 A 54-year-old male with back pain. Axial CT image (**a**) in soft tissue algorithm shows a lytic lesion that involves the left transverse process, pedicle, and posterior vertebral body (*arrows*). Axial CT image (**b**) shows coaxial placement of the biopsy needle (*arrow*) along the lateral margin of the lesion; this technique yielded both osseous and soft tissue material. The histopathology was consistent with an aneurysmal bone cyst

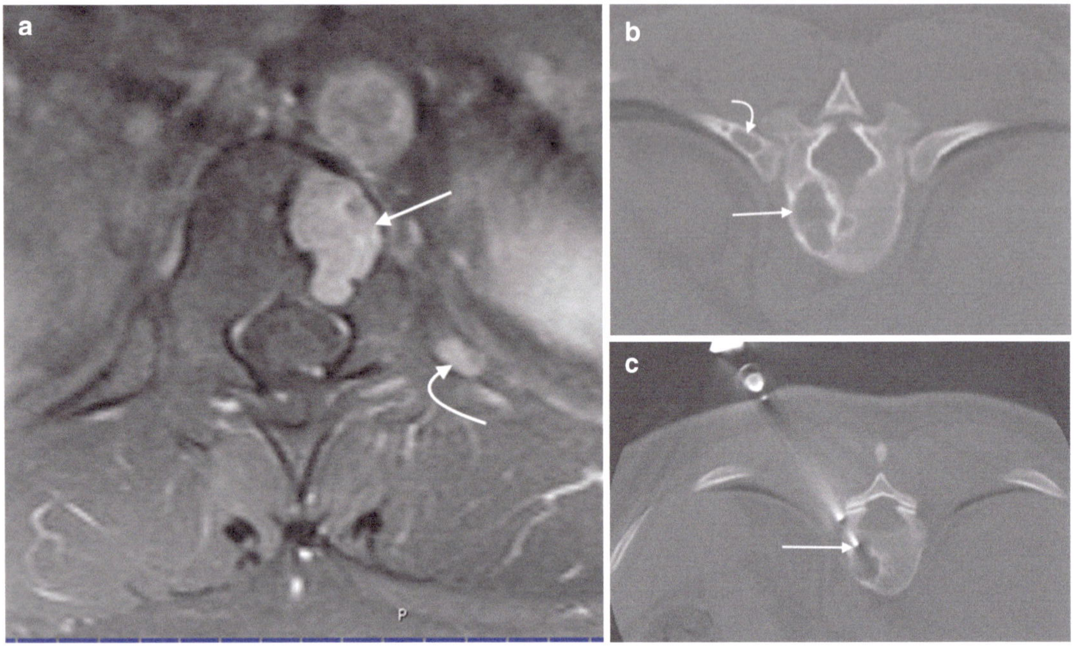

Fig. 5.17 A 31-year-old female with back pain. Fat-suppressed contrast-enhanced T1-weighted axial image (**a**) shows enhancing lesions within the left side of the vertebral body (*arrow*) and left rib (*curved arrow*). Axial CT image (**b**) in bone window algorithm shows well-circumscribed lytic lesions with sclerotic margins within the left rib (*curved arrow*) and posterior vertebra body (*arrow*). Axial CT image (**c**) shows the use of coaxial technique to sample the margin of the vertebral body lesion. The biopsy showed epithelioid hemangioma

a medial to lateral fashion such that pedicle projects over the vertebral body. Think of the pedicle as a flashlight with a cylindrical beam that shines into the vertebral body – this will be the bone needle trajectory into the vertebral body and will represent the area of the vertebral body that will be sampled. In general, mild angulation of the fluoroscope facilitates bone needle access to the anterior and lateral aspect of the vertebral body, while steeper angulations of the fluoroscope will enable placement of the bone needle into more posterior and paramedian areas of the vertebral body.

The intended needle trajectory is anesthetized with a local anesthetic agent. A cross hair incision is made at the skin entry site with a #11 scalpel blade. A bone needle, anywhere from 10 gauge in diameter or smaller, at the operator's discretion and preference, is advanced using a down-the-barrel approach with the pedicle of interest centered in the field of view of the fluoroscope. The bone needle is carefully advanced into the posterior vertebral body. The operator should check the needle position in the oblique, frontal, and lateral fluoroscopic projections during the advancement of the bone needle. This is done to ensure that the needle does not enter the spinal canal and stays within the confines of the vertebral body. In order to avoid entry into the spinal canal, the needle tip should not cross the medial pedicle margin on the frontal projection until the needle tip enters the posterior vertebral body on the corresponding lateral projection. Once the bone needle tip reaches the posterior vertebral body, the needle stylet is removed, and the bone cannula can now be used as a guide cannula for subsequent sequential coaxial bone biopsy needle placements and biopsies. With each coaxial bone needle pass, the position of the guide cannula and bone needle tip is monitored with fluoroscopy to ascertain that the needle has not extended beyond the vertebral body. An advantage of fluoroscopic technique is the opportunity that the operator has to slightly adjust the trajec-

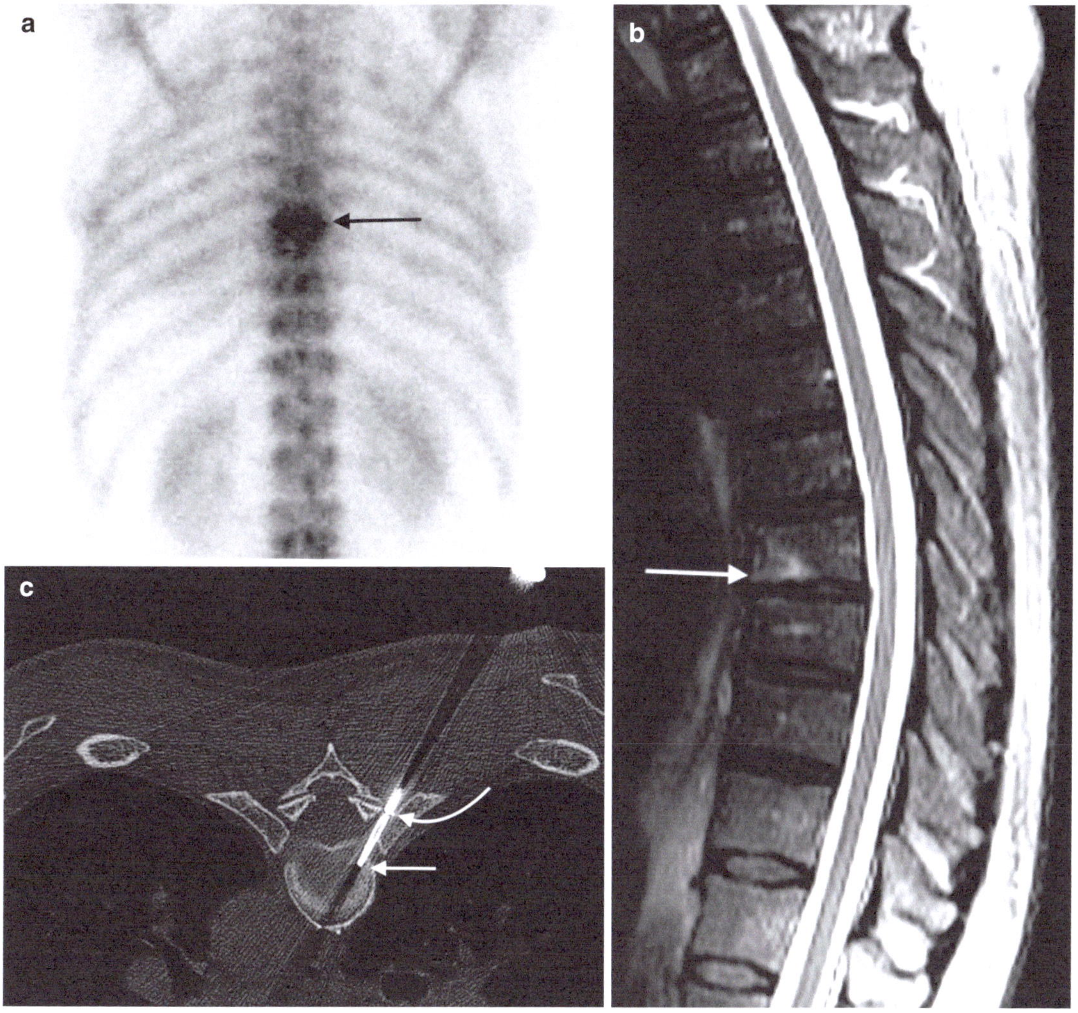

Fig. 5.18 A 64-year-old male with right rib cage pain; normal WBC, ESR, and CRP. Single posterior projection (**a**) from a bone scan shows focal radionuclide uptake (*arrow*) within the mid-thoracic spine. T2-weighted sagittal image (**b**) shows focal hyperintense signal within the anterior vertebral body (*arrow*). Axial CT image (**c**) from the biopsy procedure shows the use of a costovertebral approach (*curved needle*) with coaxial insertion of a bone needle (*arrow*) into the disk-endplate complex. The biopsy, with respect to both pathology and microbiology, was negative

tory of the initial bone needle within the pedicle. This can be readily accomplished by slowly retracting the bone needle, with stylet in place, within the pedicle under fluoroscopic guidance and redirecting the needle tip slightly. This creates a new biopsy tract and a source of additional bone samples.

In certain situations, the operator may not be able to access the vertebral body through a transpedicular route. Extrapedicular approaches can be performed in the thoracic spine using fluoroscopic guidance, especially when the pedicles of a given vertebral body level are small and cannot accommodate the bone needle. The key principle with this type of approach is to stay medial to the rib and lateral to the pedicle at the initial parapedicular entry point; the needle tip is directed medially. It is important to note that these unique approaches can be utilized only if the operator is able to visualize the key osseous anatomic landmarks of the thoracic spine with fluoroscopy. These bony radiographic landmarks include the vertebral pedicle; the oval configuration of the posterior rib, or rib head, as it articulates with the vertebral body; the posterior and anterior vertebral body margins; the spinous process; and the superior and inferior vertebral endplates. This is essentially a costovertebral approach, and it can also be used to access the disk space by aligning the vertebral endplates at the level of interest. The disk space can be initially approached either with a 20 gauge spinal needle or an 18 gauge spinal needle using this oblique fluoroscopic approach. The operator should place the disk within the center of the fluoroscope's field of view in order to facilitate advancement of the needle under fluoroscopy (Fig. 5.19). The spinal needle can also be used to inject a small amount of local anesthetic agent at the margin of the disk just prior to penetrating the annulus fibrosis. The needle tip position can be ascertained using a combination of oblique, frontal, and lateral projections. With experience the operator will note the tactile sensation of advancing a spinal needle into the disk. Once disk access is obtained, the operator can attempt needle aspirations under fluoroscopic guidance. The spinal needle in turn can be exchanged over a small guidewire in order to introduce a bone biopsy needle system for disk-endplate biopsy or to introduce a percutaneous diskectomy device. These options can be exercised at the operator's discretion; however, each needle exchange and each needle pass require meticulous fluoroscopic surveillance.

5.8.5 Post-procedure Care

Once the biopsy procedure is complete, then the guide cannula can be removed from the patient's back, and hemostasis at the skin entry site can usually be achieved with hand compression. Longer periods of hand compression may be required in larger patients, in cases where a large gauge (e.g., 10 gauge) cannula has been utilized, in patients who have been on anticoagulant and/or antiplatelet therapy, or in cases where there is a possible hypervascular lesion. In some situations it may be necessary to inject a small amount of surgifoam into the deep soft tissues of the needle tract and up to the skin surface (also refer to Chap. 2). This may be helpful in patients in whom vascular lesions have been biopsied, in patients in whom antiplatelet and/or anticoagulant medication will be resumed, or in patients with blood oozing around the guide cannula. It is helpful to apply hand compression for about 3–5 min after the surgifoam is injected and to monitor the skin entry site afterward for an additional 3–5 min prior to moving the patient off the procedure table. A sterile bandage is placed on the skin entry site. Once the patient is moved into the supine position onto a stretcher, the skin entry site should be reexamined. After the biopsy procedure, the patient will be recovered for a minimum of 2 hours. It is important not only for the staff to monitor the patient's pain level and vital signs but also to periodically look at the biopsy site for signs of active bleeding or swelling. Post-procedure care instructions are reviewed with the patient at the time of discharge (refer to Chap. 1). A contact telephone number is given to the patient should they have any further questions or should their condition deteriorate when they get home. Patients are reminded that it may take several days to receive the biopsy results and that they should follow up with the doctor who referred them for the procedure. It is very helpful for the operator to contact the requesting clinician and to update them with respect to the procedure and the patient's clinical status after the procedure.

Fig. 5.19 A 30-year-old male with back pain and chronic vertebral compression deformity from prior car accident. Lateral fluoroscopic image (**a**) shows partial T8 vertebral compression deformity (*arrow*); the disk spaces above and below T8 have been aligned by slightly angling of the fluoroscope. Frontal fluoroscopic image (**b**) shows alignment of the disk spaces (*arrows*). Oblique fluoroscopic image (**c**) with the disk aligned (*arrow*) and centered in the field of view shows the approach to the aligned T8-9 disk between the rib (*r*) and the pedicle (*p*). A spinal needle would be advanced, using a down-the-barrel approach, directly into the disk at the point indicated by the *curved arrow*. In this case, staying medial and posterior to the rib avoids the lung, and staying lateral to the pedicle avoids the spinal canal

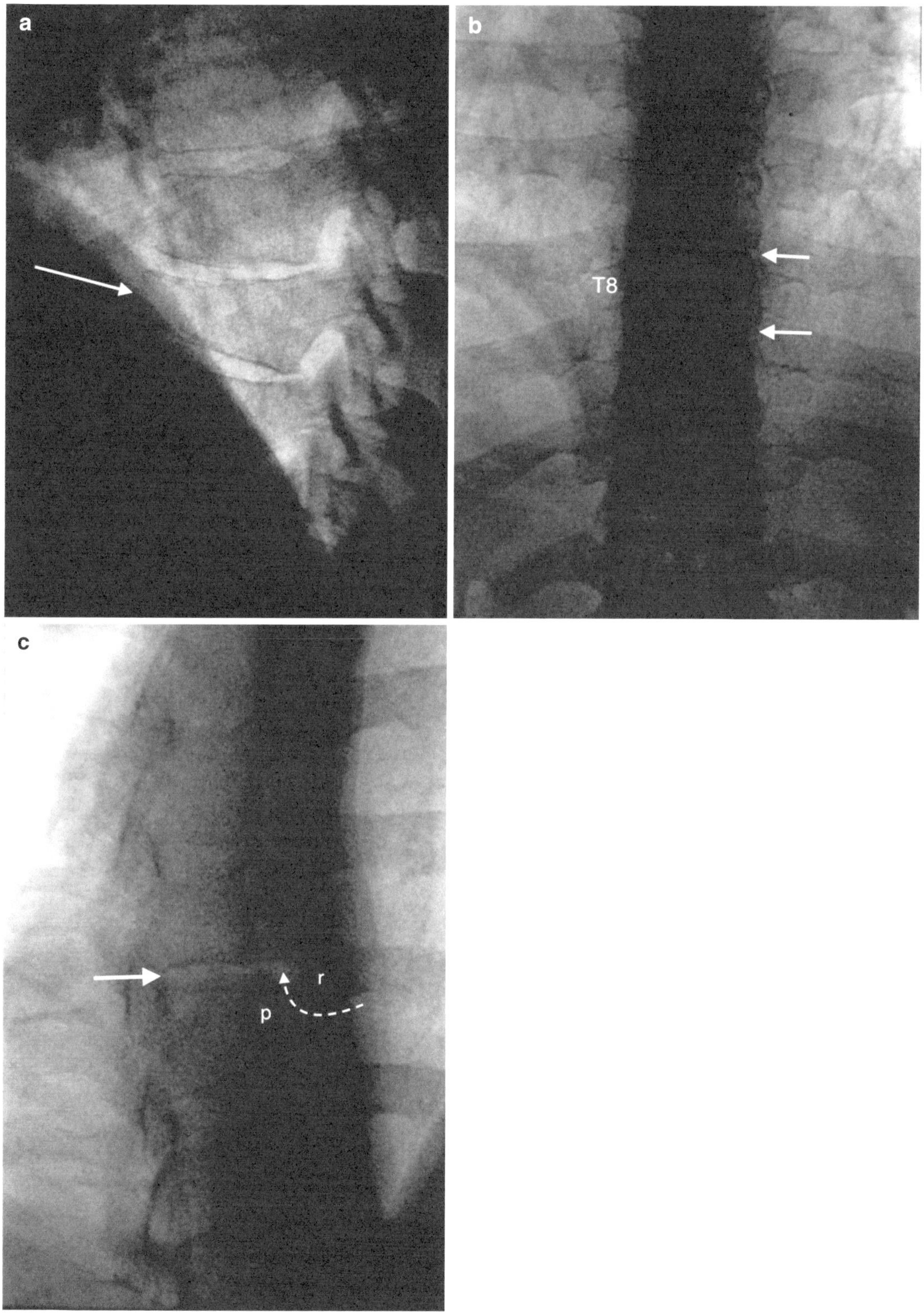
a
b
T8
c
r
p

It is extremely important to take care of the biopsy specimens. Thoracic spine biopsy specimens should be placed in properly labeled containers. For bone biopsies, the transport media is usually 10% formalin. Certain suspected pathologic diagnoses require special transport media or handling at the time of acquisition, and this should be discussed with the pathologist ahead of time. Microbiology specimens are placed in sterile containers and are immediately transported to the microbiology laboratory. All specimens should be accounted for, labeled properly, and accompanied by appropriately completed requisitions, and promptly transported by trained and qualified personnel to the appropriate laboratories. The operator should address any clinical concerns with the pathologist or microbiologist before or at the time the specimens are submitted. The operator should follow up on the biopsy results.

Key Review Points

1. Given the greater number of thoracic vertebrae, it is important to count vertebral levels carefully and to match the counting and labeling scheme with all prior studies in order to localize the correct level for a thoracic biopsy procedure.
2. Critical anatomic structures to be aware of during an image-guided percutaneous thoracic spine biopsy include the spinal cord, the lungs, and the aorta and intercostal arteries.
3. A sound radiologic understanding of osseous landmarks within the thoracic spine is a prerequisite to performing thoracic spine biopsy procedures with CT or fluoroscopic guidance.
4. Common indications for thoracic spine biopsy include a clinical concern for neoplastic involvement of one or more thoracic vertebrae, evaluation of suspected pathologic vertebral compression fractures of the thoracic spine, and the assessment of possible spine infection.
5. The approaches for thoracic spine biopsy are either transpedicular or extrapedicular; extrapedicular approaches include costotransverse, costovertebral, and intercostal techniques.
6. The use of coaxial technique in the thoracic spine facilitates procedure efficiency and safety.
7. Major determinants of specimen yield in thoracic spine biopsy procedures include lesion location relative to critical structures, lesion size, and lesion type (lytic, sclerotic, or mixed).

References

Carrino JA, Campbell Jr PD, Lin DC, Morrison WB, Schweitzer ME, Flanders AE, Eng J, Vaccaro AR. Effect of spinal segment variants on numbering vertebral levels at lumbar MR imaging. Radiology. 2011;259:196–202.

Chew F, Kline M. Diagnostic yield of CT-guided percutaneous aspiration procedures in suspected spontaneous infectious diskitis. Radiology. 2001;218:211–4.

Geremia GK, Charletta DA, Granato DB, Raju S. Biopsy of vertebral and paravertebral structures with a new coaxial needle system. AJNR Am J Neuroradiol. 1992;13:169–71.

Heyer CM, Al-Hadari A, Mueller KM, Stachon A, Nicolas V. Effectiveness of CT-guided percutaneous biopsies of the spine: an analysis of 202 examinations. Acad Radiol. 2008;15:901–11.

Lis E, Bilsky MH, Pisinski L, Boland P, Healey JH, O'Malley B, Krol G. Percutaneous CT-guided biopsy of osseous lesion of the spine in patients with known or suspected malignancy. AJNR Am J Neuroradiol. 2004;25:1583–8.

Olscamp A, Rollins J, Tao SS, Ebraheim NA. Complications of CT-guided biopsy of the spine and sacrum. Orthopedics. 1997;20:1149–52.

Onik G. Automated percutaneous biopsy in the diagnosis and treatment of infectious discitis. Neurosurg Clin N Am. 1996;7:145–50.

Ortiz AO, Zoarski G, Brook A. Image-guided percutaneous spine biopsy. In: Mathis JM, Golovac S, editors. Image-guided spine interventions. 2nd ed. New York: Springer; 2010. p. 75–106.

Pierot L, Boulin A. Percutaneous biopsy of the thoracic and lumbar spine: transpedicular approach under fluoroscopic guidance. AJNR Am J Neuroradiol. 1999;20:23–5.

Renfrew DL, Whitten CG, Wiese JA, el-Khoury GY, Harris KG. CT-guided percutaneous transpedicular biopsy of the spine. Radiology. 1991;180:574–6.

Rimondi E, Staals EL, Errani C, Bianchi G, Casadei R, Alberghini M, Malaguti MC, Rossi G, Durante S, Mercuri M. Percutaneous CT-guide biopsy of the spine: results of 430 biopsies. Eur Spine J. 2008;17:975–81.

Santiago FR, Kelekis A, Alvarez LG, Gilippiadis DK. Interventional procedures of the spine. Semin Musculoskelet Radiol. 2014;18:309–17.

Talac R, McLain RF. Biopsy principles and techniques for spinal tumors. Semin Spine Surg. 2009;21:70–5.

Tehranzadeh J, Tao C, Browning CA. Percutaneous needle biopsy of the spine. Acta Radiol. 2007;48:860–8.

Yaffe D, Greenberg G, Leitner J, Gipstein R, Shapiro M, Bachar GN. CT-guided percutaneous biopsy of thoracic and lumbar spine: a new coaxial technique. AJNR Am J Neuroradiol. 2003;24:2111–3.

Lumbar Spine Biopsy

6

Amish H. Doshi, Amit Aggarwal,
Javin Schefflein and A. Orlando Ortiz

Learning Objectives

1. To learn the pertinent radiologic anatomy, including bony, neural, and vascular anatomy, as it relates to image-guided lumbar spine biopsy
2. To review the most common indications and contraindications for image-guided lumbar spine biopsy
3. To review different approaches and techniques when planning image-guided coaxial lumbar spine biopsy

6.1 Introduction

Of all the image-guided percutaneous spine biopsy procedures that are performed along the spinal axis, lumbar spine biopsy is the most frequently performed of these procedures.

Compared to the cervical spine, percutaneous biopsy of the lumbar spine is relatively safer and technically less difficult. The thicker lumbar pedicles and larger surface area for initial needle insertion allow ease of navigation around adjacent critical nerves and vasculature. Numerous pathologic entities, including infectious and neoplastic processes, can originate from or spread to the lumbar spine and paraspinal tissues. A study of 410 biopsied lumbar spine lesions found metastatic breast and lung cancer to be the most common etiologies found in women (28% and 7%, respectively), while metastatic lung and prostate cancer were found to be the predominant etiologies in men (12% and 7%, respectively) (Lis et al. 2004). Image-guided percutaneous lumbar spine biopsy is generally useful, as the vast majority of procedures yield an adequate specimen for diagnosis (Kornblum et al. 1998). Due to the variety of pathologies affecting the lumbar spine, the diagnostic yield of a biopsy sample varies depending upon the cause of disease as well as on the internal architecture of the lesion. Lumbar spine biopsy for primary and metastatic tumors has an accuracy of approximately 90%. The reported accuracy of spine biopsy for infection is less accurate, only providing a diagnosis around 50% of attempted biopsies (Hau et al. 2002). In spite of the high rate of sample adequacy, the most frequent adverse outcome remains nondiagnostic sampling, especially for the evaluation of spine infection. Image-guided percutaneous lumbar spine biopsy possesses the lowest rate of diagnostic utility in lesions that contain a large necrotic component, diffuse vascularity, or are densely blastic (Sundaresan et al. 2004; Wu et al. 2008). Sclerotic lesions present a particular challenge compared to their lytic counterparts due to the technical difficulty denser tissue presents when extracting a sample. In addition, clinical scenarios in which the likelihood of neoplastic or infectious pathology is low, but there is an overlap in the imaging findings between neoplastic and degenerative pathologic processes or between infectious and inflammatory

A.O. Ortiz, *Image-Guided Percutaneous Spine Biopsy*, DOI 10.1007/978-3-319-43326-4_6

or traumatic processes, raise the suspicion for neoplasm or infection just enough that a biopsy is requested. For example, in an older patient, the presence of extensive degenerative changes of the spine, and a concomitant diagnosis of metastatic disease, may lead to a false suspicion of sclerotic metastases (Ghelman et al. 1991). For similar reasons, differentiating pathologic from benign osteoporotic compression fractures in an elderly patient population presents an ongoing challenge to clinicians.

Over the past several decades, due to a combination of progressive advancements in radiology imaging equipment, image-guiding technology as well as the instruments for performing these procedures, image-guided percutaneous biopsy techniques have grown in use and utility. Despite open biopsy remaining the ultimate procedure for diagnosis, percutaneous spine biopsy has become the preferred method at most institutions around the world (Hau et al. 2002). CT- and fluoroscopic-guided biopsy provides numerous advantages over open biopsy, the most notable of which is a lower morbidity (Chooi et al. 2007). Percutaneous access affords numerous benefits over open surgical techniques, including lower rates of postoperative wound infection, a lower incidence of post-biopsy pathologic fracture, and avoidance of complications from general anesthesia (Schajowicz and Derqui 1968; Murphy 1983). Furthermore, image-guided spine biopsy serves as a cost-effective diagnostic tool, due to the shorter procedure time compared with open techniques and the shorter post-procedure recovery time (Schajowicz and Derqui 1968; Murphy 1983; Peh 2006). Post-biopsy observation varies by institution, but, generally, lasts no longer than 3 h, whereas open techniques may require an overnight hospital stay (Lis et al. 2004). Percutaneous lumbar spine biopsy is an invaluable tool in establishing a diagnosis and guiding subsequent disease-specific treatment. This chapter aims to elucidate the various techniques of fluoroscopic- and CT-guided lumbar spine biopsy as well as provide an overview of different indications and complications that the operator should consider prior to performing the procedure.

6.2 Anatomic Considerations

The lumbar spine typically consists of five lumbar vertebrae and their intervening intervertebral disks (Fig. 6.1). Although biopsy at the level of the lumbar spine is often technically less demanding compared to other locations in the spine, it remains crucial to consider the anatomical structures surrounding the lumbar vertebrae and intervertebral

Fig. 6.1 CT anatomy of the lumbar spine. Midline reformatted sagittal CT image (**a**) in bone window algorithm shows five lumbar vertebral bodies (*L1–L5*) and their corresponding spinous processes (*arrows*) and the intervertebral disks (*curved arrows*); note the orientation of the most caudal disk space (*lower curved arrow*). Reformatted left parasagittal CT image (**b**) in bone window algorithm shows the vertebral pedicle (*curved arrow*) and its relationship to the posterior vertebral body and to the neural foramen (dashed oval); the aorta is partially visualized (*arrow*). Close-up of same image (**c**) in soft tissue algorithm shows the *L2* dorsal root ganglion (*curved arrow*) within the neural foramen at the *L2–L3* level; the proximity of posterior disk (*arrow*) to the nerve is also noted. Contrast-enhanced axial CT image (**d**) in soft tissue algorithm shows the vertebral body (*VB*), pedicle (*P*), transverse process (*TP*), lamina (*L*), and spinous process (*sp*). The erector spinae and multifidus muscles lie posterior to the posterior elements, and the psoas muscle lies lateral to the vertebral body. The lumbar artery (*arrows*) is segmentally visualized along the midpole of the vertebral body. The aorta (*A*) and inferior vena cava (*IVC*) lie anterior to the vertebral body, and the kidneys are seen laterally. The bowel is seen anterior to the aorta and inferior vena cava. Contrast-enhanced axial CT image (**e**) in soft tissue algorithm at the level of the intervertebral disk shows the dorsal root ganglia (*arrows*) and the base of the spinous process (*sp*). Axial CT image (**f**) in bone window algorithm shows the trabecular structure of the vertebral body (*VB*) and a small central focal defect within the posterior vertebral body cortex that corresponds to the basivertebral plexus (*curved arrow*). The spinal canal (*Sc*) is bordered anteriorly by the posterior vertebral cortex, laterally by the pedicles and posteriorly by the laminae. The laminae join to support the spinous process (*sp*). The posterior surface of the pedicle (*arrow*) lies medial to the transverse process and is the access point for a transpedicular approach. Axial CT image (**g**) in bone window algorithm at the level of an upper lumbar facet joint (*large arrow*) shows the more lateral superior articular facet (*small arrow*) that corresponds to the vertebra shown and the more medial inferior articular facet (*curved arrow*) of the vertebra above

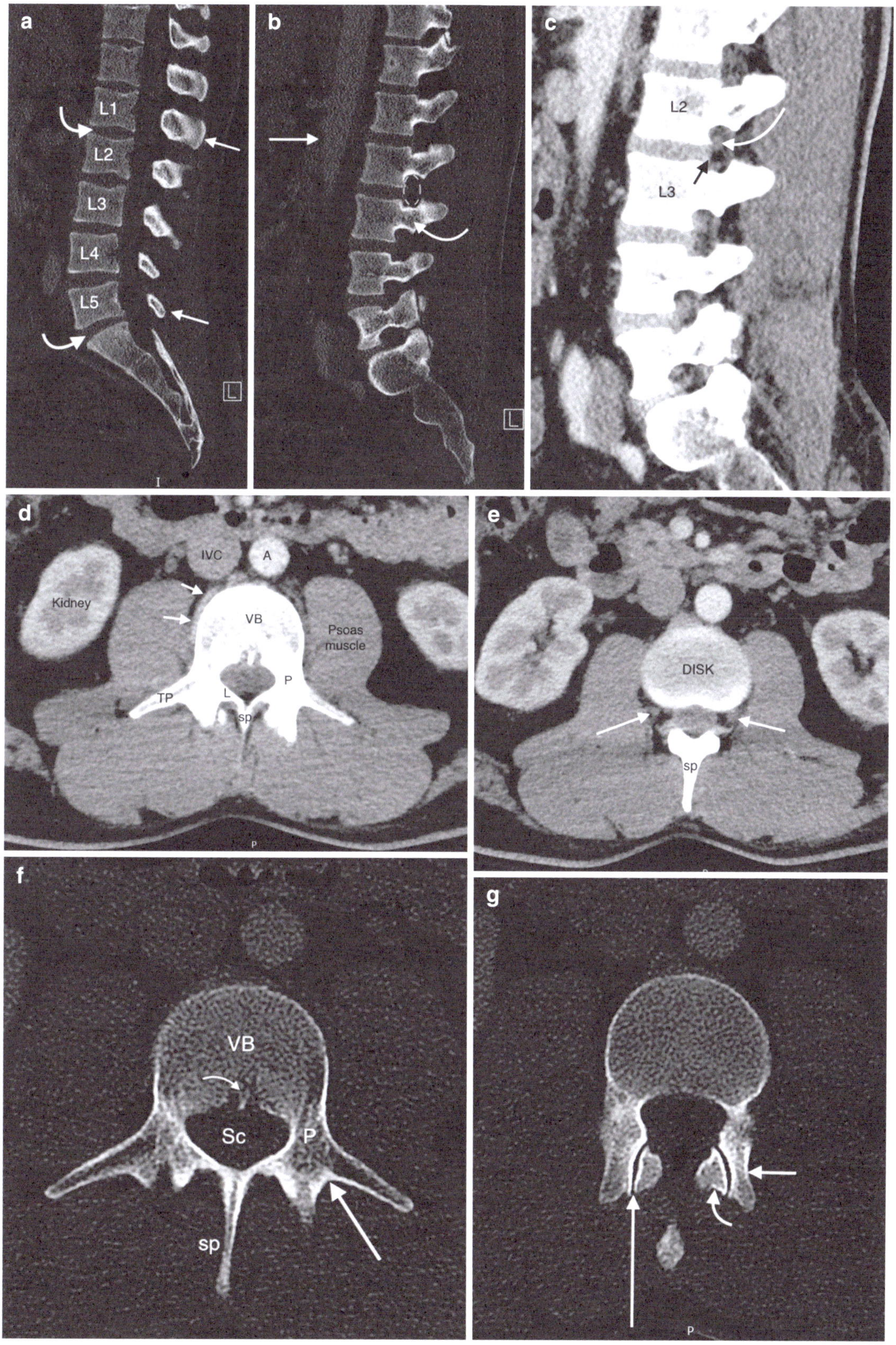
a
L1
L2
L3
L4
L5
L
b
L
c
L2
L3
d
IVC
A
Kidney
VB
Psoas muscle
P
TP
L
sp
e
DISK
sp
f
VB
Sc
P
sp
g

disks. Image-guided percutaneous lumbar spine biopsies are almost universally performed from a posterior approach. The operator must guide the needle through the posterior paraspinal musculature including the erector spinae and multifidus or quadratus lumborum muscles, in order to access the vertebral body and/or paravertebral soft tissues. Often a transpedicular approach is selected for access to a vertebral body lesion as the pedicle size within the lumbar vertebra can easily accommodate most commercially available biopsy needle systems. Access via the pedicle, if possible, can serve as a safe conduit into the vertebral body (Chooi et al. 2007). Care must be taken to ensure that the medial border of the pedicle is not breached prior to entering the posterior vertebral body in order to avoid inadvertent entrance into the spinal canal. Although the location of the needle tip must be monitored during a transpedicular approach, there is reduced risk to adjacent soft tissues, nerves, or vasculature once the needle passes within the safe channel provided by the pedicle. An alternate approach for biopsy, however, may be necessary depending upon the location of the lesion within the vertebral body. For example, smaller posterior median lesions may not be accessible via a transpedicular route. The intervertebral disk and the paraspinal soft tissues, likewise, are usually not accessed via a transpedicular approach. Posterolateral or extrapedicular approaches are optional trajectories, and an active awareness of the anatomic location of neural and vascular structures is critical toward reducing the risk of injury with these approaches. The lumbar arteries arise from the aorta and run along the equatorial or mid-portion of the vertebral body, coursing posteriorly, where they enter the neural foramina bilaterally. These arteries give rise to both vertebral nutrient arteries which supply blood to the vertebrae and radiculomedullary arteries which can contribute to the blood supply of the spinal cord and cauda equina. Visualization of these vessels is often difficult during lumbar spine biopsy, especially since the procedure is performed without the use of intravascular contrast agents when using imaging guidance. It is nevertheless important to consider and be aware of these vascular structures when using a posterolateral approach.

Often a transpedicular approach is selected for access to a vertebral body lesion as the pedicle size within the lumbar vertebra can easily accommodate most commercially available biopsy needle systems.

The spinal cord terminates as the conus medullaris usually at the L1–L2 level of the spinal canal. This critical structure must be accounted for when considering lumbar spine biopsy procedures within the upper lumbar spine. The cauda equina, a constellation of sensory and motor nerve roots, arises from the conus medullaris. These nerve roots are named for the vertebra bordering the superior portion of the neural foramen through which they pass (e.g., the L2–L3 neural foramen contains the L2 nerve root). These nerves enter the proximal neural foramina bilaterally above the level of the disk space at their respective intervertebral level and course along the superior portion of the foramen. As the nerve roots exit the foramen, they course inferiorly. The L1–L4 nerve roots join to form the lumbar plexus which runs along and within the psoas musculature. The operator must consider the location of the nerve roots when performing a posterolateral approach. These approaches are frequently performed with CT guidance and therefore allow direct but segmental visualization of the nerve with respect to needle trajectory.

CT guidance can offer more direct visualization of anatomic structures related to the lumbar spine which may be particularly helpful when using a posterolateral approach.

The aorta runs along the anterior margin of the lumbar spine, almost always on the left side; the inferior vena cava is located on the right side (Fig. 6.1). A lesion may occasionally extend to and penetrate the anterior cortex of the vertebral body. Identification of the lesion's extension with respect to the aorta and inferior vena cava is important in preventing potential injury to these vital structures. Injury to the aorta is rare, as most lesions are confined to the vertebral bodies. It may be appropriate to utilize CT guidance in these cases to ensure proper visualization of the aorta and inferior vena cava in relation to the biopsy needle. If fluoroscopic guidance is considered, the use of lateral imaging is necessary during advancement of the biopsy needle to prevent penetration of the anterior cortex of the vertebral body or the anterior aspect of the intervertebral disk. The lumbar sympathetic plexus is located bilaterally along the anterior and lateral aspect of the lumbar vertebral column. Fortunately, no significant injuries to this structure with lumbar spine biopsy have been reported. The other critical organs, however remote, that must always be considered when performing lumbar spine biopsy include the inferior aspects of the lungs and pleura, the kidneys, and the bowel.

Once a request for percutaneous image-guided lumbar spine biopsy has been received, all available and pertinent imaging studies must be reviewed and a planned needle trajectory formulated bearing in mind the aforementioned anatomic structures. Consideration of needle approach will be required to ensure proper sampling of the lesion within the vertebral body, intervertebral disk, or paraspinal soft tissue. All approaches rely on a careful review of the available imaging examinations and the assessment of anatomic structures, lesion location, and lesion size in order to ensure that the optimal needle trajectory is chosen.

> Knowledge of the critical anatomy of the lumbar spine is extremely important in planning needle trajectory for image-guided percutaneous lumbar spine biopsy and for avoiding complications.

6.3 Indications

Image-guided percutaneous biopsy of the lumbar spine allows access to the vertebral body, posterior elements, intervertebral disks, as well as surrounding soft tissues. Requests for lumbar spine biopsies are most frequently a result of imaging (i.e., CT, MRI, PET-CT, bone scan) that shows the possible presence of a neoplastic or infectious process (Peh 2003; Hodge 1997). A list of most common indications for image-guided percutaneous lumbar spine biopsy is provided in Table 6.1. Histopathologic identification of malignancy plays an important role in the management of newly diagnosed malignancy, modification of current treatment, and assessment of prognosis in metastatic disease of a known primary malignancy (Sundaresan et al. 2004; Herkowitz and Wesolowski 1986). In particular, tissue identification of specific etiologies of malignancy may change oncologic management – a patient previously planned for surgery may be discovered to have a plasmacytoma or lymphoma involving the spinal canal and thus would benefit from other treatments such as chemotherapy or radiation. Even after treatment, patients many times require lumbar biopsy to exclude disease recurrence when a new lesion is identified on an imaging study (Peh 2003; Hodge 1997). More recent advances in medical therapy have reinforced the importance of biopsy, such as evaluating active lesions demonstrated on PET imaging. Emerging concepts such as tailoring specific treatment regimens to the inherent

Table 6.1 Indications for image-guided percutaneous lumbar spine biopsy

1. Infection
   - Spondylitis-diskitis
   - Paraspinal abscess
2. Neoplasm
   - Primary osseous neoplasm
   - Evaluation of solitary bone lesion
   - Secondary osseous neoplasm
     - Osseous metastatic disease or involvement by systemic malignancy
   - Diffuse marrow replacement process
   - Evaluation of neoplastic lesions with diffusion restriction or FDG-PET avidity posttreatment to assess for treatment response
   - Paraspinal soft tissue mass
   - Pathologic vertebral body compression fracture
3. Pretreatment (including the above categories)
   - Tissue characterization prior to treatment initiation

biologic heterogeneity of a neoplasm requires biopsy for accurate tissue sampling and subsequent genetic analysis (Talac and Mclain 2009).

Lumbar spine biopsy may be requested in patients who were initially considered to have benign disease, but subsequent clinical evaluation suggests otherwise. For example, in patients with back pain secondary to what is initially thought to be an osteoporotic vertebral compression fracture, when symptoms worsen or concerning imaging characteristics such as progressive tumor growth or pathologic abnormality emerge, tissue sampling may be beneficial to exclude malignancy (Herkowitz and Wesolowski 1986). Additionally, equivocal imaging findings or patient anxiety from uncertainty may result in a request for image-guided biopsy. Another common indication for lumbar spine biopsy is for definitive diagnosis of vertebral osteomyelitis and/or diskitis (Peh 2003; Hodge 1997; Herkowitz and Wesolowski 1986). Occasionally, the clinical presentation raises suspicion for spinal infection, which can be confirmed with MR imaging of the spine. In this setting, lumbar spine biopsy plays an important role in identification of the infectious organism, which enables antimicrobial therapy to be tailored specific to the infectious pathogen. Alternatively, both imaging and clinical findings may not be specific for spinal infection, which then requires biopsy with surgical pathology evaluation of core tissue from the disk and/or vertebral body for diagnostic confirmation or exclusion.

6.4 Contraindications

Image-guided percutaneous lumbar spine biopsy is a relatively safe procedure with few contraindications (Table 6.2). A major contraindication, however, is uncorrected coagulopathy (Santiago et al. 2014). This is often the result of anticoagulant therapy, but may also be seen in patients who have intrinsic coagulopathy due to underlying malignancy or other disease states. When possible, it is important to hold anticoagulation therapy prior to procedure to reduce risk of hemorrhage (refer to the Chap. 2). Consultation with the provider managing this therapy is often necessary to ensure that holding this medication does not produce additional risk to the patient due to a thromboembolic event. In patients with intrinsic coagulopathy, it may be necessary to infuse platelets or administer vitamin K prior to the procedure, such as when platelet counts fall below 50,000/mcL (Peh 2006). Again, the operator should discuss the appropriate management of the coagulopathy with the responsible patient care provider(s). Occasionally, consultation with a hematologist may provide additional insight into the appropriate management.

Table 6.2 Contraindications to image-guided percutaneous lumbar spine biopsy

Absolute
Uncorrected coagulopathy
Untreated infection in patient with suspicious mass lesion
Relative
Patient factors
Combative or uncooperative patient
Clinically unstable patient
Lesion type
Vascular lesion
Probable benign lesion
Lesion size
Discretion must be exercised with smaller lesions (< 5 mm in diameter)
Limited or no specimen yield may result in false negative biopsy
Lesion location
Defer biopsy for lesions located adjacent to critical structures or inaccessible locations

Preexisting infection at the skin site, such as a cellulitis or a decubitus ulcer, can sometimes occur near the intended area for possible percutaneous biopsy. Infection at the skin site or within the soft tissues surrounding a tumor can be considered a contraindication to percutaneous biopsy (Peh 2003; Hodge 1997; Ghelman 1998). Although unlikely, the spread of the infection into deep soft tissues, tumor, or within the vertebral body can occur if a soft tissue infection, such as a cellulitis, is not treated prior to biopsy. Consultation with an infectious disease specialist may be necessary to optimize antibiotic therapy and provide medical clearance prior to biopsy.

Patients who are uncooperative or unstable are not candidates for image-guided lumbar spine biopsy (Peh 2006). If a patient is clinically unstable, it is prudent to wait until the patient is medically stabilized as well as to consult with the patient's clinical providers in order to assess for the urgency and clinical need for a biopsy. With respect to uncooperative patients, after discussion with the appropriate patient representative and requesting provider, a clinically necessary lumbar spine biopsy can be performed under general anesthesia or monitored anesthesia care. The risk and benefits of the anesthesia and the need for tissue diagnosis must be carefully assessed in order to appropriately triage candidates for the procedure. The type of lesion may also influence whether or not a biopsy gets performed. Hypervascular lesions may dissuade an operator for fear of a hemorrhagic event. The operator should try to avoid performing biopsy procedures in cases where the radiographic features are highly suggestive or pathognomonic of a benign lesion (Figs. 6.2 and 6.3). Very small (less than 5 mm diameter) lesions may not be amenable to biopsy; it just may not be possible to obtain tissue. Lesions, especially small lesions, that are located near critical structures such as the spinal cord, lung, or aorta may also not be amenable to percutaneous biopsy.

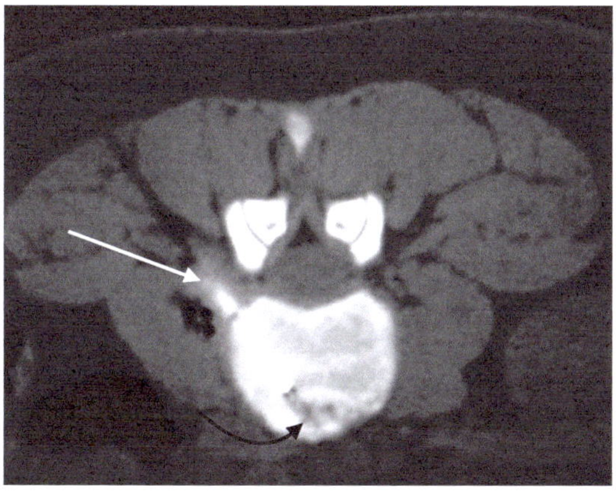

Fig. 6.2 Axial CT image shows posterolateral approach with bone biopsy needle (*arrow*) for biopsy of a round sclerotic lesion with a lucent center at the vertebral endplate. This is a Schmorl's node and a biopsy was not necessary

6.5 Risks and Complications Associated with Lumbar Spine Biopsy and How to Minimize Them

It is important for the operator to be aware of the potential complications that have been associated with lumbar spine biopsy in order to help reduce the overall risk to the patient during this procedure (Ortiz et al. 2010) (Table 6.3). Complications from image-guided percutaneous lumbar spine biopsy are relatively uncommon, with a reported rate of less than 1–3% (Tehranzadeh et al. 2007). Although image-guided lumbar spine biopsy is safely performed on a routine basis, operators must be aware of potential complications in order to first prevent and avoid them and, second, to acutely manage such situations in order to avoid further injury to the patient. Lumbar spine biopsy complications can be divided into acute and delayed or late complications (Tehranzadeh et al. 2007). Acute complications after lumbar spine biopsy include subcutaneous hemorrhage or hematoma formation, hemorrhage from biopsy of hypervascular lesions, neurologic injury, dural puncture, and vertebral fracture. Specifically, renal cell carcinoma and thyroid carcinoma are well-known examples of hypervascular tumors that are prone to hemorrhage when biopsied (Talac and McLain 2009). An acute or even subacute complication that is often overlooked by operators is the occurrence of a thromboembolic event (myocardial ischemia in a patient with coronary artery stents or stroke in a patient with atrial fibrillation) in a patient when anticoagulant or antiplatelet medication has been transiently discontinued. Late complications, which can arise weeks to months after the spine biopsy procedure, include infection and tumor seeding along the needle tract. Risk of infection is low in the setting of percutaneous biopsy when performed with appropriate sterile preparation of the biopsy entry/access site. In one study, no post-procedural infections were reported out of 94 CT-guided spine biopsy cases (Olscamp et al. 1997). Needle tract seeding by tumor is also a late complication and is rare when utilizing specific coaxial techniques and the smaller gauge

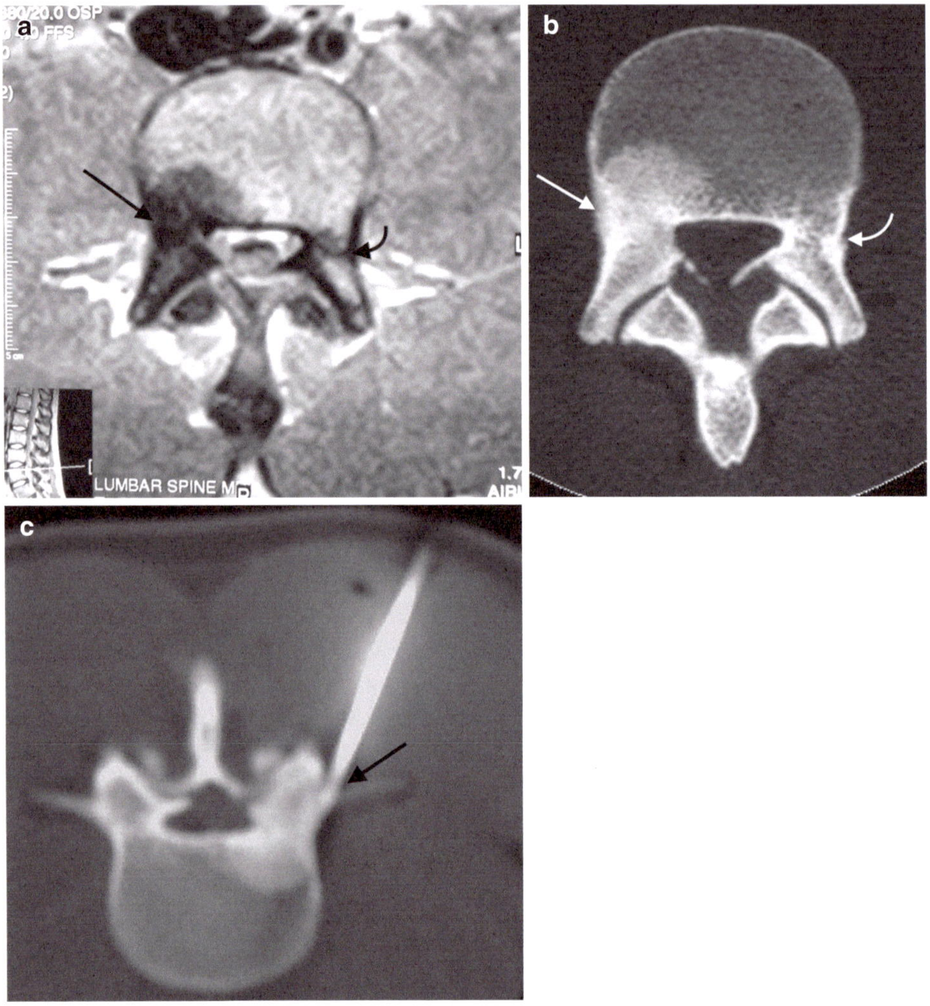

Fig. 6.3 A 20-year-old male with chronic low back pain. T1-weighted axial image (**a**) shows a hypointense lesion within the pedicle (*arrow*) and a linear hypointense defect within the opposite pedicle (*curved arrow*). The clinicians and family insisted upon a biopsy procedure for what is obviously a stress fracture. Axial CT image (**b**) in bone window algorithm shows sclerosis in the right pedicle (*arrow*) and a fracture line (*curved arrow*) in the left pedicle. Axial CT image (**c**) shows biopsy of the sclerotic pedicle with a bone needle (*arrow*). The biopsy was negative

needle sizes that are typically used for spine biopsy (Saghieh et al. 2010; Davies et al. 1993).

Hemorrhage can occur with any invasive procedure, and a minimal amount is often unavoidable. Therefore, correction of coagulopathy is important to help reduce the risk of significant hemorrhage during lumbar spine biopsy. As previously mentioned, a coaxial approach minimizes the need for multiple passes through the skin, subcutaneous soft tissues, and muscles when accessing the vertebral body or paravertebral soft tissues. Reduced manipulation of the adjacent soft tissue results in reduced risk of injury to vascular structures. In the lumbar spine, the lumbar arteries typically pass along the equatorial plane of the vertebral body and traverse the anterior margin of the neural foramen to enter the posterior vertebral body as the nutrient supply to the vertebral body (Fig. 6.1). Although there are multiple periosteal arteries that originate along the course of the lumbar artery, it is not usually necessary to identify these vessels since access into the vertebral body is transpedicular or parapedicular, avoiding injury to these vascular structures.

Table 6.3 Percutaneous lumbar spine biopsy: potential risks and complications

Tissue injury
Vascular injury
Neural injury
Pneumothorax
Hemorrhage
Superficial or subcutaneous
Deep – hemorrhage into a tumor and/or spinal canal can result in acute neurologic changes, or retroperitoneal hemorrhage can result in hypotension or severe pain
Infection (superficial or deep) in those cases being performed to assess for neoplasm
Inappropriate needle placement
Breach of the anterior vertebral body or medial pedicle cortex
Needle placement within the spinal canal
Wrong level
Inadequate tissue sampling
Technical failure – biopsy system failure, lost specimen
Tumor seeding along the biopsy tract
Radiation exposure
Anesthesia complications
Aspiration, airway compromise, respiratory depression
Thromboembolic events in patients with reversed anticoagulation/antiplatelet therapy

Biopsy of hypervascular tumors can result in excessive bleeding. Typically, waiting 5–10 min with the stylet placed in the introducer needle when using a coaxial needle system will result in hemostasis. Occasionally, it may be necessary to inject Gelfoam or Surgifoam into the introducer needle along the biopsy tract to achieve hemostasis (Talac and McLain 2009). The use of a smaller needle in these types of lesions also can reduce the risk of hemorrhage. An alternative to core needle biopsy of suspected hypervascular lesions is fine-needle aspiration. This technique allows for the placement of a small needle, typically 25 or 27 gauge, and can often yield enough cellular tissue to establish a histologic diagnosis.

Injury to the lumbar nerve roots, as well as the thecal sac (dura mater), can be avoided with the use of CT guidance. Visualization of these structures in relation to the advancing needle tip can allow the operator to modify needle trajectory or establish a new path of needle placement if there is concern for injury to neural structures. It is important to be able to identify important bony landmarks when performing spine biopsy under fluoroscopic guidance as direct visualization of neural structures is not possible with this imaging modality. Specifically, when using a transpedicular approach, it is necessary to ensure that the biopsy needle does not penetrate the medial margin of the pedicle as seen on the anterior-posterior fluoroscopic projection prior to reaching the posterior margin of the vertebral body as seen on the simultaneous lateral fluoroscopic projection. Confirmation of this precise needle positioning will ensure that the needle does not penetrate the medial border of the pedicle and advances into the spinal canal (Fig. 6.4).

6.6 Imaging Guidance

The most commonly utilized modalities for image-guided percutaneous lumbar spine biopsies are CT, CT fluoroscopy, and fluoroscopy. A meta-analysis of 25 studies revealed accuracy rates of 90.2% and 88.1% for CT- and fluoroscopic-guided biopsies, respectively, when compared to the subsequent clinical confirmation of the diagnosis (Nourbakhsh et al. 2008). The use of other modalities, such as MRI and ultrasound, is limited in the setting of lumbar spine biopsies. It is often challenging to use MRI for imaging guidance due to limited scanner availability, procedure time, and the need for specialized MRI-compatible biopsy equipment. Additionally, patients with certain types of implants (e.g., certain aneurysm clips and non-MRI conditional pacemakers) cannot be placed in MR scanners. Ultrasound can be used for superficial soft tissue biopsy or aspiration of subcutaneous fluid collections, but cannot be reliably utilized for deep bone lesions due to the significant shadowing that occurs with cortical bone.

CT guidance is often the preferred modality for sampling discrete lesions in lumbar spine biopsy (Fig. 6.5). It provides visualization of important anatomic structures, excellent spatial resolution, and the ability to help guide the biopsy needle into small focal lesions within the vertebral body (Lis et al. 2004; Peh 2006; Ortiz et al.

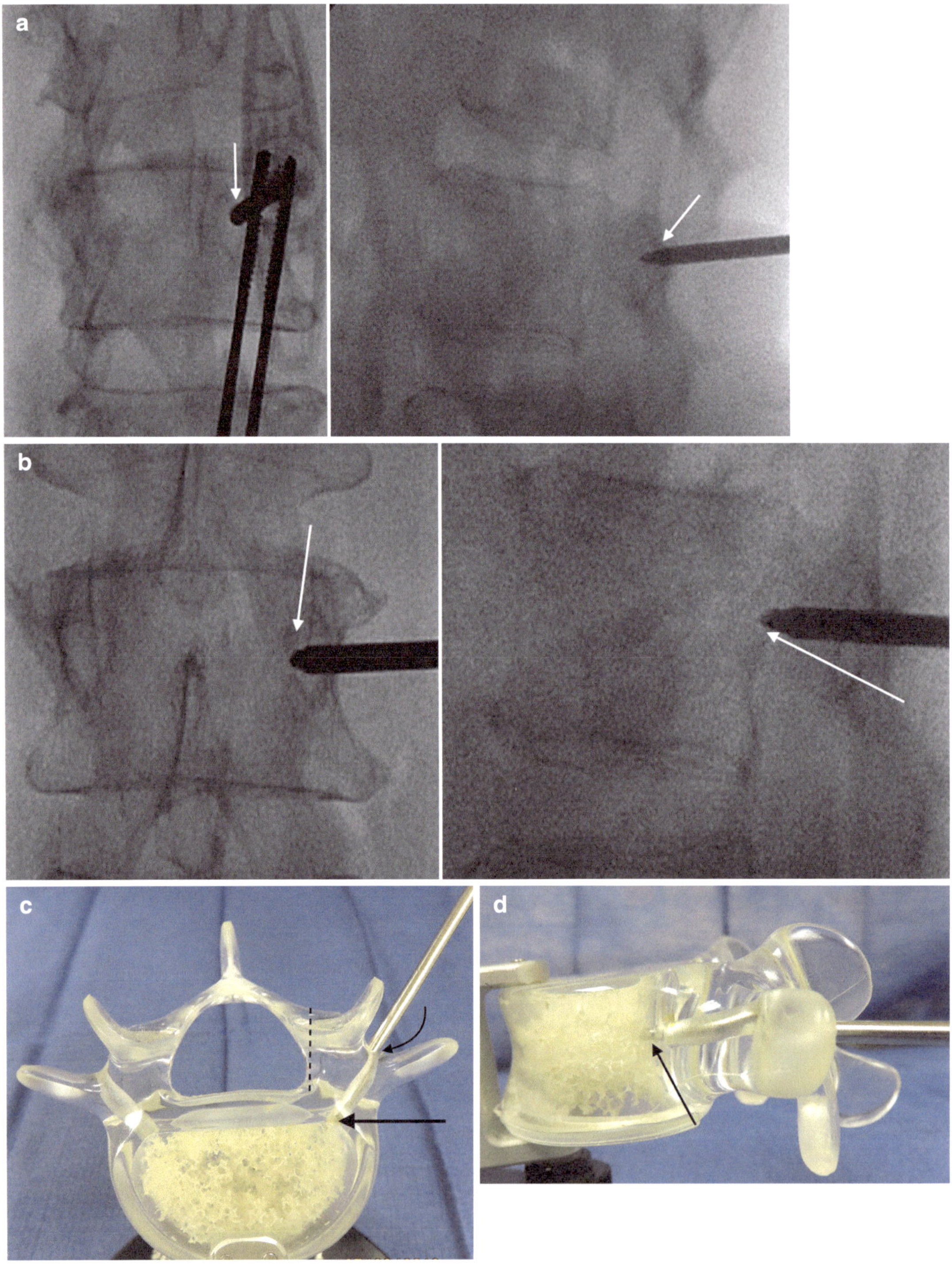
a
b
c
d

2010). The operator can obtain images at multiple time points throughout the procedure in order to guide the biopsy needle into the desired location while simultaneously evaluating the needle position relative to critical organs and vascular and neural structures. Imaging confirmation of biopsy needle placement within the lesion will document that the appropriate abnormality was sampled in the event that a "nondiagnostic" pathology result is obtained. This can be seen on occasion with lesions treated with prior radiation, cystic lesions, and necrotic lesions. The CT gantry can also be angled to parallel the area of interest, such as the disk space or vertebral body, to allow visualization of a possible or actual needle path in a single plane (Fig. 6.6). Some CT fluoroscopy systems enable the operator to obtain axial and sagittal reconstructions during needle advancement. Moreover, for lesions where resection may eventually be performed, including resection of the biopsy tract, CT better documents the path of the biopsy needle and the skin entry point for the surgeon to later follow when resecting residual tumor (Lis et al. 2004).

Although radiation is required for CT and fluoroscopic procedures, the operator can employ lower-dose techniques to reduce radiation dose to the patient without affecting diagnostic yield (Shpilberg et al. 2014). Strategies that can be used to reduce the patient's radiation exposure during a spine biopsy procedure include reviewing the prior studies to optimize the procedure before you perform it, limiting the scan volume to the area of interest (e.g., focusing on two or three vertebral levels instead of the entire lumbar spine), adjusting CT scanner parameters such as tube current modulation (mAs) and tube potential (kV) based upon patient and body part size, and using automatic exposure control features of the CT scanner and radiation dose monitoring. CT fluoroscopy also reduces procedure time by allowing sequential imaging of needle placement while the operator remains in the procedural suite. Typically, after the operator presses a foot pedal, a set of three images are obtained, which include an image below, at, and above the level of imaging. The operator can use this information to modify trajectory in order to ensure appropriate needle placement into the vertebral lesion. Although radiation exposure through this technique is reduced for the patient, it is important for the operator to be actively aware of their own radiation exposure during these procedures. Modern CT fluoroscopy scanners typically have a leaded area along the outside of the scanner which allows for minimal operator exposure when scanning. Alternatively, the operator can stand behind a portable lead shield a short distance away from the gantry; this exploits the benefit of the inverse square law for reducing radiation exposure to the operator and the benefit of added radiation shielding.

Fluoroscopic guidance can be employed in the setting of more diffuse vertebral body disease and suspected spinal infections. This modality allows real-time imaging of needle placement and advancement into the vertebral body or disk space (Pierot and Boulin 1999). Some major

Fig. 6.4 Initial needle positioning for the transpedicular approach. Oblique and lateral fluoroscopic images (**a**) obtained simultaneously with a bone needle docked on the posterior surface of the pedicle (*arrows*). The oblique orientation shows the needle tip within the "eye of the Scotty dog" (*arrow*). Frontal and lateral fluoroscopic images (**b**) obtained simultaneously show advancement of the bone needle through the pedicle to the margin of the posterior vertebral body as shown on the lateral image (*arrow*). It is very important to observe that the needle tip has not crossed the medial pedicle cortex (*arrow*) as shown on the frontal projection (if it had, then the needle tip would be in the spinal canal!). A photograph of a plastic see-through vertebral body model (**c**) from an overhead view with a bone needle (*curved arrow*) inserted to the same position as in (**b**) shows the tip of the needle (*large arrow*) at the junction of the anterior pedicle and posterior vertebral body. Note that the needle tip has not crossed the medial pedicle cortex (*dashed arrow*); compare to the frontal fluoroscopic image in **b**. A photograph of the model from a lateral view (**d**) with the needle in the same position shows the needle tip at the pedicle-vertebral body junction (*arrow*); compare to the lateral fluoroscopic image in **b**

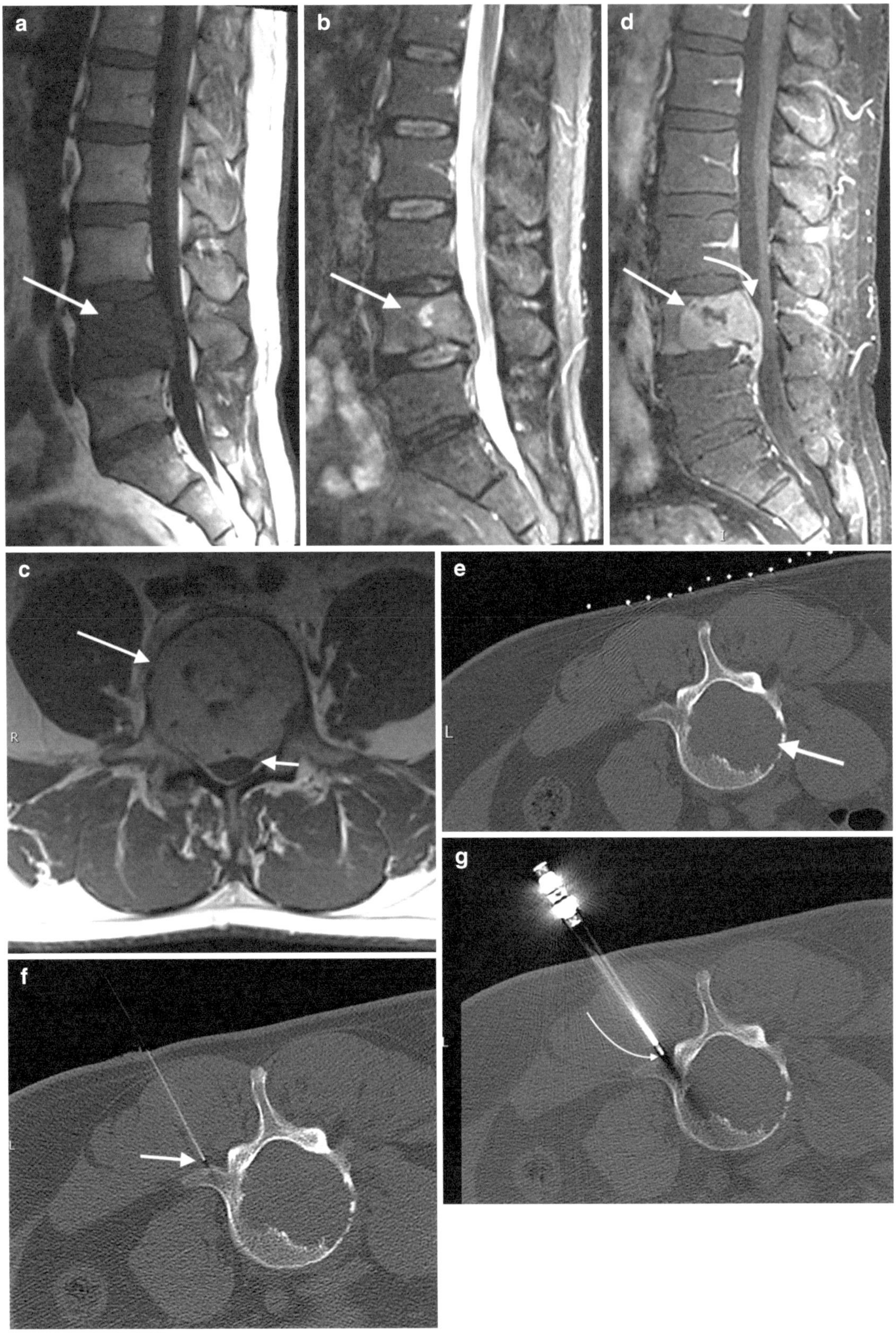
a
b
d
c
R
e
L
f
L
g

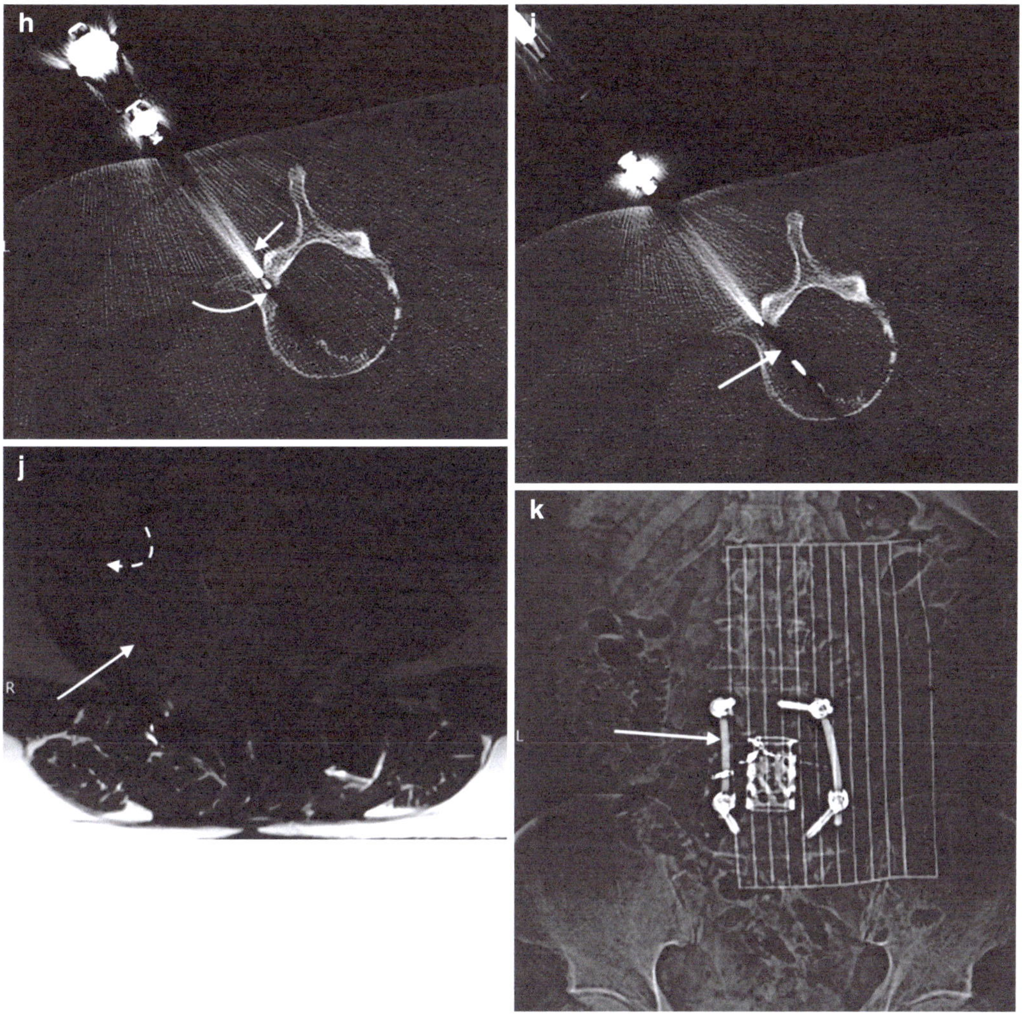

Fig. 6.5 (continued)

Fig. 6.5 A 47-year-old male with low back pain. T1-weighted sagittal image (**a**) shows a hypointense lesion within the L4 vertebral body; the lesion has a thin hypointense anterior margin (*arrow*). T2-weighted sagittal image (**b**) shows a moderately hyperintense lesion (*arrow*) that encroaches upon the spinal canal. Contrast-enhanced T1-weighted axial image (**c**) shows a diffusely enhancing lesion (*large arrow*) with ventral epidural encroachment (*small arrow*). The fat-suppressed contrast-enhanced T1-weighted sagittal image (**d**) better delineates the mass (*arrow*) and shows the epidural encroachment (*curved arrow*). Axial CT image (**e**) during the spine biopsy procedure shows a large lytic vertebral body lesion (*arrow*). Axial CT image (**f**) shows a spinal needle (*arrow*) that is used to infiltrate the posterior pedicle with local anesthetic. Axial CT image (**g**) shows a coaxial bone biopsy needle system docked (*arrow*) into the posterior pedicle cortex. Axial CT image (**h**) shows advancement of the bone needle (*curved arrow*) through the pedicle with the guide cannula (*arrow*) in place. Axial CT image (**i**) shows coaxial placement of a cutting needle (*arrow*) through the guide cannula; this was possible once the initial bone needle pass created an access channel to the lytic lesion. Follow-up contrast-enhanced T1-weighted axial image (**j**) obtained 1 year after L4 corpectomy and anterior and posterior fusion; the patient is asymptomatic. A solid moderately enhancing mass (*arrow*) displaces the psoas muscle laterally (*curved arrow*). Scout frontal CT image (**k**) from a biopsy procedure shows a skin grid partially overlying the area of instrumentation from L3 to L5 (*arrow*). Axial CT image (**l**) shows insert needle (*arrow*) used to anesthetize the margin of the large soft tissue mass. Axial CT image (**m**) shows coaxial advancement of a guide needle (*arrow*). Axial CT image (**n**) shows soft tissue cutting needle (*arrow*) that was inserted via coaxial technique. Axial CT image (**o**) shows sequential advancement of the biopsy needle through the lesion. The initial biopsy provided a pathologic diagnosis of giant cell tumor, and the follow-up biopsy confirmed the presence of a recurrent tumor

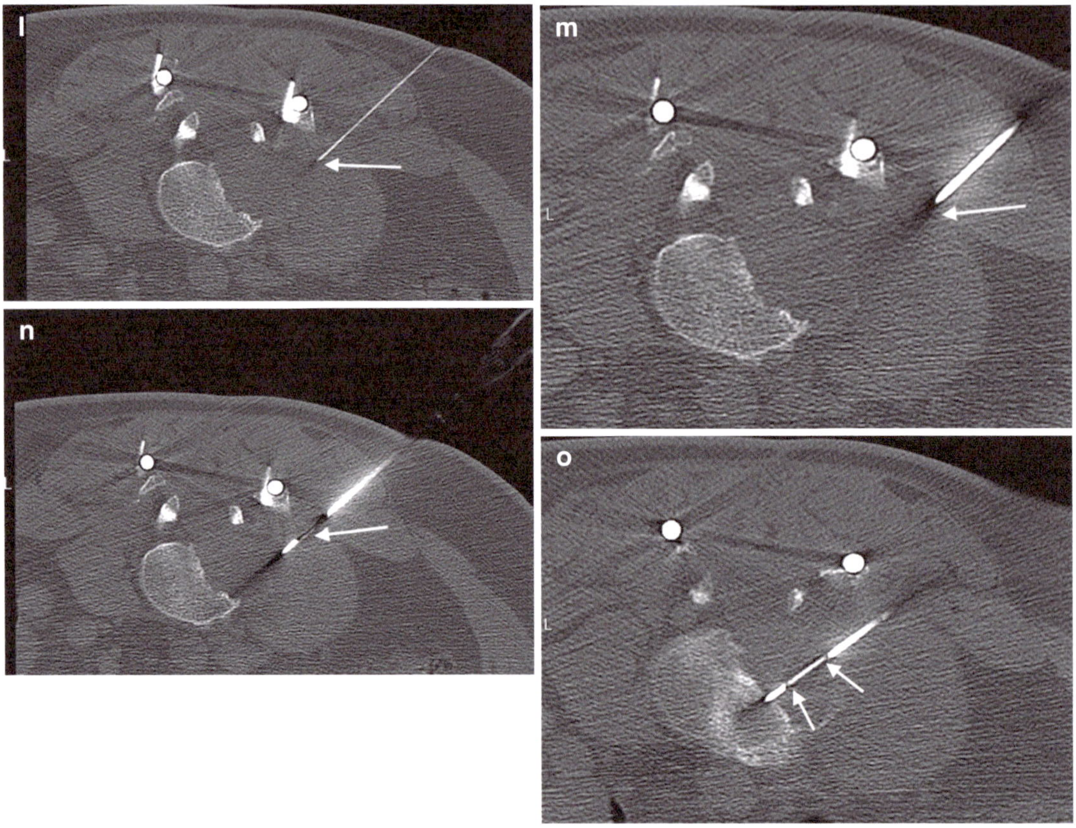

Fig. 6.5 (continued)

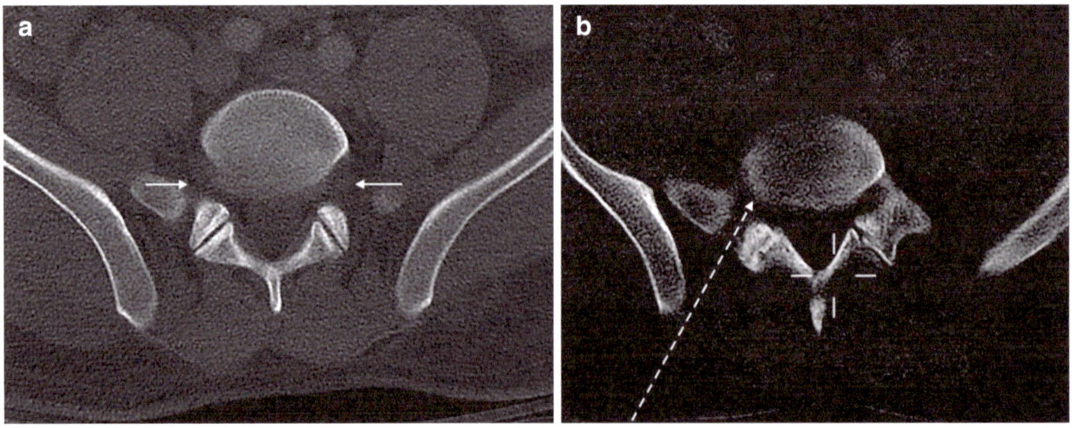

Fig. 6.6 Axial CT image (**a**) at L5–S1 shows a compromised approach to the L5–S1 disk; the dorsal root ganglia (*arrows*) essentially block access to the disk. This reformatted axial CT image (**b**) shows the effect of gantry angulation; the L5–S1 disk can now be accessed with this superomedial approach (*dashed arrow*)

advantages of fluoroscopy over CT are reduced procedure and imaging time needed to access the biopsy site, and immediate access to a procedural suite if a complication occurs (Nourbakhsh et al. 2008). Lateral fluoroscopy enables the operator to safely advance the needle into the anterior column of the vertebral body with real-time imaging. In addition, fluoroscopy can often provide quick access to the intervertebral disk space (Fig. 6.7). Some of the physical limitations of a CT scanner can be overcome by fluoroscopic imaging, such as when sampling the L5–S1 disk space and endplate complex. The steep angulation of the disk space at L5–S1 often limits access when using CT guidance, as the gantry angle is typically limited in paralleling the imaging slice to the disk space. Oblique and caudal angulation with fluoroscopy allows for appropriate visualization of the L5–S1 vertebral endplates and disk space; the greater angulation and positioning capacity of fluoroscopy provides more direct access for needle insertion into the L5–S1 disk. Identification of bony landmarks in this projection is critical for proper needle positioning in order to avoid neural structures, in particular, the exiting nerve root. Patient exposure to radiation during fluoroscopy-guided lumbar spine biopsy procedures can be reduced by utilizing appropriate fluoroscopy techniques such as low-dose pulsed fluoroscopy, automatic exposure control, collimation and last-image hold features, fluoroscopy time monitoring with alarm functions, and radiation dose monitoring. The operator's exposure to radiation during the procedure can similarly be reduced by optimizing fluoroscopy time and distance and by using appropriate shielding techniques (Luchs et al. 2005).

6.7 Approaches

As previously discussed, the transpedicular and posterolateral approaches are the two most commonly utilized approaches for image-guided percutaneous needle biopsy in the lumbar spine (Fig. 6.8). The most important factor that influences which approach to use is the lesion location within the lumbar spine. The inability to directly access the lesion via the pedicle eliminates the transpedicular approach as an option (Fig. 6.9). Typically, lesions located in the anterior or lateral margins of the vertebral body, disk space, or within paraspinal soft tissues require an extrapedicular or posterolateral approach (Pierot and Boulin 1999). This allows appropriate angulation of the needle trajectory in order to access the lesion (Fig. 6.10). We again must emphasize that it is important for the operator to be aware of the location of neural and vascular structures using this approach. CT guidance is often necessary to visualize soft tissue structures in relation to needle placement. For lesions located within the posterior elements, a biopsy of one or more of these structures may be necessary. Posterior element structures that can be successfully biopsied with CT guidance include the facet joint, the vertebral pedicle, the lamina, and the spinous process (Fig. 6.11). These are smaller structures as compared to the vertebral body; hence, CT guidance is often necessary to ensure accurate placement into these structures and to avoid complications. Often, the needle trajectory parallels the long access of the posterior element in order to allow for needle purchase into the bone and sufficient tissue sampling (Fig. 6.12). Diffuse vertebral body pathology or large focal lesions can be biopsied through a transpedicular approach if the lesion can be easily reached through the vertebral pedicle (Ashizawa et al. 1999). Transpedicular approaches can be performed with fluoroscopic or CT guidance, as bony landmarks are also clearly visible with the former modality (Fig. 6.13).

Careful pre-procedure review of available CT/MR imaging is crucial to planning a needle approach. This step is emphasized as careful planning will decrease intraoperative procedure time and complications.

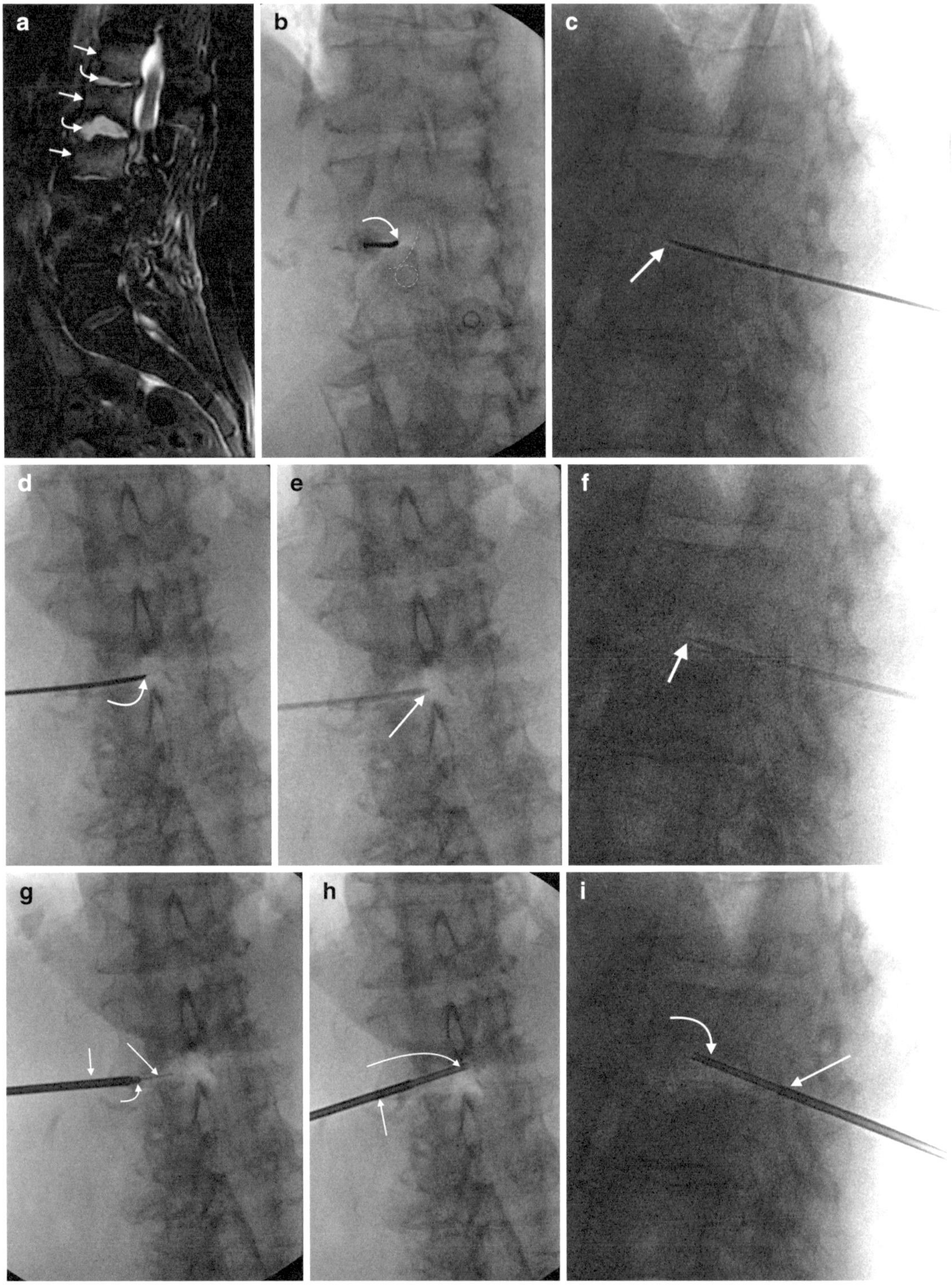
a
b
c
d
e
f
g
h
i

6.8 The Lumbar Spine Biopsy Procedure

6.8.1 General Considerations

6.8.1.1 Patient Factors

Percutaneous lumbar spine biopsies are performed to establish or confirm a diagnosis in both healthy and ill patients. A clear clinical picture of the patient's overall mental and physical health status should be considered prior to performing a procedure. Patients who present with altered mental status and significant comorbidities may not be candidates for lumbar spine biopsy; this may require consultation with the appropriate provider to determine the need and feasibility of a safe biopsy procedure. For clinically stable, yet uncooperative patients or younger patients, it may be necessary to perform the procedure with monitored anesthesia care or general anesthesia in order to ensure that the patient remains still during the procedure. Certain patient factors such as severe pain, recent abdominal or thoracic surgery, or respiratory challenges may not allow for patients to lie in the prone position. In these circumstances, decubitus or oblique positioning may be necessary. Intravenous pain medication and sedation with appropriate patient monitoring can be helpful in order to keep the patient comfortable during the procedure.

Prior to the procedure, the operator should reconcile medications, review allergies, and check the coagulation profile, such as platelet count, prothrombin time, activated partial thromboplastin time, and international normalized ratio (INR). The patient should be NPO after midnight the evening prior to the procedure if they are receiving intravenous sedation and analgesia. Patients who have eaten before the procedure cannot receive conscious sedation, but can still be considered for the procedure if local anesthesia is determined to be sufficient for pain control. A review of the imaging and order request should also be performed to identify and document that the appropriate lumbar level and lesion are being sampled and to confirm if any additional test is required such as flow cytometry. Informed con-

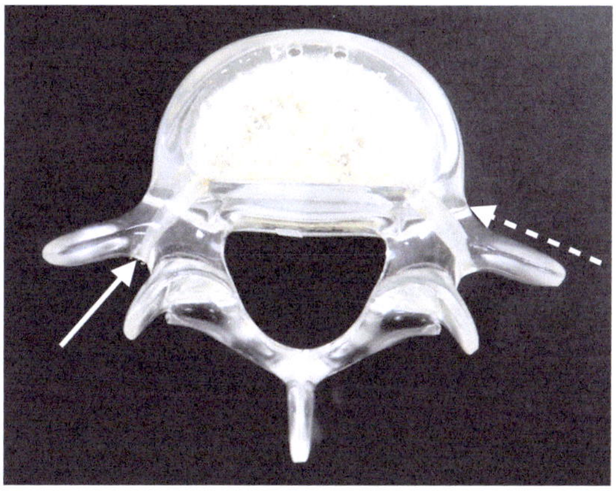

Fig. 6.8 Photograph of plastic vertebrae model shows the two basic approaches for lumbar spine biopsy, either through the pedicle (transpedicular) (*solid arrow*) or lateral to the pedicle (extrapedicular or posterolateral) (*dashed arrow*)

Fig. 6.7 An 86-year-old female with severe back pain. Fat-suppressed T2-weighted sagittal image (**a**) shows hyperintense signal within three consecutive vertebral bodies (*arrows*) and abnormal signal within the intervening disks (*curved arrows*) at T12–L1 and L1–L2. Oblique fluoroscopic image (**b**) shows advancement of a 17 gauge spinal needle (*curved arrow*) just lateral to the superior articular process (*dashed line*); the pedicle is outlined by a dashed oval. Lateral fluoroscopic image (**c**) shows advancement of the spinal needle into the center of the abnormal L1–L2 disk space (*arrow*); note the loss of the vertebral endplates at this level. Corresponding frontal fluoroscopic image (**d**) shows the needle tip within the center of the disk (*arrow*). Frontal fluoroscopic image (**e**) shows exchange of the needle stylet for a percutaneous diskectomy device (*arrow*). The lateral fluoroscopic image shows the tip of the diskectomy device within the disk (*arrow*). This device is moved in short excursions under fluoroscopic monitoring in order to extract tissue from the disk. Frontal fluoroscopic image (**g**) shows exchange of the percutaneous diskectomy system for a bone biopsy guide cannula (*small arrow*) and introducer (*curved arrow*) over a guidewire (*long arrow*). Frontal fluoroscopic image (**h**) shows that a trephine bone needle (*curved arrow*) has been advanced into the guide cannula (*arrow*) after removal of the introducer and guidewire; the bone biopsy system is angled cephalad in order to sample osseous tissue. Lateral fluoroscopic image (**i**) shows the bone biopsy needle (*curved arrow*) within the inferior L1 vertebral body; the guide cannula (*arrow*) is situated near the posterior aspect of the disk

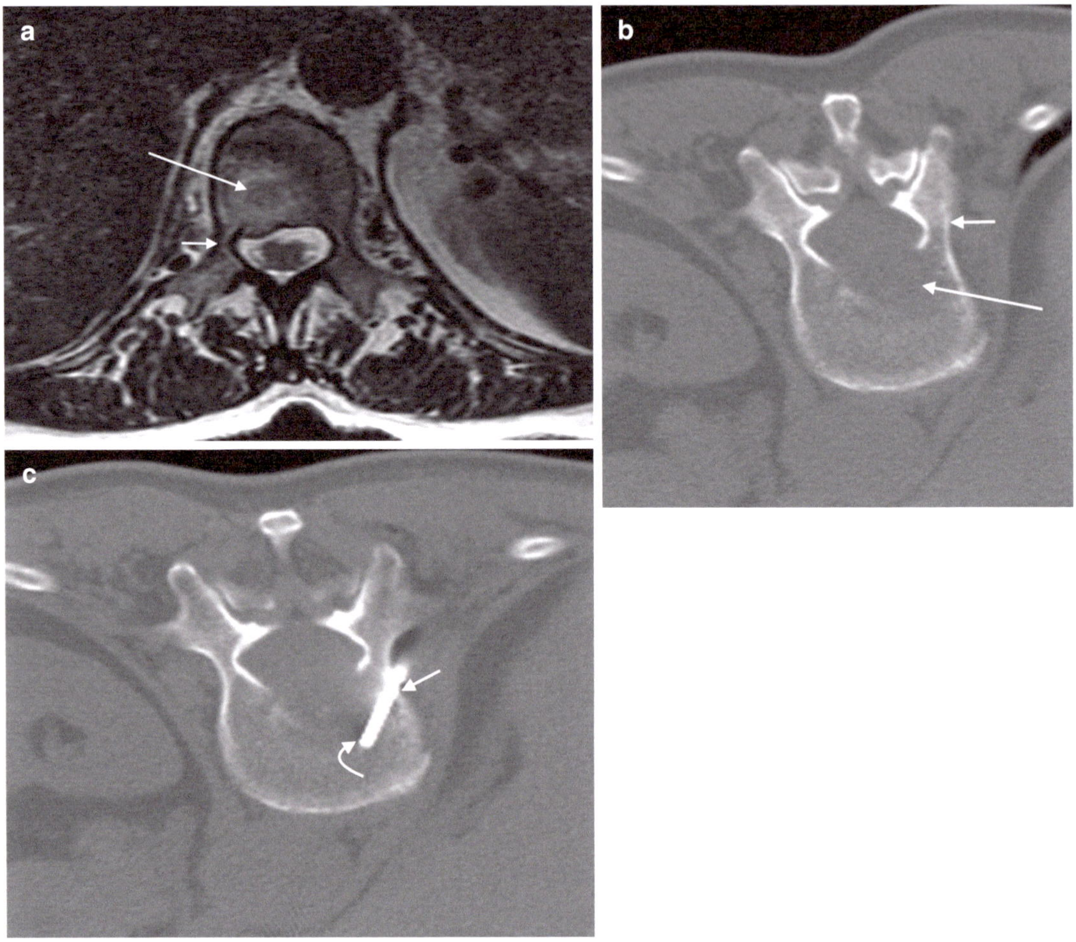

Fig. 6.9 A 77-year-old female with diffuse back pain. T2-weighted axial image (**a**) shows a focal slightly hyperintense lesion within the posterior aspect of the vertebral body (*large arrow*); the pedicles (*small arrow*) are small in size. Axial CT image (**b**) in bone window algorithm shows the posterior and paramedian location of the lytic lesion (*large arrow*); again note the small pedicles (*small arrow*). Axial CT image (**c**) shows biopsy needle (*curved arrow*) inserted into the lesion via an extrapedicular approach (arrow)

Fig. 6.10 A 65-year-old male with sclerotic L1 vertebral body lesion. Axial CT image (**a**) with skin grid in place shows a small round sclerotic lesion (*arrow*) within the L1 vertebral body. Axial CT image (**b**) shows the use of a spinal needle (*arrow*) for the injection of a local anesthetic agent. Given the proximity of the needle to the dorsal root ganglion (*curved arrow*), the trajectory of the subsequent needle placement is adjusted. Axial CT image (**c**) shows a bone needle (*arrow*) that is introduced using an extrapedicular approach. This trajectory was chosen to avoid the small pedicle (*curved arrow*) and to maximize the sampling volume of what is already a small lesion. Axial CT images (**d**, **e**) show careful advancement of the bone needle to the margin of the lesion (*arrows*). Axial CT image (**f**) shows the bone needle just beyond the distal margin of the lesion (*arrow*) and stopping just before the anterior vertebral body cortex (*curved arrow*); note the aorta (**a**). Post-procedure axial CT image (**g**) shows a lucent biopsy tract (*arrows*) through the sclerotic lesion, a pathologically proven prostate metastasis

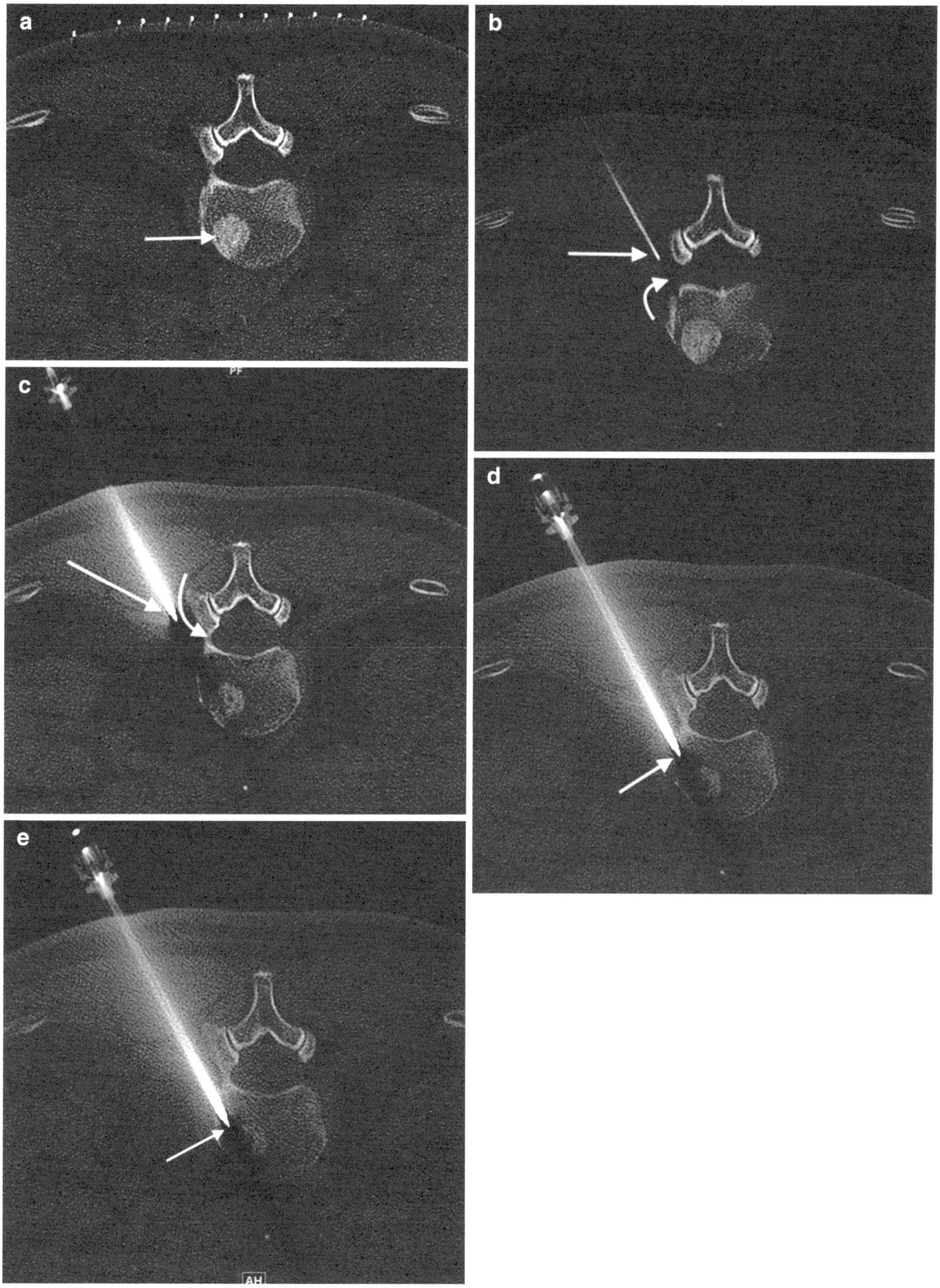
a
b
c
PF
d
e
AH

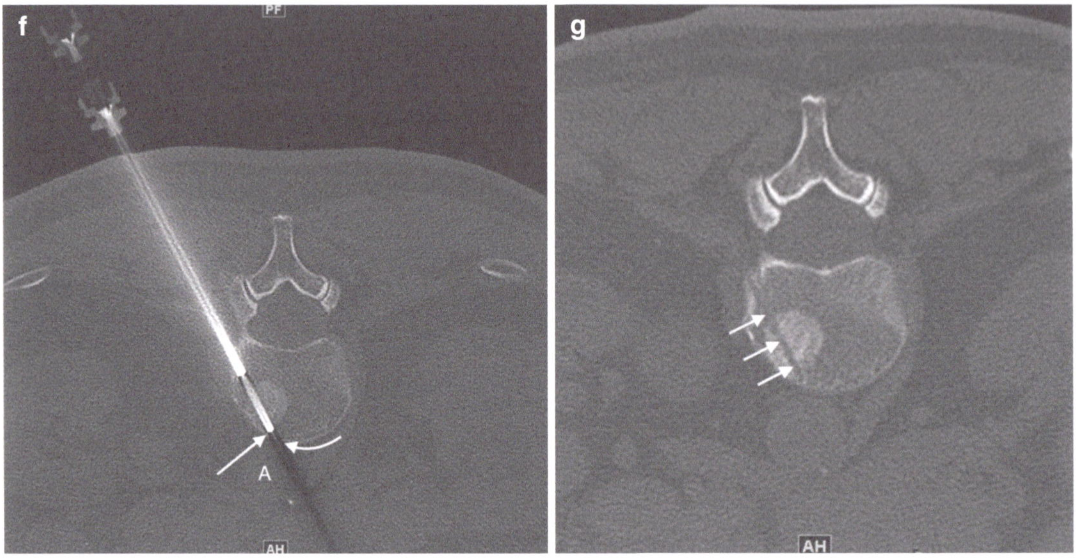

Fig. 6.10 (Continued)

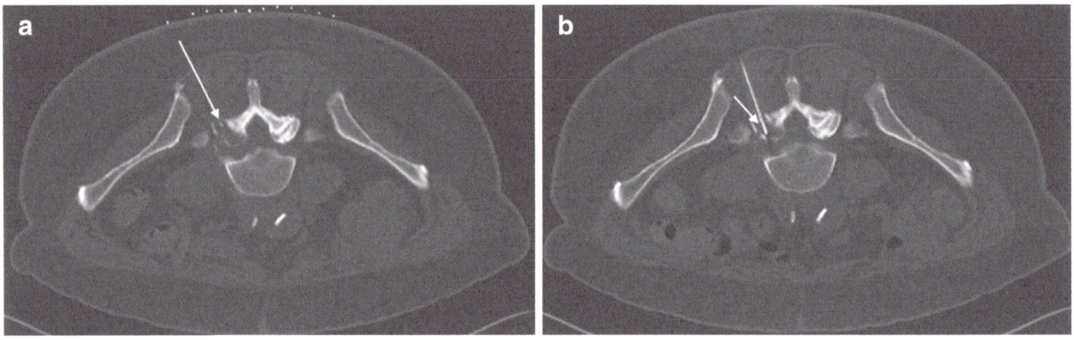

Fig. 6.11 Posterior element (facet joint) biopsy. Axial CT image (**a**) shows a destructive lesion of the left L5–S1 facet joint (*arrow*). Axial CT image (**b**) shows direct fine-needle aspiration (*arrow*) of the joint to evaluate for infection or infiltrative mass

Fig. 6.12 An 18-year-old male with chronic severe back pain, worse at night. Scout frontal radiograph (**a**) from CT scan shows skin grid in place over five lumbar vertebra and mild levoscoliosis. Axial CT image (**b**) in bone window algorithm with a skin grid in place shows a small round hypodense lesion (*arrow*) with a small sclerotic center and sclerotic reaction within the right L4 pedicle. Axial CT image (**c**) shows the use of a 22 gauge needle (*arrow*) to infiltrate the deep soft tissues and posterior pedicle cortex with a local anesthetic agent. Axial CT image (**d**) shows docking (*arrow*) of the coaxial bone biopsy system on the posterior aspect of the pedicle. Sequential axial CT images (**e**–**g**) show coaxial sequential advancement of a bone biopsy needle (*curved arrow*) through the guide cannula (*arrow*) that is docked into the posterior pedicle cortex; samples of the lesion are obtained from the lesion with each sequential advancement of the bone needle. The position and location of the bone needle is monitored with each movement. The pathologic evaluation was consistent with osteoid osteoma. This lesion was successfully treated with radiofrequency ablation immediately after the biopsy

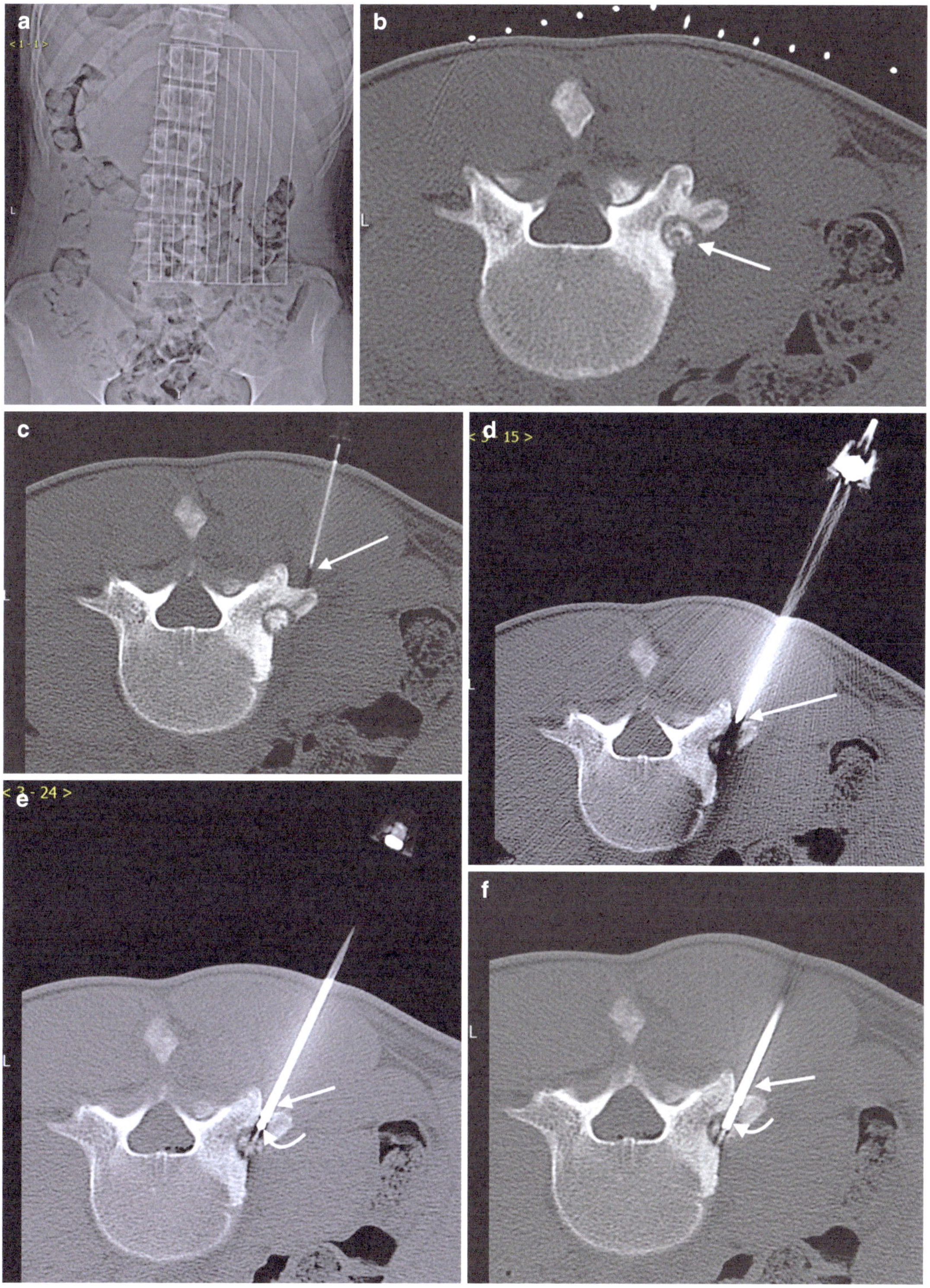
a
b
c
d
e
f

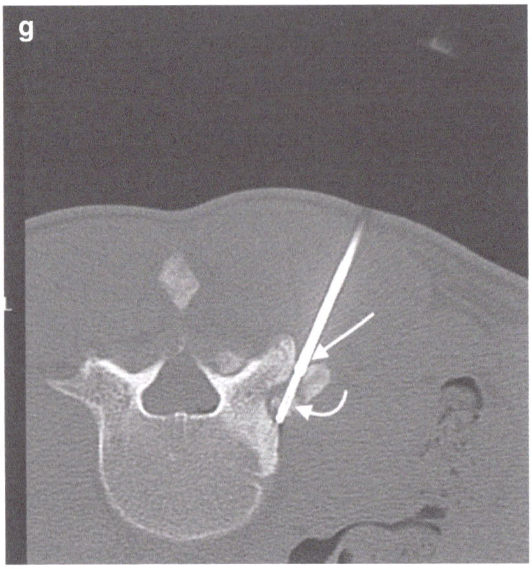

Fig. 6.12 (continued)

sent must be reviewed and signed by the patient or appropriate patient representative. The risks, benefits, and alternatives of the procedure should be discussed, including the option of open biopsy. The patient and patient representatives should have an opportunity to ask questions. Postoperative wound care should be discussed with the patient and, when necessary, the designated caretaker.

6.8.1.2 Staff Factors

As with any image-guided biopsy, it is necessary to inform the staff (such as technicians, nurses, and anesthesiologists) of the type of spine biopsy that will be performed. The biopsy team should perform patient and procedure verification. Discussion of patient positioning for optimal imaging and biopsy site access is important so as to reduce the need to reposition the patient during the procedure. Specifically, it is important to note on which side of the patient the operator will be working and whether to place the patient in the gantry head or feet first. This will allow nursing and ancillary staff to position the procedure table and monitoring equipment in the most optimal locations and allow the technologist to select the appropriate imaging position on the scanner. Nursing should be informed of the level of the anesthesia plan so as to allow appropriate monitoring and support as well as access to medications.

6.8.1.3 Anesthesia

Both local and intravenous anesthesias are commonly employed for lumbar spine biopsy. Local anesthesia with 1% or 2% lidocaine is administered at the skin surface and within the deep soft tissues. It is important to aspirate prior to injection of anesthetic to ensure that a blood vessel is not inadvertently injected. When necessary and clinically appropriate, intravenous medications such as midazolam and fentanyl can be administered to decrease procedure-related anxiety and reduce patient pain, respectively. Occasionally, it may be necessary to perform a lumbar spine biopsy with an anesthesiologist present when intravenous or general anesthesia is required for the case. Situations that require general anesthesia are intractable pain in adult patients and spine biopsy procedures in the pediatric population.

Fig. 6.13 An 80-year-old male with a lung mass. Axial fused PET-CT image (**a**) shows focal FDG uptake (*arrow*) within the left side of the L2 vertebral body. Scout frontal CT image (**b**) with skin grid in place shows a large body habitus. Axial CT image (**c**) with skin grid in place shows large lytic lesion within the left side of the vertebral body (*arrows*). Due to the patient's large size, the biopsy system could not be safely placed within the CT scanner gantry, and the patient was transferred to the fluoroscopy suite. Lateral fluoroscopic image (**d**) shows the use of a spinal needle to anesthetize the periosteal surface of the left pedicle. Lateral fluoroscopic image (**e**) shows the bone needle entering the posterior pedicle (*arrow*). Lateral fluoroscopic image (**f**) shows coaxial insertion of a trephine bone biopsy needle (*curved arrow*) via a guide cannula (*arrow*) into the anterior aspect of the left pedicle. Simultaneously acquired frontal fluoroscopic image (**g**) shows the guide cannula (*arrow*) and the position of the biopsy needle tip relative to the medial pedicle margin. Now that an adequate transpedicular position of the needle has been confirmed, the bone biopsy needle can be safely advanced into the vertebral body (*arrows*) as shown on the lateral (**h**) and frontal (**i**) fluoroscopic images. This biopsy confirmed the presence of metastatic lung cancer

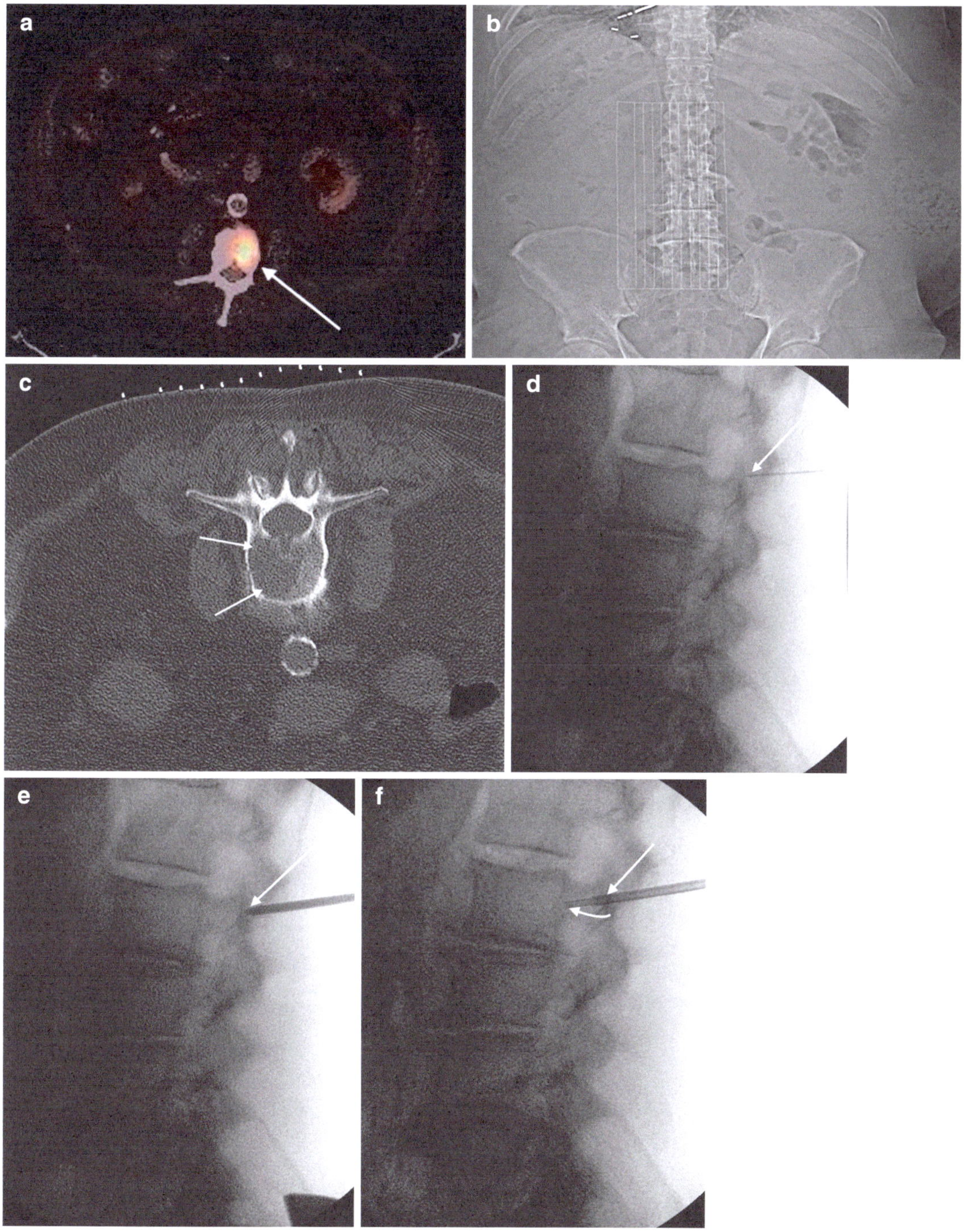
a
b
c
d
e
f

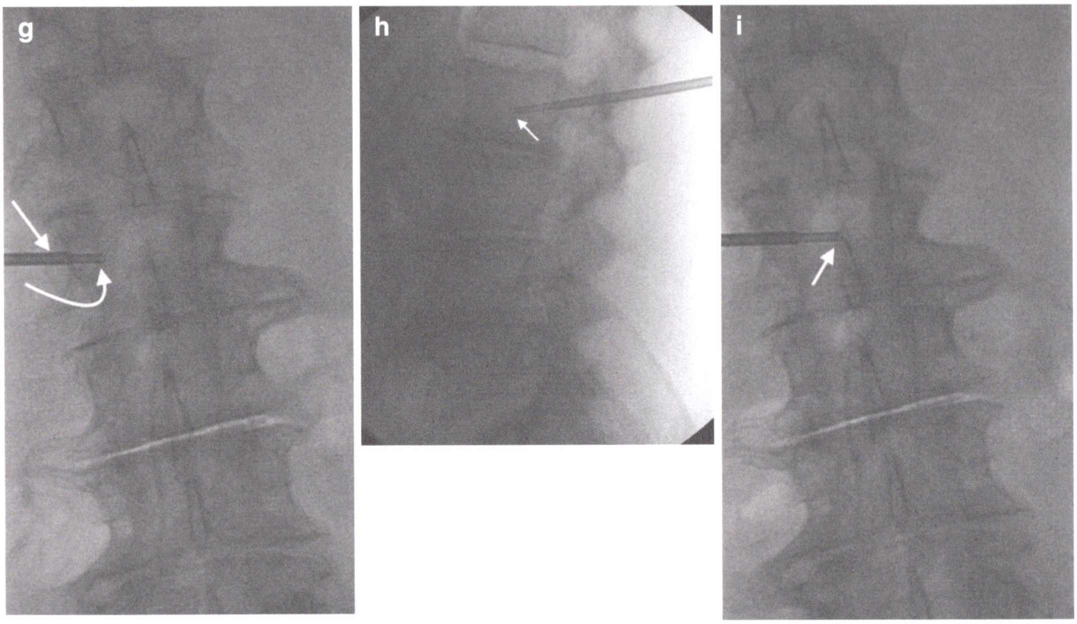

Fig. 6.13 (continued)

Regardless of the type of systemic anesthesia, appropriate monitoring of blood pressure, oxygen saturation, heart rate, and cardiac activity with electrocardiography is essential.

6.8.1.4 Patient Preparation

Before the procedure, certain medications may need to be stopped, such as anticoagulants, which should be ideally suspended several days prior or bridged based on provider and pharmaceutical recommendations (refer to the Chap. 2). Antibiotic therapy might be required for prophylaxis in immunocompromised patients (Santiago et al. 2014). When the biopsy procedure is concerned with identifying infectious pathogens, antibiotic therapy should be initiated after the biopsy procedure is performed in order to maximize the chances of isolating the microorganism

The patient is most commonly placed on the procedure table in the prone position. An oblique or decubitus position may be necessary if the patient cannot tolerate the prone position, such as in patients with excruciating pain in the prone position, recent abdominal surgery, or an abdominal ostomy site. Once positioned, a skin grid can be placed over the lumbar region at the desired level prior to CT imaging in order to select and mark the skin entry site. If performing the procedure with fluoroscopy, a radiopaque instrument, such as a towel clamp or hemostat, can be used to identify the desired biopsy location with imaging and marking the skin before or after sterile prepping. Once an entry site has been marked for biopsy, the back is prepped with using strict aseptic technique. A sterile drape is then placed around the skin entry site in order to provide a larger sterile field (Fig. 6.14).

> Careful pre-procedural attention to patient positioning and needle trajectory will decrease the need for patient and needle repositioning at the time of biopsy.

6.8.2 Technique

6.8.2.1 CT Guidance

Initial assessment of the needle path trajectory is typically performed with a radiopaque skin grid placed over the lumbar region at the desired level for biopsy. Scout CT images in both the frontal

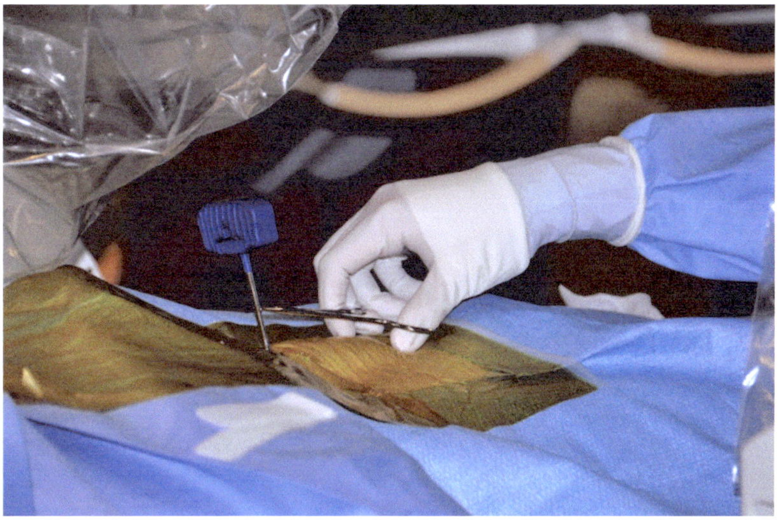

Fig. 6.14 Photograph obtained during a fluoroscopic biopsy procedure shows the sterile field

and lateral projections should be obtained. Always count the vertebra on the scout images to confirm the region of interest; this will help to prevent a wrong level biopsy. The operator should instruct the CT technologist to focus the field of view (FOV) over the region of interest and ensure that the skin surface is included in order to visualize the grid. If the desired trajectory is at a cranial or caudal angle to routine axial imaging, the FOV can be angled to allow for gantry angulation, if available, simulating the needle path on the lateral scout (Fig. 6.15). This typically requires axial scanning mode rather than helical or spiral scanning. Slice thickness less than or equal to 3 mm is important to ensure proper visualization of bony anatomy with respect to the lesion. CT scanning of the region of interest is then performed. Images can be reconstructed with soft tissue and/or bone algorithm to allow visualization of the biopsy site (Fig. 6.16). In general, soft tissue windows are necessary for soft tissue lesions and bone windows for lesions within the vertebral bodies or posterior elements (Fig. 6.17). Once the intended biopsy site is identified, the operator can choose the slice positioning and draw a line from the radiopaque marking on the image to the lesion, establishing the needle trajectory and depth. Depth measurement of the lesion from the skin site allows for proper selection of the biopsy needle length. The number of the radiopaque mark can then be ascertained by counting from either end of the visualized markings. Once the position is determined, the table can be moved into the desired slice position, and a red line can be illuminated over the skin surface with the CT laser alignment system, corresponding to the axial CT image at the skin entry site. This allows appropriate marking of the grid at the corresponding slice position. The grids used for CT-guided biopsies are porous, and, therefore, a skin marker will transfer an ink mark from the grid to the patient's skin. The grid can then be removed, and the table moved out of the gantry to allow access for sterile preparation of the patient's back.

> Always count the vertebra on the scout images to confirm the vertebral level of interest; this will help to prevent a wrong level biopsy.

Once the back has been prepped with Betadine scrub and/or chlorhexidine scrub and appropriately draped, the skin at the marking site is anesthetized with a local anesthetic agent, such as 1 or 2% lidocaine. Deep soft tissue anesthetic is administered at this time. A 22 or 20 gauge spinal needle is advanced through soft tissues to the level of the periosteum or deep soft tissue adjacent to the biopsy site. It is important to periodically

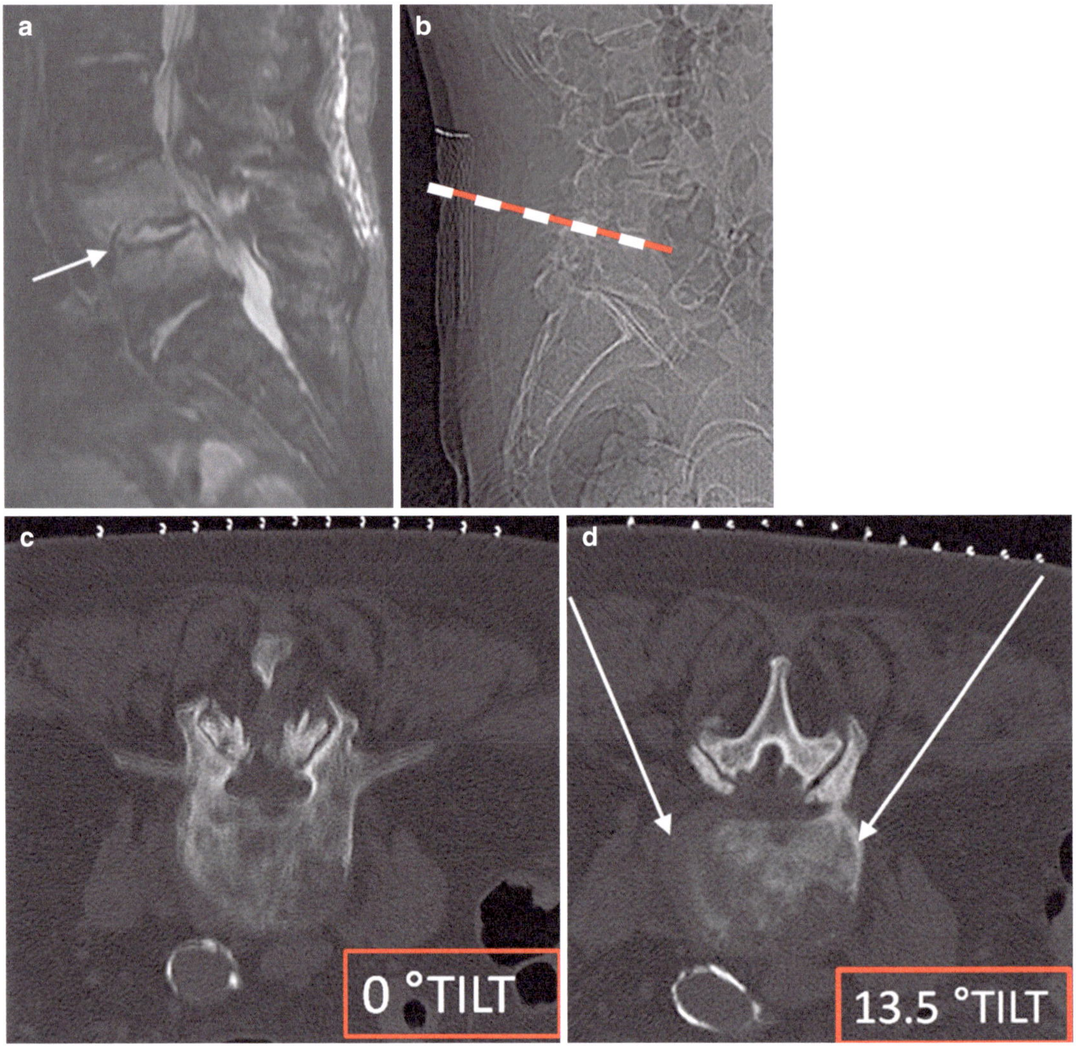

Fig. 6.15 Use of CT gantry angulation. T2-weighted sagittal image (**a**) shows findings compatible with L4–L5 disk infection (*arrow*). Scout lateral CT image (**b**) shows the angulation (*dashed line*) that the gantry is adjusted to in order to access the disk. Axial CT image (**c**) with no gantry angulation; the disk is not accessible. Axial CT image (**d**) with 13.5° of gantry angulation provides a trajectory to the disk (*arrows*)

image during needle advancement to ensure a safe advancement as well as proper position and depth of the spinal needle. Once in the desired location, an anesthetic agent can be administered to anesthetize the periosteum, allowing significant reduction in pain related to bony entry with a bone biopsy needle (Fig. 6.12). Once deep anesthesia has been administered, the needle can be left in place to serve as a guide for the bone biopsy needle or can itself be used for coaxial technique if a guide needle was used (Fig. 6.18).

CT-guided percutaneous lumbar spine biopsy can be performed with tandem needle technique or with direct coaxial technique.

If the operator chooses to use a trephine needle for biopsy, a dermatotomy made with a number 11 scalpel is required at the skin entry site. Manual blunt dissection at the dermatotomy allows easier passage of the needle through the

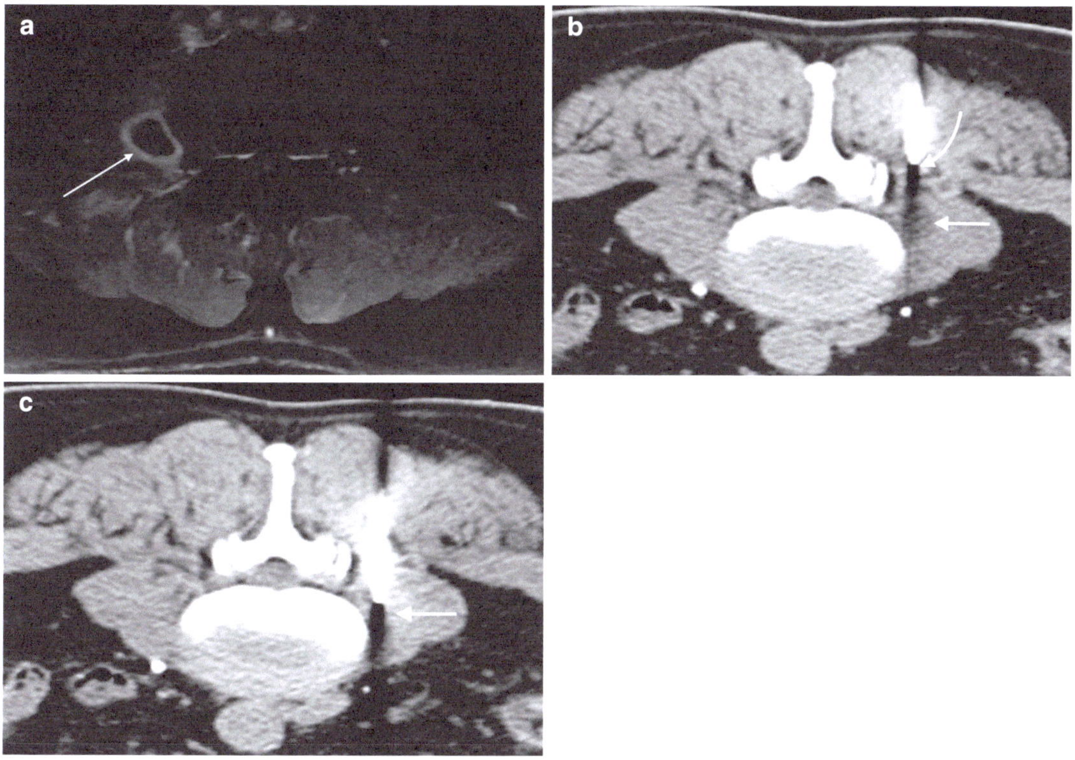

Fig. 6.16 A 43-year-old male with low back pain, fever, and elevated ESR. Fat-suppressed contrast-enhanced T1-weighted axial image (**a**) shows a ring-enhancing lesion (*arrow*) within the right psoas muscle. In the clinical context, this was thought to be a psoas abscess. Axial CT image (**b**) obtained with soft tissue algorithm in order to better visualize the right psoas abscess (*arrow*) so that the biopsy needle (*curved arrow*) could be readily advanced to the target. Axial CT image (**c**) in soft tissue algorithm shows the needle within the abscess collection (*arrow*); purulent material was aspirated from the abscess

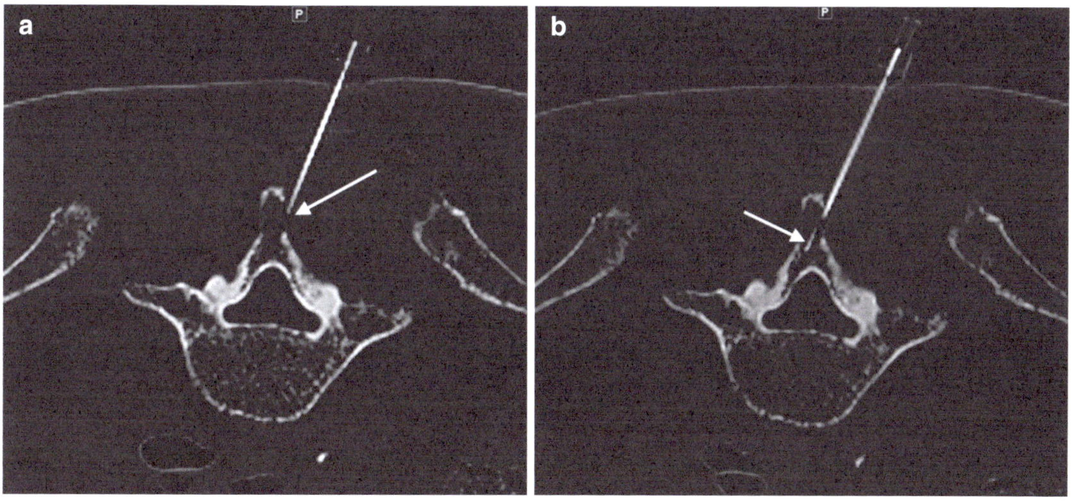

Fig. 6.17 Use of bone window algorithm for a posterior element (spinous process) lesion. Axial CT image (**a**) shows 18 gauge spinal needle (*arrow*) at the margin of a lytic spinous process lesion. Axial CT image (**b**) shows coaxial insertion of 25 gauge spinal needle for fine-needle aspiration of the lesion (*arrow*). The cytology was positive for myeloma

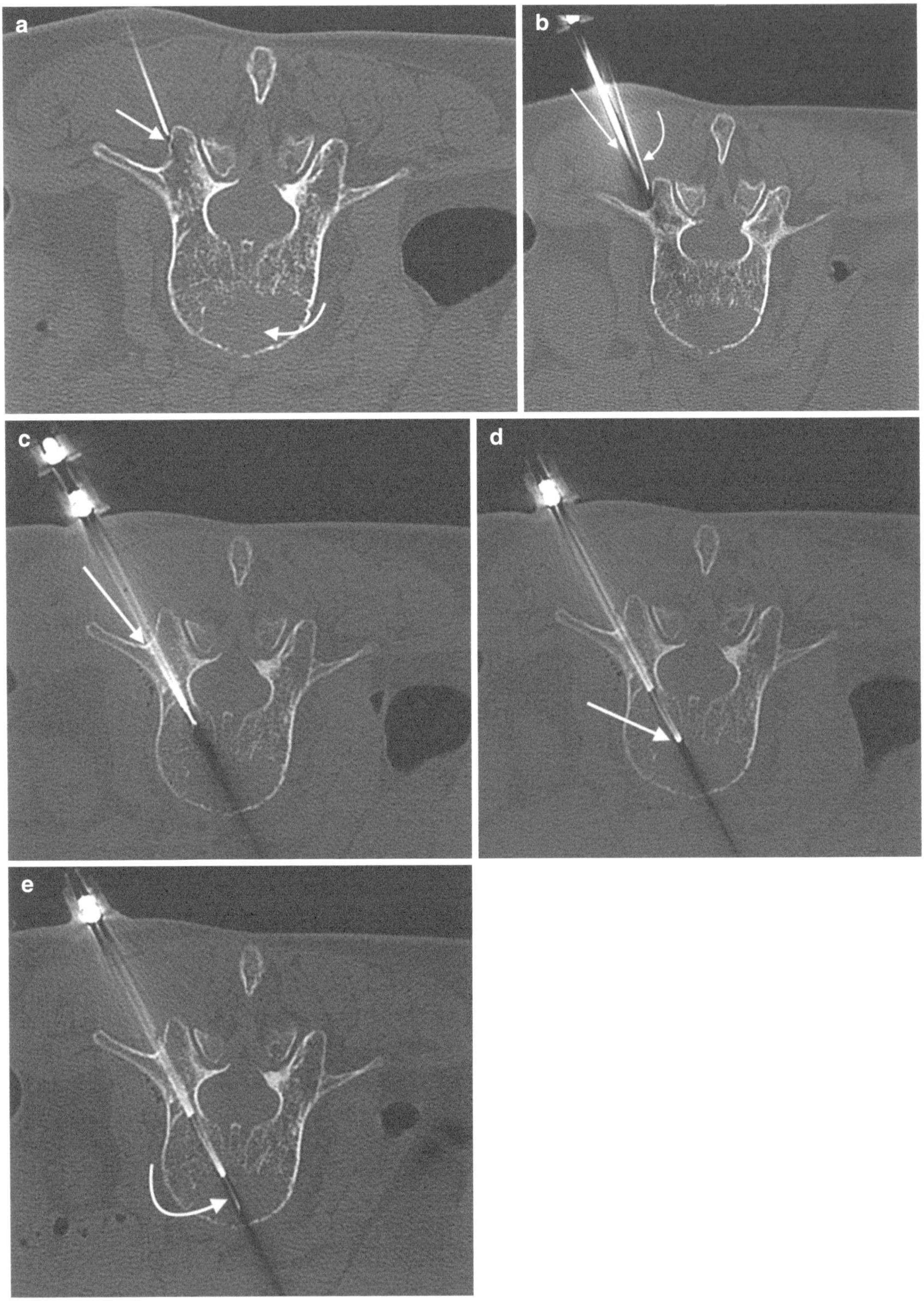
a
b
c
d
e

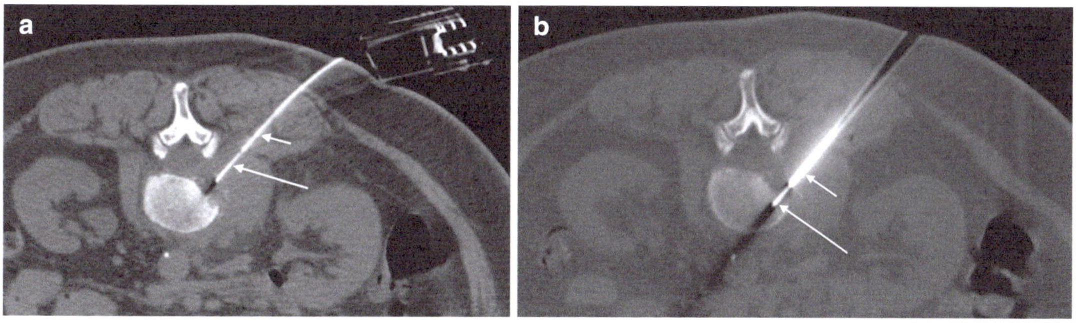

Fig. 6.19 A 64-year-old female with focal upper low back pain. Axial CT image (**a**) shows use of coaxial guide cannula (*small arrow*) and cutting needle (*large arrow*) in order to biopsy a large paraspinal soft tissue component of this lumbar mass. Once sufficient soft tissue cores were obtained, the guide cannula was advanced closer to the vertebral body (*small arrow*) as shown on the axial CT image (**b**). A bone biopsy needle (*large arrow*) was then used to obtain bone cores from this lesion. The bone cores show histopathologic evidence of acute inflammation consistent with acute osteomyelitis. The soft tissue cores, which were sent to both pathology and microbiology, were positive for bacterial growth on the microbiologic analysis. This case reinforces the useful practice of submitting specimens for both pathologic and microbiologic analysis, whenever the diagnosis is in question

soft tissues. Alternatively, a dermatotomy may not be necessary if an 18 or larger gauge needle is used, as these needles can easily pass through the skin. Once the needle enters the patient's body, it is advanced in the trajectory established on initial planning of site selection and needle path. For access to the lumbar vertebral body or disk space, this is often at a 20–40 ° oblique trajectory from midline and may include cranial or caudal angulation of the needle. When advancing the needle, it is again important to utilize periodic CT imaging to ensure safe and appropriate placement in regard to both obliquity and depth.

Once the needle reaches the bone, disk, or soft tissue that is to be biopsied, further advancement for sampling of the lesion depends on needle type, such as trephine, cutting, and fine needle (Fig. 6.19). For access into the vertebral body, a trephine needle is preferred. This type of needle allows for penetration of cortical bone and easy advancement through the vertebral body. Progression through the cortex can be achieved by manually twisting the needle or with the use of a mallet or hammer. Some trephine biopsy systems provide a drill, which can be coaxially inserted into the introducer needle and used to drill through the cortex and bone. The drill creates a path anterior to the introducer needle to allow for needle advancement manually along this path. Coaxial cutting needles can be used for sampling of disk space and soft tissue lesions, which tend to be smaller gauge needles that allow for core sampling (Yaffe et al. 2003). Biopsy of some lesions may not be feasible with trephine or cutting needle systems and may instead require fine-needle aspiration (FNA). The operator may prefer FNA for small soft tissue lesions or highly vascular lesions for accuracy and safety, respectively (Fig. 6.20).

Once the needle position is confirmed by CT imaging to be at the margin or within the lesion, measurements can be taken on imaging from the anterior margin of the needle to the anterior mar-

Fig. 6.18 Tandem needle technique. Axial CT image (**a**) shows use of a 20 gauge spinal needle (*arrow*) to anesthetize the posterior pedicle surface in order to facilitate transpedicular access to an anterior lytic L3 vertebral body lesion (*curved arrow*). Axial CT image (**b**) shows insertion of a bone biopsy needle (*arrow*) alongside the spinal needle (*curved arrow*). Axial CT image (**c**) shows removal of the spinal needle and advancement of the biopsy needle via a transpedicular approach (*arrow*). Axial CT image (**d**) shows coaxial advancement of a core biopsy needle to the proximal margin of the lytic lesion (*arrow*). Axial CT image (**e**) shows coaxial placement of a 25 gauge spinal needle (*curved arrow*) into the lesion; FNA was performed because there was a clinical concern for a hypervascular lesion. Pathology yielded a diagnosis of multiple myeloma

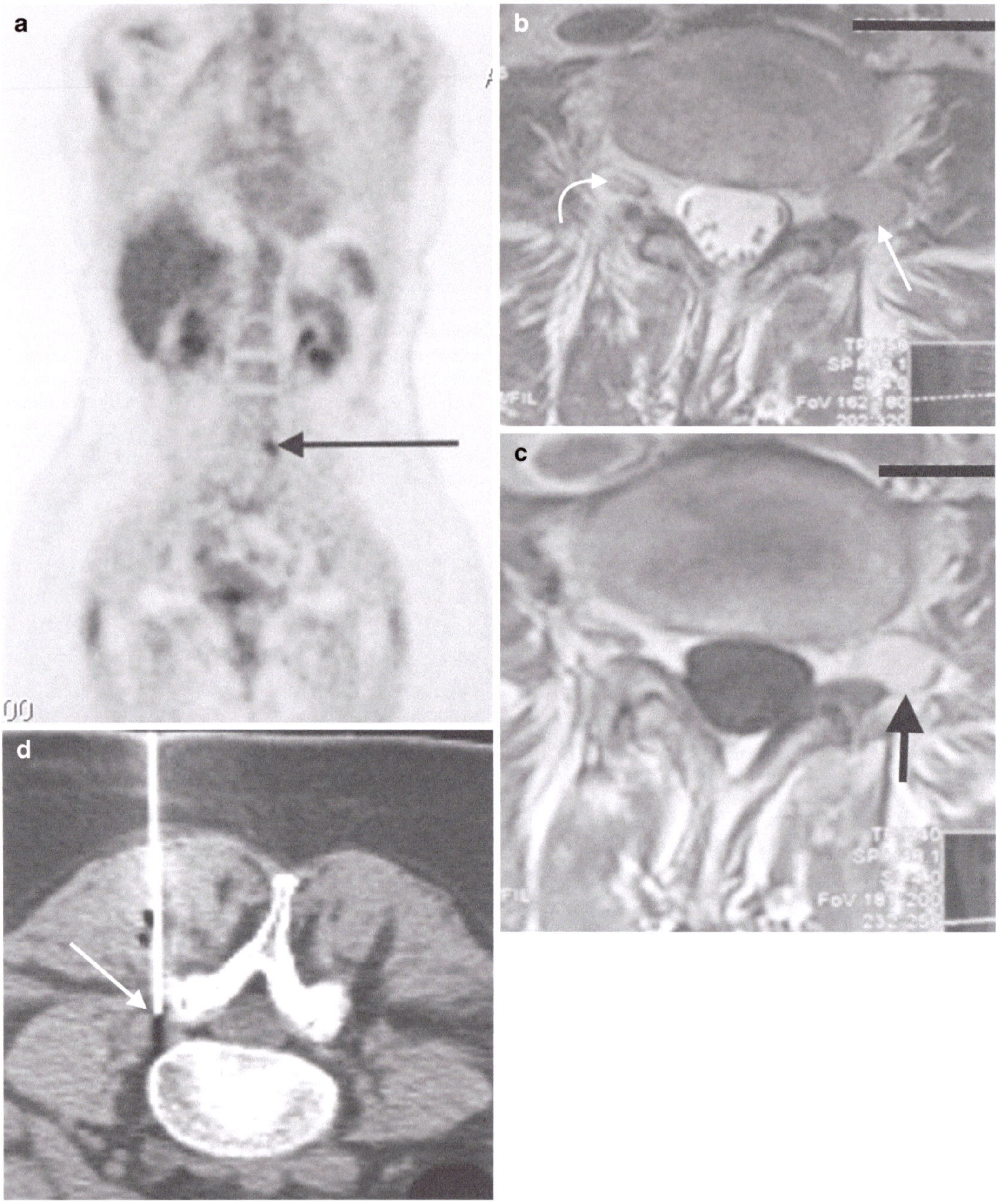

Fig. 6.20 A 51-year-old female with breast cancer and left L4 radiculopathy. Posterior projection from PET examination (**a**) shows focal FDG uptake in the lower left lumbar spine (*arrow*). T2-weighted axial image (**b**) shows focal enlargement and hyperintensity within the left L4 dorsal root ganglion (*arrow*); compare to the normal right dorsal root ganglion (*curved arrow*). Close-up view of contrast-enhanced T1-weighted axial image (**b**) shows intense enhancement (*arrow*) within the dorsal root ganglion. Axial CT image (**c**) in soft tissue algorithm shows the placement of a guide needle (*arrow*) at the proximal margin of the enlarged dorsal root ganglion for the purpose of performing FNA. Two passes with a 25 gauge needle confirmed the presence of metastatic breast carcinoma

gin of the lesion, vertebral body, or disk space. This allows the operator to determine the approximate depth that the biopsy needle can be advanced through the introducer needle in order to ensure both accurate sampling and to avoid incorrect needle placement through the anterior margin of the spine or soft tissue lesion. The biopsy needle is then advanced into the lesion. Many biopsy systems, including both trephine and cutting needles, provide markings or measurements on the needle to allow the operator to determine the position of the biopsy needle tip in relation to the anterior margin of the introducer needle.

When the biopsy needle is advanced to the desired depth, a CT image is obtained to confirm needle placement (Fig. 6.12). In a trephine biopsy system, the biopsy needle is then removed, usually with slight aspiration to ensure that the sample remains in the needle chamber upon extraction. The sample can then be pushed out of the biopsy needle with a needle pusher, which is provided with most biopsy systems. In cutting needle systems, the needle can be directly removed after a core sample has been taken. The core is then transferred to the appropriate solution, such as formalin, for future analysis. With coaxial biopsy systems, the introducer or guide needle can remain in place at the lesion margin such that additional biopsy needles can be sequentially and safely inserted as needed in order to obtain additional biopsy specimens. In the setting of FNA, the samples can be provided to an on-site cytopathologist or cytopathology technician for assessment of adequate cellularity. Sampling of vertebral body, disk space, or soft tissue lesions should be performed several (approximately three times) to ensure appropriate volume of tissue for analysis. In the setting of core biopsy of the vertebral body, this may not always be possible. If the core is visualized to be large enough, only one sample may be required. Alternatively, when FNA is performed, it is often necessary to make three to five passes with 22–25 gauge needles for adequate diagnostic cellularity. Once the pathologist or cytotechnologist is satisfied that they have adequate specimen for diagnosis, the FNA procedure can be stopped. When sampling the paraspinal soft tissues for suspected infection, needle aspiration is performed first, especially if there is a fluid collection. If necessary, a drainage catheter can be placed (Fig. 6.21). In those cases where no material can be aspirated, a small amount of normal sterile saline or local anesthetic can be infiltrated into the area and re-aspirated. A core needle biopsy can also be utilized to obtain tissue, and this too can be sent for microbiologic analysis (Fig. 6.22).

6.8.2.2 Fluoroscopic Guidance

Fluoroscopic guidance can often be used to biopsy vertebral body and disk space pathology. In the setting of diffuse pathologic involvement of the vertebral body, fluoroscopy is a preferred modality due to the real-time assessment of needle advancement and reduced procedure time (Fig. 6.23). Additionally, fluoroscopy provides excellent visualization of and prompt access to the disk space. One advantage fluoroscopic guidance has over CT is the ability for significant craniocaudal angulation as well as right and left obliquity, allowing for positioning of the image intensifier over the desired bone or disk space in order to facilitate a needle trajectory that may not be possible with CT imaging and with decreased need for patient repositioning. This is most helpful when a biopsy of the L5–S1 disk space is required. A major disadvantage of fluoroscopy is the inability to visualize and evaluate soft tissues, and therefore, CT must be utilized when the target lesion is located within the paraspinal soft tissues. When smaller, focal lesions are present or there is need for confirmation of biopsy needle placement within the lesion, CT guidance is preferred.

Slight differences in patient preparation are required when performing lumbar spine biopsy with fluoroscopy when compared to CT. Prior to sterile prep, the entry site can be established by rotating the image intensifier to the desired location in the frontal projection. The tip of a hemostat is pressed over the skin with simultaneous

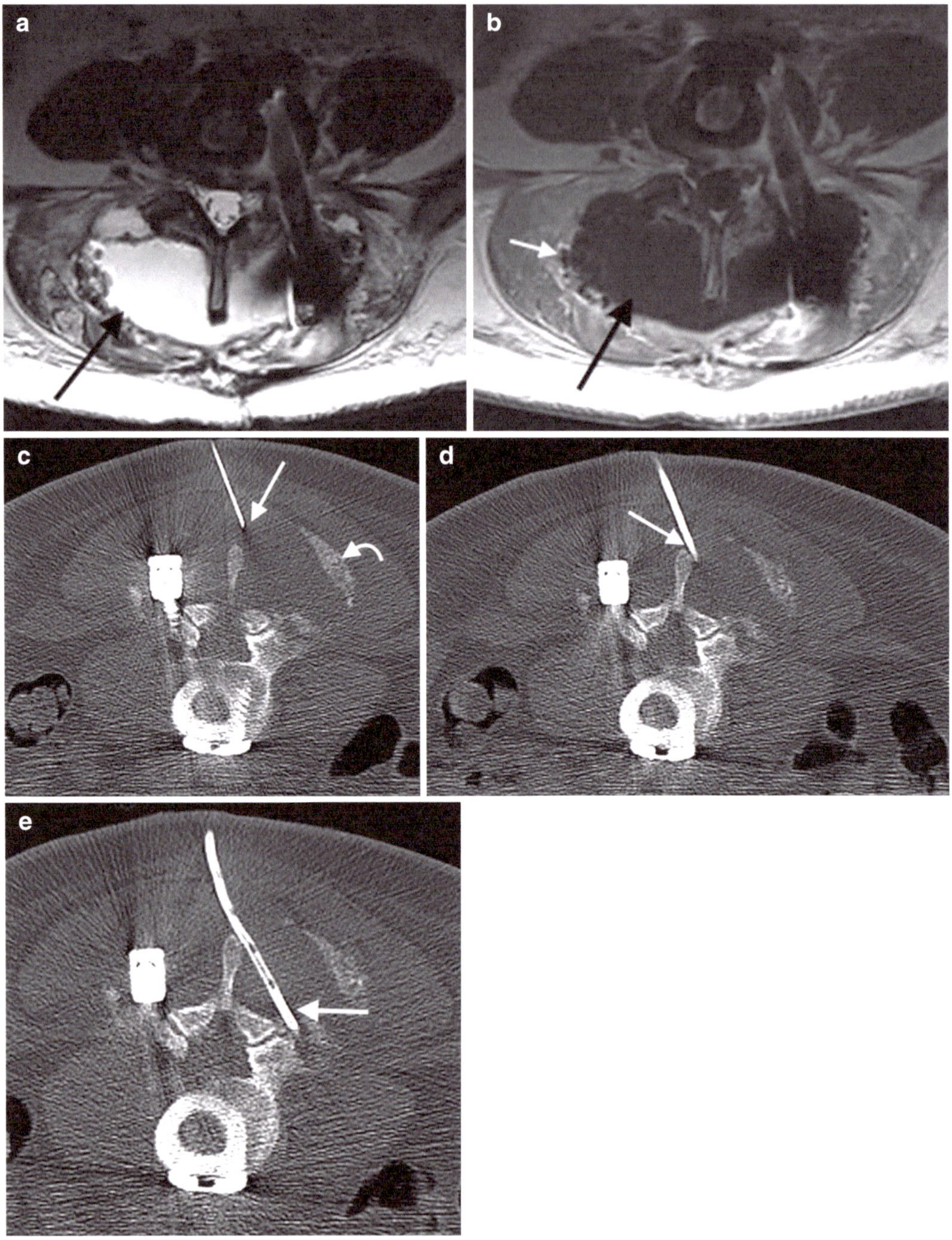

Fig. 6.21 A 37-year-old female with back discomfort following an anterior and posterior lumbar spinal fusion procedure. T2-weighted axial image (**a**) shows a large hyperintense posterior paraspinal fluid collection (*arrow*). Contrast-enhanced T1-weighted axial image (**b**) shows a hypointense fluid collection (*large arrow*) with no abnormal enhancement; note the multiple small punctate hypointense foci (*small arrow*) at the periphery of the collection. Axial CT image (**c**) shows an introducer needle at the periphery of the collection (*arrow*) from which a few milliliters of clear straw-colored fluid were initially aspirated; peripheral heterotopic bone formation (*curved arrow*) accounts for the low-signal foci on the MRI. Bone morphogenic protein was used in the posterior fusion surgery. Axial CT image (**d**) shows advancement of a trocar-bearing multi-sidehole catheter (*arrow*) into the collection. Axial CT image (**e**) shows drainage catheter in place (*arrow*). The microbiologic analysis was negative

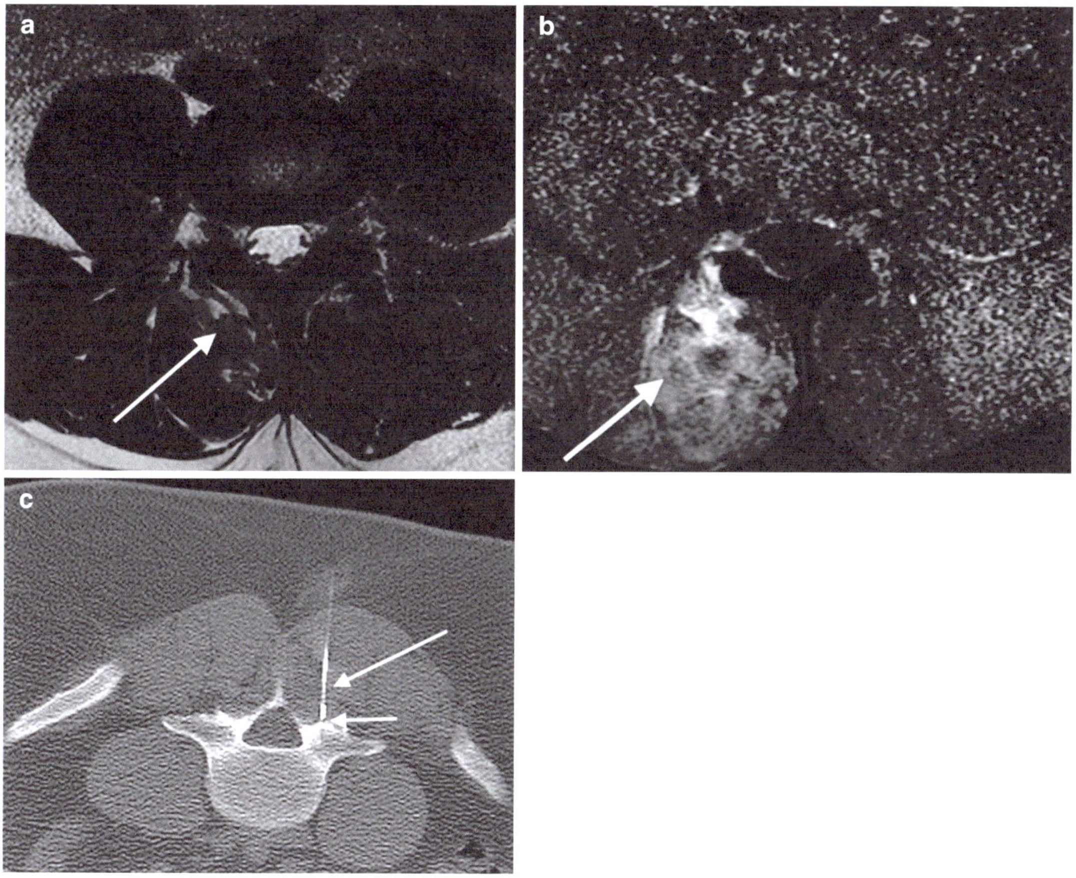

Fig. 6.22 A 31-year-old male with low back pain and elevated ESR (68) and CRP (300). T2-weighted axial image (**a**) shows increased signal intensity within the right posterior paraspinal musculature (*arrow*). Fat-suppressed contrast-enhanced T1-weighted axial image (**b**) shows patchy focal enhancement in this location (*arrow*). Axial CT image (**c**) shows a small cutting needle placed at the level of the soft tissue abnormality (*large arrow*) and advanced to the margin of the facet joint (*small arrow*). This small core of soft tissue was positive for coagulase-negative *Staphylococcus*, and the patient was immediately started on the appropriate antibiotic therapy

imaging to determine the point of needle entry at the skin. A mark is then made at this site and allows the operator to prep a field around this location. Once the back has been prepped with sterile technique, anesthesia and dermatotomy can be performed in a similar fashion as with the CT technique. The needle is then advanced under fluoroscopic guidance. It is important to keep the needle and osseous landmarks within the center of the field of view of the fluoroscope as the needle is advanced. This reduces parallax error and improves targeting of the needle. A hemostat can be used to hold the needle in place while imaging with fluoroscopy so as to avoid radiation exposure to the operator's hand. The needle should parallel the plane of frontal imaging and be seen as a "dot." This allows directed advancement of needle along the established trajectory. When the needle has advanced to a depth several centimeters away from the pedicle or disk space, the tube can be rotated to the lateral position to assess needle depth. Once the needle has been advanced to the disk space or pedicle, it can be further advanced into the desired location with continuous lateral imaging. It may be necessary to rotate the tube from the frontal and lateral projections several times through needle advancement to confirm both needle placement within the vertebral body or disk space as well as the depth of the needle and the location of the needle tip relative

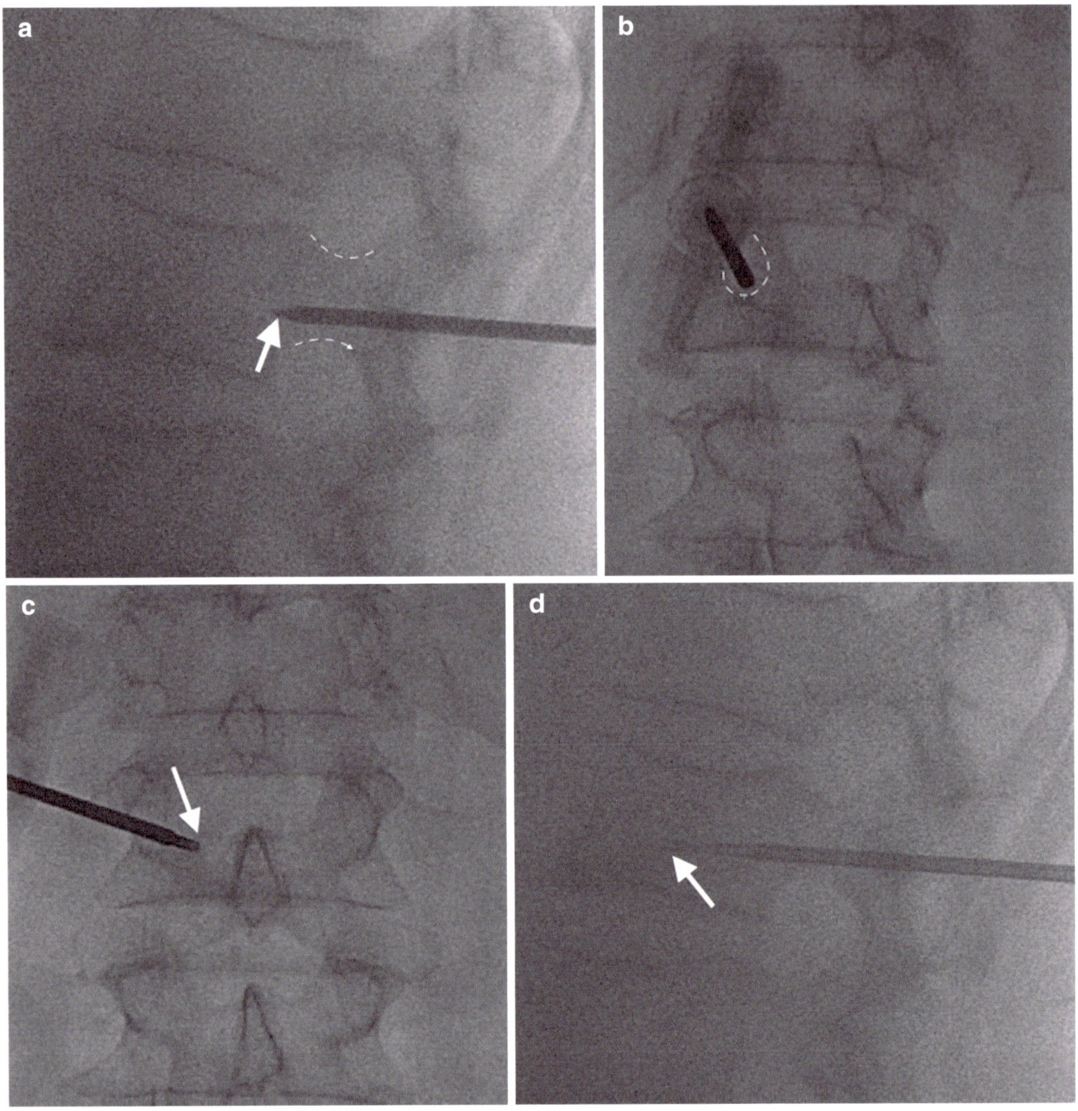

Fig. 6.23 A 76-year-old male with history of lung cancer and a diffusely abnormal L1 vertebra on a PET-CT study. Lateral fluoroscopic image (**a**) shows transpedicular needle placement (*arrow*), not the superior and inferior margins (*dashed lines*) of the pedicle. Oblique fluoroscopic image (**b**) shows the position of the needle within the pedicle (dashed semicircle). Frontal fluoroscopic image (**c**) shows coaxial advancement of a bone needle (*arrow*) into the vertebral body. Lateral fluoroscopic image (**d**) shows the position of the needle (*arrow*) within the vertebral body. Four bone cores were obtained, and the biopsy was positive for metastatic adenocarcinoma

to critical structures (Fig. 6.23). A biplane fluoroscopy unit, if available, can eliminate the necessity for these multiple movements of the multidirectional fluoroscope.

6.8.2.3 Fluoroscopic Vertebral Body Biopsy

Percutaneous access into a lumbar vertebral body is often performed through a transpedicular approach (Fig. 6.23). Pre-biopsy imaging review is essential to determine if the lesion can be accessed with fluoroscopic guidance. Diffuse involvement of the vertebral body allows for sampling within any portion of the vertebrae without great concern for missing the lesion. Similarly, fluoroscopic guidance may be used to access a large vertebral body lesion or a sclerotic lesion. A transpedicular approach is performed by rotating the fluoroscopic tube approximately 30° from midline. This allows visualization of the "Scotty dog" within the lumbar spine. The eye of the Scotty dog represents the pedicle, which can be overlapped with a portion of the vertebral body (Fig. 6.23). This creates a needle trajectory that passes from the skin though the pedicle into the vertebral body. Lateral and frontal imaging during needle advancement will confirm the correct needle path into the pedicle as well as needle depth once with the vertebral body (Fig. 6.24). A coaxial approach with a biopsy needle system, similar to what is used with CT guidance, can also be utilized with fluoroscopic guidance. In certain situations, for example, a more posterior and paramedian location of a lesion, it may be necessary to access the lumbar vertebral body with an extrapedicular approach such as a parapedicular approach. This facilitates steeper angulation of the biopsy needle into the vertebral body and allows for access to the posterior and median portion of the vertebral body.

6.8.2.4 Fluoroscopic Disk Space Biopsy

In the setting of suspected diskitis and/or osteomyelitis, biopsy may be requested to confirm the diagnosis of spine infection and to provide information on the type of organism involved in order to optimize antibiotic therapy (refer to the Chap. 9). Although CT can be used to biopsy the disk space and paraspinal fluid collections, fluoroscopy offers several advantages over CT. Oblique and craniocaudal angulation on fluoroscopy allows the operator to directly visualize the disk space and vertebral endplates. The fluoroscopy tube is rotated so that the disk space and endplates are parallel and the position of the superior articular process of the vertebral body below the disk space overlaps the midportion of the disk space in this projection. The needle is advanced in a path that lies lateral to the superior articular process (Fig. 6.7). The extent of medial-lateral or oblique angulation will place the superior articular process anywhere from one-third to half-way across the full extent of the disk as visualized on the oblique-frontal view. Steeper angulations of the fluoroscope allow for needle placement along the median aspect of the disk space, whereas a less steep approach allows for access to the lateral aspect of the disk space. This technique allows for safe passage of the needle into the disk space and avoids the exiting lumbar nerve root. It may be necessary to sample both vertebral body/endplate and intervertebral disk in order to establish a diagnosis of infection. Core material in this setting can and, whenever possible, should be sent for both microbiology and surgical pathology analysis. Tissue assessment for both microorganism and histologic evidence of infection has been shown to provide a greater diagnostic yield than either alone (Michel et al. 2006). Fluoroscopic guidance allows for transpedicular access into the disk-endplate complex. The tube is rotated to allow for overlap of the pedicle of either vertebral body bordering the disk space with the adjacent vertebral body. This provides an angulated needle trajectory which will allow passage of the needle through both endplates and the intervertebral disk.

Core samples can be divided, as necessary, and should be placed in sterile containers for microbiologic analysis. It is important to avoid placement of microbiology samples in formalin to avoid reducing the ability to analyze the tissue for microorganisms. Any aspirated fluid or pus should be sent for microbiologic assessment only. For histology, core samples are placed in a formalin container. Special stains for microorganisms can also be performed with histological assessment of the tissue.

> Fluoroscopy can be used to guide percutaneous biopsy of the lumbar spine in the setting of diffuse pathologic infiltration of the vertebral body or to access an abnormal lumbar intervertebral disk, allowing for real-time assessment of biopsy needle advancement and potentially reduced procedure time.

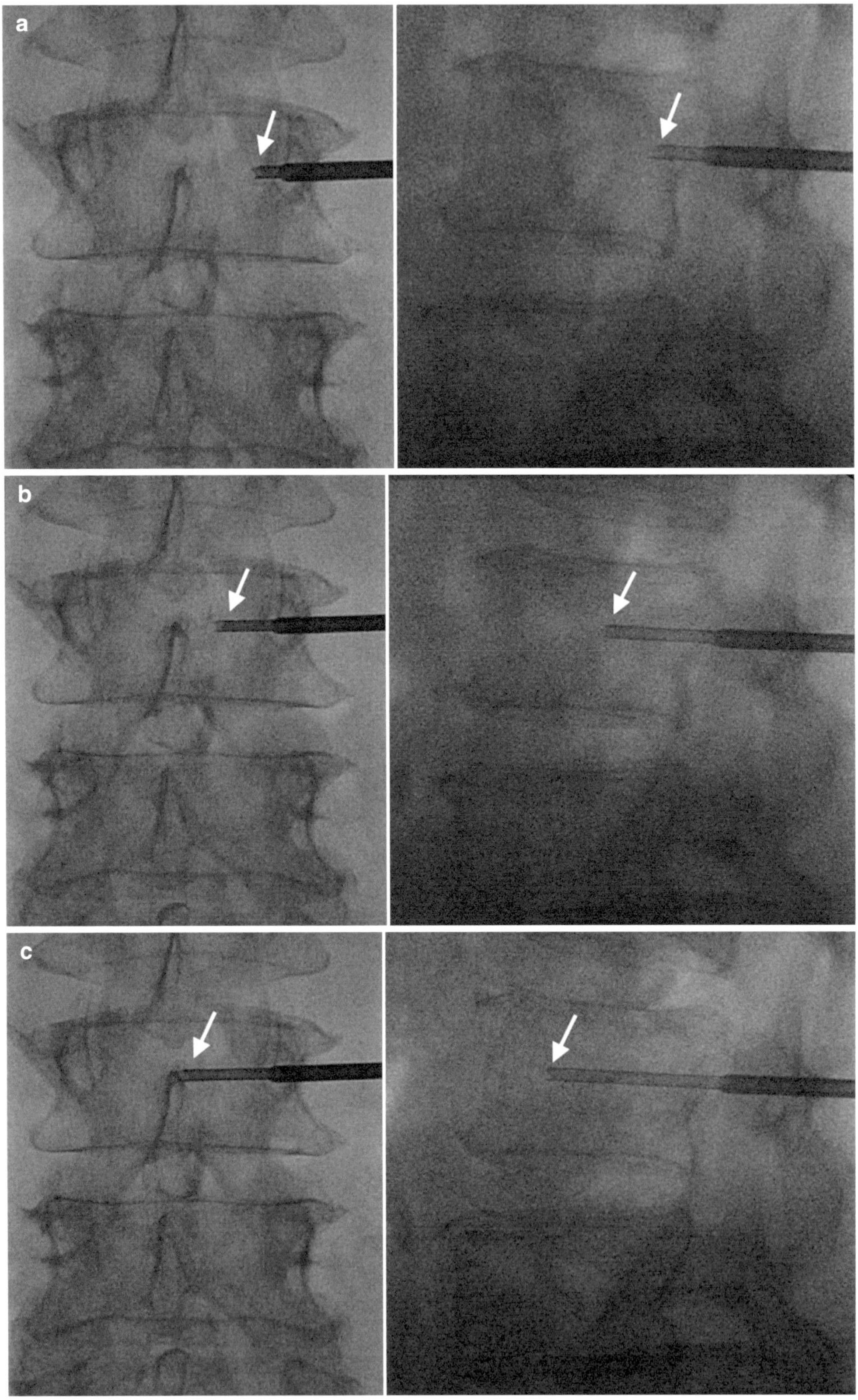
a
b
c

6.9 Post-procedure Care

Following image-guided percutaneous lumbar spine biopsy, the patient is transferred to a recovery area and observed and monitored for a minimum of 2 h. During this time, vital signs are recorded, and the biopsy site is examined as per the instructions of the operator. Continued close monitoring is necessary immediately after the procedure to assess for acute complications. Oral or intravenous acetaminophen may be administered for pain relief. If pain is persistent or significant, opiates can be considered. A progressive increase in pain level, however, requires clinical evaluation by the operator. Once stable, the patient can be discharged home with an adult companion, while inpatients can return to their hospital room. Notification of completion of the procedure is to be communicated with the ordering provider. This is especially true of collaborating surgeons, who will need to know the biopsy entry site and pathway, since these are considered contaminated with tumor and may need to be removed at later resection (Davies et al. 1993). The patient should be provided with the appropriate follow-up contact telephone number in case of questions or concerns and should also be instructed to go to emergency room if they experience severe symptoms, such as fever, increasing pain, or bleeding, which are not resolved with conservative measures. A follow-up communication on the day after the procedure is important to ensure that no clinically significant changes have occurred since discharge and to address any patient concerns or questions. The operator or a designated staff member should follow up on all biopsy results to ensure that the sample has been received, tissue or microbiologic diagnosis established, and the appropriate provider(s) notified.

Key Review Points

1. Image-guided lumbar spine biopsy allows sampling of the vertebra, disk, and paraspinal lesions with lower morbidity as compared to open biopsy procedures.
2. The goal of image-guided percutaneous lumbar spine biopsy is to sample the target lesion while avoiding injury to nearby critical anatomic structures.
3. Careful pre-procedure review of all available imaging studies with planning of the patient's position, biopsy approach, and needle trajectory will decrease the procedure time and reduce the likelihood of a complication.
4. Indications for percutaneous lumbar spine biopsy include the evaluation of possible neoplastic or infectious processes in order to establish a diagnosis and guide the patient's clinical management.
5. Complications related to lumbar spine biopsy can be minimized with careful and thorough patient pre-procedure screening and medical optimization, with particular attention to procedure indications and contraindications.
6. Multiple approaches and techniques are available for image-guided percutaneous lumbar spine biopsy depending upon the lesion type, location, and extent.
7. Optimizing diagnostic efficacy can be enhanced with multiple biopsy needle passes, thereby increasing sample size.
8. CT and fluoroscopy can be used for imaging guidance in lumbar spine biopsy procedures, depending on lesion location, size, and extent.

Fig. 6.24 A 63-year-old female with history of breast cancer and low back pain. Frontal and lateral fluoroscopic images (**a**) show the tip of bone biopsy needle (*arrows*) at the junction of the pedicle and posterior vertebral body; the bone needle is temporarily removed in order to dislodge the specimen that has accumulated within the bone needle, into the appropriate container. Frontal and lateral fluoroscopic images (**b**) show advancement of the bone needle (*arrows*); this forward movement again fills the bone needle lumen with additional specimen that is then removed and, in this case, submitted for pathologic analysis. Frontal and lateral fluoroscopic images (**c**) show further advancement of the bone needle (*arrows*) to the anterior and paramedian aspect of the vertebral body in order to obtain additional specimen in this patient with metastatic breast cancer

References

Ashizawa R, Ohtsuka K, Kamimura M, Ebara S, Takaoka K. Percutaneous transpedicular biopsy of thoracic and lumbar vertebrae—method and diagnostic validity. Surg Neurol. 1999;52:545–51.

Chooi YS, Kamil OI, Kob SC. Percutaneous transpedicular biopsy of the spine. Med J Malaysia. 2007;62:46–8.

Davies NM, Livesley PJ, Cannon SR. Recurrence of an osteosarcoma in a needle biopsy track. J Bone Joint Surg Br. 1993;75:977–8.

Ghelman B, Lospinuso MF, Levine DB, O'Leary PF, Burke SW. Percutaneous computed-tomography-guided biopsy of the thoracic and lumbar spine. Spine. 1991;16:736–9.

Ghelman B. Biopsies of the musculoskeletal system. Radiol Clin North Am. 1998;36:567–80.

Hau MA, Kim JI, Kattapuram S, Hornicek FJ, Rosenberg AE, Gebhardt MC, Mankin HJ. Accuracy of CT-guided biopsies in 359 patients with musculoskeletal lesions. Skeletal Radiol. 2002;31:349–53.

Herkowitz HN, Wesolowski DP. Percutaneous biopsy of the spine: indications, techniques, results, and complications. Update Spinal Disord. 1986;1:1–9.

Hodge JC. Musculoskeletal Imaging: Diagnostic and Therapeutic Procedures. Basel: Karger Landes Systems; 1997.

Kornblum MB, Wesolowski DP, Fischgrund JS, Herkowitz HN. Computed Tomography-Guided Biopsy of the Spine: A Review of 103 Patients. Spine. 1998;23:81–5.

Lis E, Bilsky MH, Pisinski L, Boland P, Healey JH, O'Malley B, Krol G. Percutaneous CT-guided biopsy of osseous lesion of the spine in patients with known or suspected malignancy. AJNR Am J Neuroradiol. 2004;25:1583–8.

Luchs JS, Rosioreanu A, Gregorius D, Venkataramanan N, Koehler V, Ortiz AO. Radiation safety during spine interventions. J Vasc Interv Radiol. 2005;16:107–11.

Michel SC, Pfirrmann CW, Boos N, Hodler J. CT-guided core biopsy of subchondral bone and intervertebral space in suspected spondylodiskitis. AJR Am J Roentgenol. 2006;186:977–80.

Murphy WA. Radiologically guided percutaneous musculoskeletal biopsy. Orthop Clin North Am. 1983;14:233–41.

Nourbakhsh A, Grady JJ, Garges KJ. Percutaneous spine biopsy: a meta-analysis. J Bone Joint Surg Am. 2008;90:1722–5.

Olscamp A, Rollins J, Tao SS, Ebraheim NA. Complications of CT-guided biopsy of the spine and sacrum. Orthopedics. 1997;20:1149–52.

Ortiz AO, Zoarski G, Brook A. Image-guided percutaneous spine biopsy. In Mathis JM, Golovac S, editors. Image-guided spine interventions. 2nd ed. New York: Springer; 2010. p. 75–106.

Peh W. CT-guided percutaneous biopsy of spinal lesions. Biomed Imaging Interv J. 2006;2:e25.

Peh WC. Imaging-guided bone biopsy. Ann Acad Med Singapore. 2003;32:557–61.

Pierot L, Boulin A. Percutaneous biopsy of the thoracic and lumbar spine: transpedicular approach under fluoroscopic guidance. AJNR Am J Neuroradiol. 1999;20:23–5.

Saghieh S, Masrouha KZ, Musallam KM, Mahfouz R, Abboud M, Khoury NJ, Haidar R. The risk of local recurrence along the core-needle biopsy tract in patients with bone sarcomas. Iowa Orthop J. 2010;30:80–3.

Santiago FR, Kelekis A, Alvarez LG, Gilippiadis DK. Interventional procedures of the spine. Semin Musculoskelet Radiol. 2014;18:309–17.

Schajowicz F, Derqui JC. Puncture biopsy in lesions of the locomotor system: review of results in 4050 cases, including 941 vertebral punctures. Cancer. 1968;21:531–48.

Shpilberg KA, Delman BN, Tanenbaum LN, Esses SJ, Subramaniam R, Doshi AH. Radiation dose reduction in CT-guided spine biopsies does not reduce diagnostic yield. AJNR Am J Neuroradiol. 2014;35:2243–7.

Sundaresan N, Boriani S, Rothman A, Holtzman R. Tumors of the osseous spine. J Neurooncol. 2004;69: 273–90.

Talac R, McLain RF. Biopsy principles and techniques for spinal tumors. Semin Spine Surg. 2009;21:70–5.

Tehranzadeh J, Tao C, Browning CA. Percutaneous needle biopsy of the spine. Acta Radiol. 2007;48:860–8.

Wu JS, Goldsmith JD, Horwich PJ, Shetty SK, Hochman MG. Bone and soft-tissue lesions: what factors affect diagnostic yield of image-guided core-needle biopsy? Radiology. 2008;248(3):962–70.

Yaffe D, Greenberg G, Leitner J, Gipstein R, Shapiro M, Bachar GN. CT-guided percutaneous biopsy of thoracic and lumbar spine: a new coaxial technique. AJNR Am J Neuroradiol. 2003;24:2111–3.

7 Sacral Biopsy

Todd Miller, Allan L. Brook, and A. Orlando Ortiz

Learning Objectives

1. To understand the value and importance of radiologic anatomy as it pertains to sacral biopsy
2. To review the indications and contraindications for biopsy of the sacrum and adjacent structures
3. To learn the approaches and techniques for image-guided percutaneous sacral biopsy

7.1 Introduction

The sacrum, as a unit, is the largest "bone" within the spinal axis. This makes it a likely site for metastatic tumor involvement. Primary tumors can also occur within the sacrum. In terms of development of the spinal column, notochordal rests predispose the sacrum to the development of chordomas (the other common location for this lesion is the clivus at the skull base). Its articulation with the pelvic bones may also predispose to the sacrum, via the sacroiliac joints, to inflammatory and/or infectious processes. The location at the level of the pelvis may also predispose the sacrum to infectious and neoplastic processes that occur in this part of the body. Biomechanically, the sacrum can be affected by traumatic and weight-bearing loads that compromise its structural integrity. Therefore, with respect to size, embryologic developmental influences, location, and role in spine biomechanics, the sacrum can be affected by several pathologic conditions that may require image-guided percutaneous biopsy in order to establish a diagnosis and facilitate clinical management. The close proximity to the skin surface can create a misconception that a sacral biopsy is a straightforward procedure. The sacrum has an intricate anatomic relationship with the neuraxis, and an image-guided percutaneous sacral biopsy must always be performed using thorough preparation and meticulous technique.

7.2 Anatomic Considerations

The sacrum is a large complex triangular osseous structure that is located at the caudal aspect of the spinal axis between the lumbar spine and coccyx (Fig. 7.1) (Diel et al. 2001). The sacrum consists of five vertebrae, but unlike the more cephalad components of the spine, these vertebrae are fused anteriorly (vertebral bodies) and posteriorly (neural arches). A residual or persistent intervertebral disk is occasionally observed at the S1–S2 level. Additionally, transitional vertebral anatomy is not uncommon at the lumbosacral junction, with either a partially lumbarized S1 or a sacralized L5 vertebra present (Carrino et al. 2011). The superior aspect or S1 portion of the sacrum has more mass or bulk, and the sacrum thins or tapers down progressively from S1 to S5. The largest sacral vertebral body, S1, possesses a prominent anterior superior end plate, or promontory, with which

A.O. Ortiz, *Image-Guided Percutaneous Spine Biopsy*, DOI 10.1007/978-3-319-43326-4_7

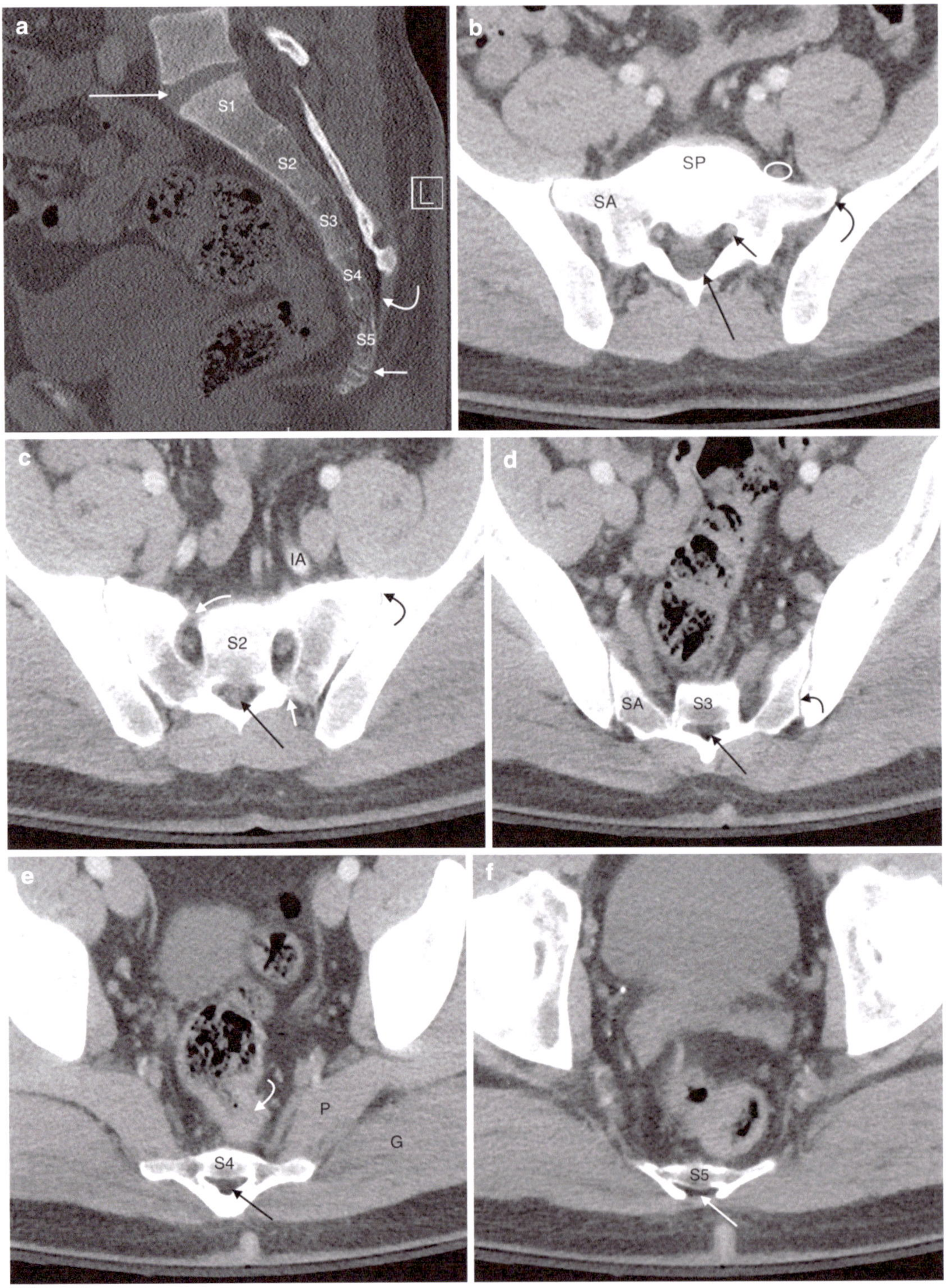
a
S1
S2
S3
S4
S5
L
b
SP
SA
c
IA
S2
d
SA
S3
e
P
G
S4
f
S5

Fig. 7.1 Cross-sectional CT anatomy of the sacrum. Reformatted midline sagittal CT image (**a**) of the sacrum shows five fused sacral vertebrae bordered superiorly by the L5–S1 intervertebral disk (*large arrow*) and inferiorly by the sacrococcygeal joint (*small arrow*). The sacral hiatus (*curved arrow*) is seen at the *S4–S5* level and defines the caudal extent of the sacral canal. Axial CT image (**b**) at the S1 level shows the sacral promontory (*SP*) and the sacral ala (*SA*). The sacral canal (*large arrow*) and S1 nerve root (*small arrow*) are seen at this level. The lumbosacral trunk is seen anterior to the sacral ala (*oval*). The upper sacroiliac joint (*curved arrow*) is seen between the sacral ala and the iliac bone. Axial CT image (**c**) at the *S2* level shows the ventral (*curved white arrow*) and dorsal (*small arrow*) aspects of the neural foramina. The sacral canal (*large arrow*) is smaller in diameter at this level, while the sacroiliac joint (*curved black arrow*) is more prominent. The internal iliac artery (*IA*) is seen anterior to the sacral ala. Axial CT image (**d**) at the *S3* level shows the smaller size of all sacral components, including the sacral canal (*large arrow*), as the sacrum tapers. The synovial portion of the sacroiliac joint (*curved*) arrow is seen at this level. Axial CT image (**e**) at *S4* shows a small sacral vertebra and canal (*arrow*). The pyriformis (*P*) and gluteus (*G*) muscles form the anterior and lateral relations of the sacrum as does the rectosigmoid portion of the large intestine (*curved arrow*). Axial CT image (**f**) at the *S5* level shows an aperture in the dorsal sacrum, the sacral hiatus, which is bordered by bony prominences, the sacral cornu

to support the lumbar spine at the L5–S1 distal articulation. The spinous processes of the sacral neural arches are fused to form the median sacral crest. Unlike the other spine segments, the sacrum does not contain transverse processes. Instead, a continuous lateral osseous mass, the sacral ala, lies lateral to and is in continuity with the sacral vertebra and neural arches. A prominent marrow-containing space is present within the sacral ala, though the trabecular network is somewhat reduced as compared to other osseous structures within the spinal axis. The sacral ala articulates with the iliac bones at the sacroiliac joints. These large joints have a superior component that is fibrous and an inferior component that consists of a synovial joint space. The sacrum articulates caudally with the coccyx at the sacrococcygeal joint.

The lumbar spinal canal continues within the center of the sacrum as the sacral canal. The sacral canal courses through the center of the sacrum and contains the caudal aspect of the dural sac. The latter usually terminates at the S2 or S3 level. The remainder of the sacral canal contains epidural fat and an epidural venous plexus. The sacral canal terminates at the sacral hiatus, a small dorsal aperture at the caudal aspect of the sacrum which is bordered dorsally by two bony protuberances that are palpable on physical examination, the sacral cornu. The sacral canal communicates with the sacral foramina from S1 to S4. These sacral foramina are unique in that they possess ventral and dorsal apertures. The dorsal apertures of these foramina transmit sensory nerves which form a fibrous meshwork over the dorsum of the sacrum as they primarily innervate the sacroiliac joints. Motor nerves course through the anterior sacral foramina. The sacral plexus is formed by the ventral rami of the L4–S4 nerves and consists of a large upper band, or lumbosacral trunk, which derives neural contribution from L4, L5, and S1 and a small inferior band that includes branches from S2, S3, and S4.

The major ventral anatomic relations of the sacrum include the pelvis and pelvic contents. The presacral space contains fat. The rectum is located just anterior to this space. The iliac vessels, arteries, and veins are seen bilaterally anterior to the ventral sacral cortex at the level of the sacral ala. The lumbar plexus or lumbosacral trunk is also located adjacent to these structures. The sacral sympathetic plexus is located at the L5–S1 level between the common iliac vessels. The impar or sacrococcygeal ganglion is located anterior to the sacrococcygeal joint. The major lateral anatomic relations of the lower sacrum include the gluteal musculature and pyriformis muscles.

The critical anatomic sacral structures to be aware of for sacral biopsy include the sacral canal and foramina and the anterior sacral cortex.

7.3 Indications and Contraindications

Sacral biopsies are indicated to evaluate mass lesions within the sacrum and/or adjacent soft tissue structures (Table 7.1). These lesions may represent primary tumors in this location such as chordoma, giant cell tumor, or sarcoma (Figs. 7.2 and 7.3). More commonly, however, mass lesions of the sacrum are often due to metastatic disease from other primary sites (Fig. 7.4) (Rajeswaran et al. 2013). Infiltrative lesions of the sacrum may also require biopsy for definitive diagnosis. Infiltrative lesions may represent sacral involvement by multiple myeloma or lymphoma. When unilateral, sacral insufficiency fractures may show features that resemble an infiltrative lesion on MRI; this may require biopsy for clarification (Fig. 7.5) (Sudhir et al. 2016). Infection, or sacral osteomyelitis, is uncommon but may be seen in bedridden patients with sacral decubitus ulcers. Infection may also involve the sacroiliac joint, and this tends to present with unilateral involvement. Suspected infection in the sacrum, sacroiliac joint, or adjacent portions of the pelvis may require biopsy in order to confirm the diagnosis and identify the causative microorganism (such as *Staphylococcus* species).

Sacral biopsies are strictly contraindicated in patients with uncorrected coagulopathy (Table 7.1). The procedure cannot be performed without informed or administrative consent. Relative contraindications to sacral biopsy include an uncooperative patient or an unstable patient. With respect to metastatic tumor, in situations where neoplastic lesions are present in both the sacrum and iliac bone, the operator may consider performing the iliac bone biopsy instead (Fig. 7.6).

Table 7.1 Indications/contraindications: image-guided percutaneous sacral biopsy

Indications
Sacral mass
Infiltrative sacral lesion
Unable to distinguish unilateral sacral insufficiency fracture from infiltrative lesion
Sacral osteomyelitis
Contraindications
Absolute
Uncorrected coagulopathy
Unable to obtain informed consent for the procedure
Relative
Uncooperative patient
Unstable patient

7.4 Risks and Complications Associated with Sacral Biopsy and How to Minimize Them

A sacral biopsy is an invasive procedure, and the possibility of a complication, though uncommon, should not be ignored (Table 7.2). Prerequisites that will help to minimize the complication rate when performing image-guided percutaneous spine biopsy procedures such as sacral biopsy are based upon fundamental surgical principles and consist of four major concepts. First, patient selection is important. The procedure should be indicated, and the contraindications to the procedure should be adhered to. If there are relative contraindications to the procedure, then they should be reconciled, with patient safety at the forefront of this decision, prior to moving forward with the procedure. Second, patient preparation must take place, including a review of the patient's medical record, an understanding of the patient's medical condition(s), and their ability and willingness to have the procedure. Medications and medical allergies must be known ahead of time and the appropriate steps taken to temporarily adjust medication regimens when necessary. Third, operator preparation is essential to a successful and safe procedure. This concept not only reflects the operators training, abilities, and knowledge with respect to image-guided percutaneous biopsy techniques (including a sound understanding of the imaging modalities, tools, and techniques for performing these procedures) but also emphasizes the basic questions of should I perform this biopsy, when do I perform this biopsy, and how should I perform this biopsy (Carberry et al. 2016)? At the clinical level, thorough preparation should reflect careful patient evaluation, image review, and communication with the referring clinician. Fourth, the value of an organized team

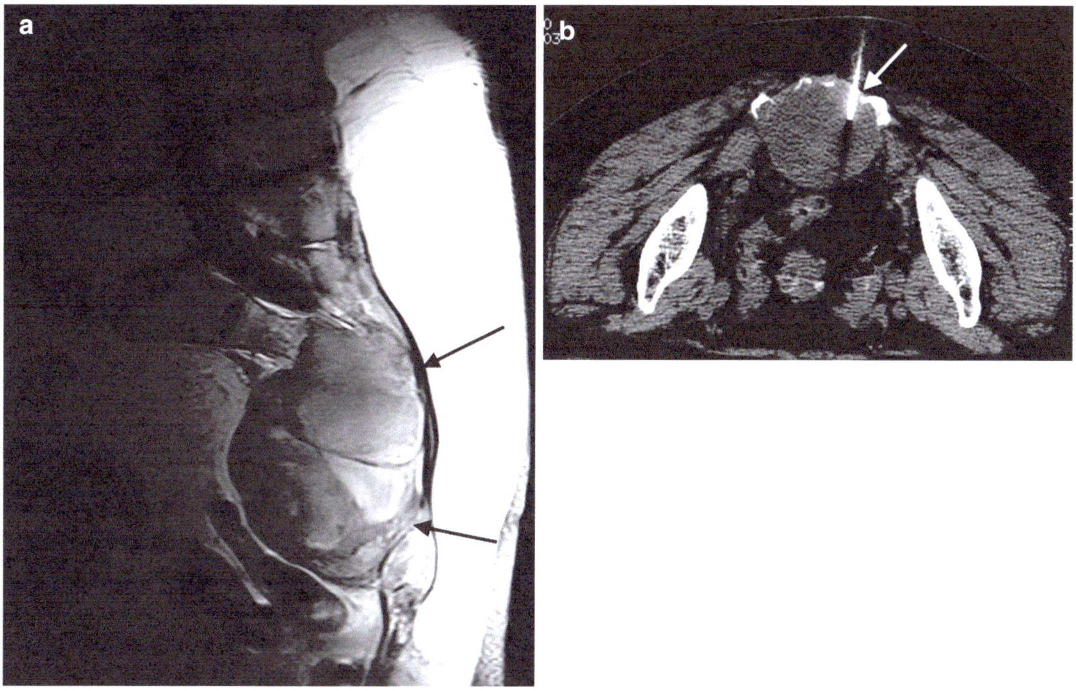

Fig. 7.2 Chordoma. Contrast-enhanced T1-weighted sagittal image (**a**) shows large moderately enhancing septated mass within the distal sacrum (*arrows*); the mass projects ventrally. Axial CT image (**b**) shows the biopsy needle (*arrow*) within this expansile mass that is centered within the sacrum and erodes the surrounding bone

approach toward performing the procedure is a major determinant in the success of the procedure and in a safe patient outcome. This includes all aspects of the procedure from patient intake, evaluation, preparation, procedure (inclusive of all appropriate procedural suite protocols such as sterile technique, patient and procedure verification), post-procedure care, and patient follow-up. The premise that everyone's role, including the patient and their family, in patient safety is equally important, and the actual practice of this credo improves the likelihood of a successful outcome.

7.5 Imaging Guidance

Given the local anatomic constraints related to the sacral canal and foramina as well as the close proximity of prominent neural and vascular structures to the ventral sacral cortex, computed tomographic guidance is the preferred imaging guidance tool for performing sacral, presacral, or parasacral percutaneous biopsy procedures. CT guidance can also be used for aspirating a suspected infected sacroiliac joint. CT fluoroscopy improves the efficiency of these biopsy procedures. With CT it is possible to establish safe trajectories to access the target lesion, avoid critical structures including the sacral canal and foramina, limit the needle excursion such that there is not a breach of the ventral sacral cortex, and monitor the position of the needle and needle tip throughout the biopsy procedure. Conventional fluoroscopy is generally not used to perform sacral biopsies but can be used to perform an aspiration of the sacroiliac joint (Fig. 7.7). Reports of successful sacral biopsy with cone beam fluoroscopic-CT (CBCT) describe the advantages of the combination of real-time needle orientation and the spatial resolution of CT fluoroscopy (Carrafiello et al. 2012).

7.6 Approaches

A posterior approach is used to biopsy the sacrum, a posterior structure. The trajectory that is used consists of a needle trajectory that is somewhat

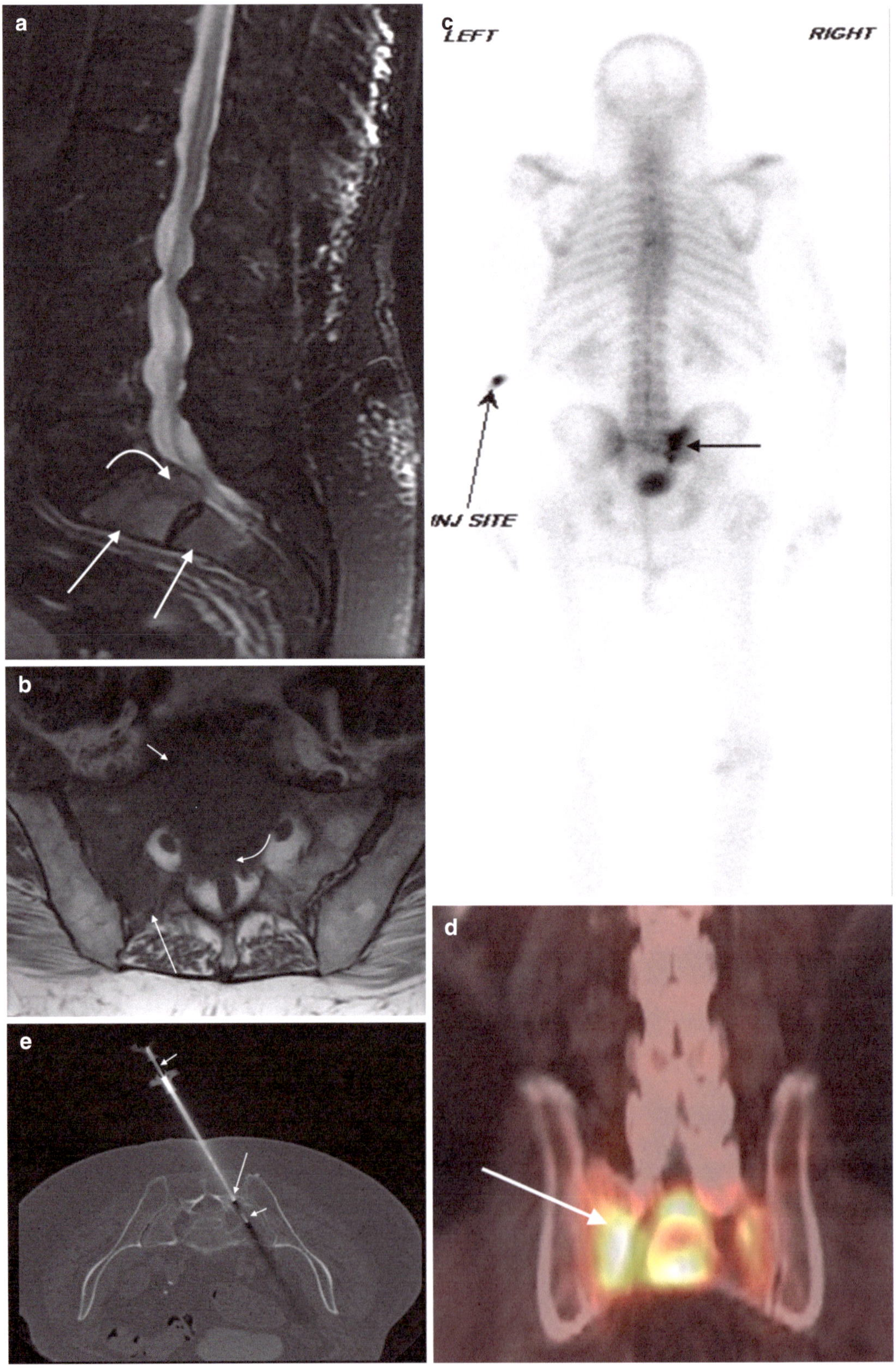
a
b
c
LEFT
RIGHT
INJ SITE
d
e

Fig. 7.3 An 81-year-old male with low back and right leg pain. Fat-suppressed T2-weighted sagittal image (**a**) shows a marrow replacement process at S1 and S2 (*arrows*) and a ventral epidural soft tissue component (*curved arrow*). T1-weighted axial image (**b**) shows an infiltrative hypointense lesion within the right sacral ala (*large arrow*) and sacral vertebral body (*small arrow*) with a hypointense epidural soft tissue component (*curved arrow*). Single posterior projection (**c**) from a bone scan shows intense focal radionuclide uptake within the right side of the sacrum. Coronal reformatted fused image (**d**) from a PET-CT examination shows intense FDG uptake within the lesion (*arrow*). Axial CT image (**e**) obtained during the biopsy procedure shows a coaxial bone biopsy needle system with a guide cannula (*large arrow*) oriented in a standard short-axis oblique approach between the sacral foramina and right sacroiliac joint. The biopsy needle (*short arrows*) has been inserted into the right sacral ala. Subsequent pathologic evaluation of the biopsy specimens showed a high-grade fibroblastic sarcoma

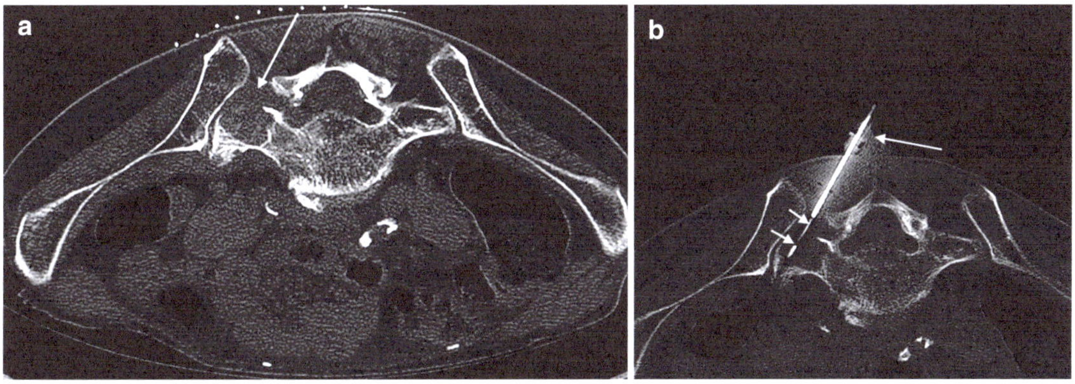

Fig. 7.4 A 73-year-old female with prior medical history of melanoma, breast cancer and a recently detected lung mass presents with lesions in the sacrum and calvarium. Axial CT image (**a**) during biopsy procedure with skin grid in place shows a lytic soft tissue mass (*arrow*) that extends posteriorly. The arrow also indicates the desired trajectory for a posterior approach to this lesion. Axial CT image (**b**) shows a coaxial soft tissue biopsy system inserted with this oblique trajectory and with the guide cannula supported by gauze at the skin entry site (*large arrow*). The biopsy chamber (*small arrows*) of the cutting needle has been exposed within the substance of the lesion. The pathology showed metastatic lung adenocarcinoma

perpendicular to the dorsal surface of the sacrum. This is referred to as a short-axis approach (Fig. 7.8). This allows for direct access to most focal or infiltrative sacral lesions. Given the oblique orientation of the sacral foramina relative to the sacrum, the needle tip may have to be angled obliquely in order to avoid the sacral foramina (Fig. 7.8). This oblique angulation of the needle tip serves a second purpose; it maximizes the traverse of the needle tip through the lesion prior to reaching the anterior sacral cortex. This technique provides an opportunity to obtain more tissue samples and simultaneously adds a margin of safety to the procedure. Because of the presence of the lumbosacral trunk, the iliac vessels, and the rectum adjacent to the anterior sacral cortex, this latter structure is a boundary that must not be crossed with the biopsy needle. Steep ipsilateral oblique approaches, which angle the needle tip toward the midline, or even lateral approaches across the sacroiliac joint may be required to access the S1 vertebral body or sacral promontory lesions (Fig. 7.9) Case reports document success obtained using recent advances in curved needle technology to access the sacral promontory and adjacent structures (Murphy et al. 2012).

The posterior approach to parasacral soft tissue masses or fluid collections will be determined by the exact location of the lesion and by the proximity to adjacent critical structures. The approaches can range from posterior and tangential to posterior with very steep ipsilateral or contralateral angulation of the needle tip (Fig. 7.10). The approach to the sacroiliac joint, a posterior structure, is also

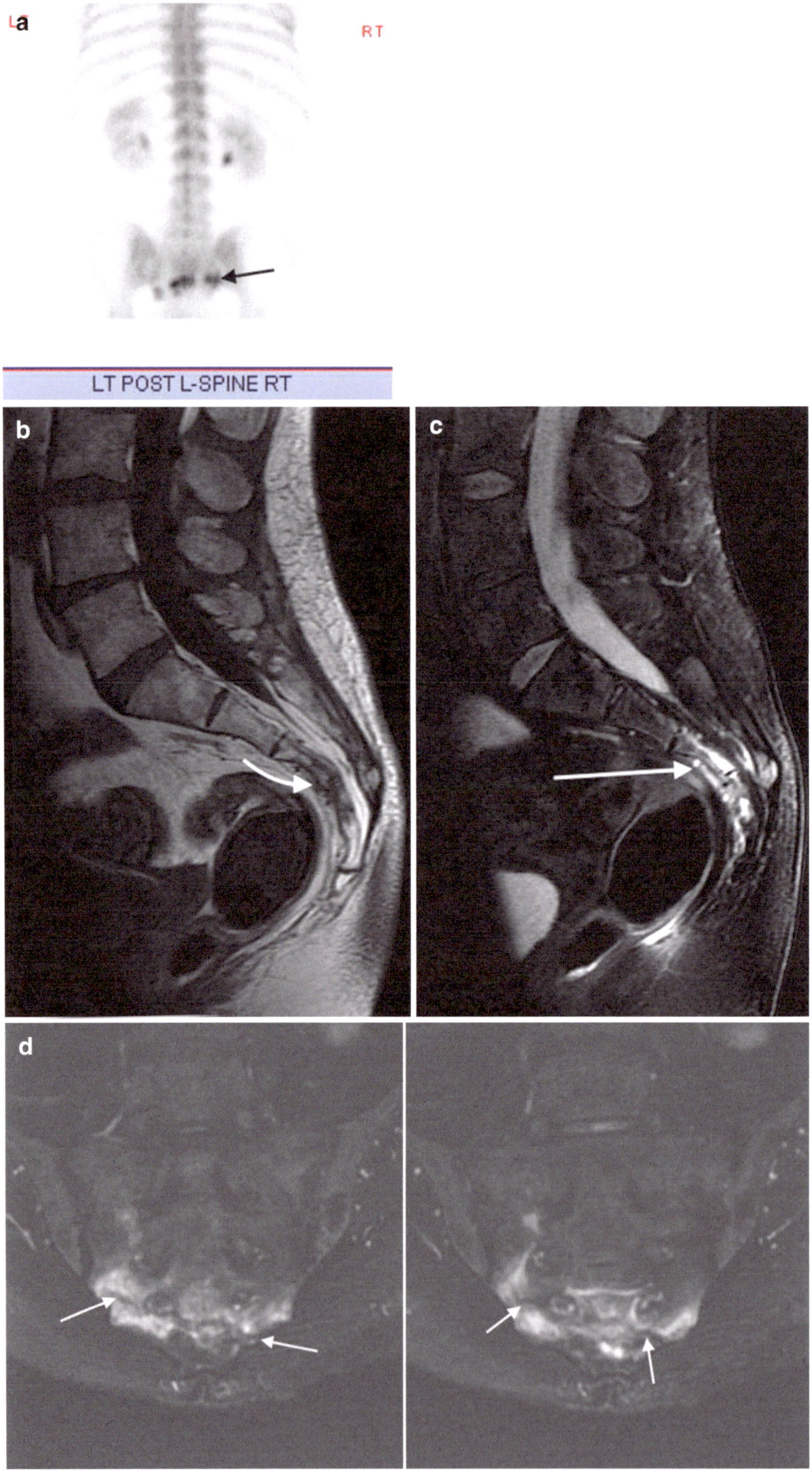
a
RT
LT POST L-SPINE RT
b
c
d

Fig. 7.5 A 47-year-old female with gait disturbance. Posterior frontal projection (**a**) from bone scan shows focal spotty radionuclide uptake within the lower sacrum (*arrow*). T1-weighted sagittal image (**b**) shows focal hypointensity at S3 and S4 (*arrow*) with corresponding hyperintensity (*arrow*) on the T2-weighted sagittal image (**c**). Fat-suppressed contrast-enhanced T1-weighted coronal images (**d**) show focal enhancement within the lower sacrum as well as the presence of a fracture line (*arrows*). In retrospect, the irregular linear pattern of the sacral insufficiency fracture line is shown on the bone scan

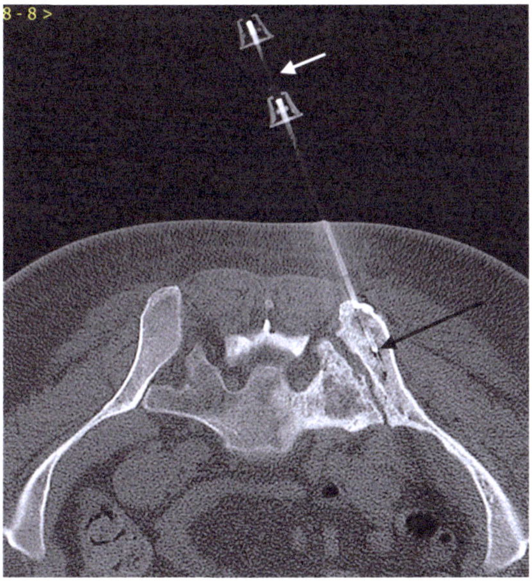

Fig. 7.6 A 51-year-old female with lower low back pain. Axial CT image obtained during biopsy procedure shows sampling of a sclerotic lesion within the iliac crest (*large arrow*) with a coaxial bone biopsy needle system (*short arrow*). This iliac crest was biopsied instead of the sclerotic lesion within the adjacent sacral ala in this patient with breast metastases

posterior. Because of its oblique orientation away from the midline, the inferior sacroiliac joint is often accessed with a contralateral oblique approach with fluoroscopy (Fig. 7.7). Some anatomic variation in the orientation of the inferior sacroiliac joint does occur, and in this situation, a more direct tangential approach is required to access the joint.

> It must be emphasized that review of the pre-biopsy imaging studies allows the operator to plan a safe and effective posterior trajectory to the target lesion, whether it is located in the sacrum, parasacral soft tissues, or sacroiliac joint.

Table 7.2 Sacral spine biopsy procedure risks and complications

Hemorrhage
Superficial – at puncture site
Deep – potential pelvic hematoma formation
Needle injury
Artery or vein puncture
Spinal canal or foramen breach
Sacral nerve root or lumbosacral trunk puncture
Other
Nondiagnostic biopsy
Wrong side biopsied
Infection (cellulitis, osteomyelitis)
Tumor seeding along the biopsy tract
Systemic – anesthesia complication
Increased pain
Radiation exposure
Equipment failure – broken needle

7.7 The Sacral Biopsy Procedure

7.7.1 General Considerations

7.7.1.1 Patient Factors

Sacral biopsy procedures can be performed on inpatients or outpatients and should only be performed on cooperative patients. Therefore, it is necessary to evaluate and examine the patient. This clinical evaluation can be accomplished at the time of the informed consent process. The operator should obtain a complete medical and surgical history and review and/or obtain hematologic, coagulation, and renal laboratory profiles as necessary. For patients with suspected infection, the operator should also obtain or review the infectious disease profile (WBC with differential, ESR, and CRP; *please refer to the* Chap. 9). The patient's medication list is reviewed and all patient medical allergies are documented. The patient consultation allows the operator to assess

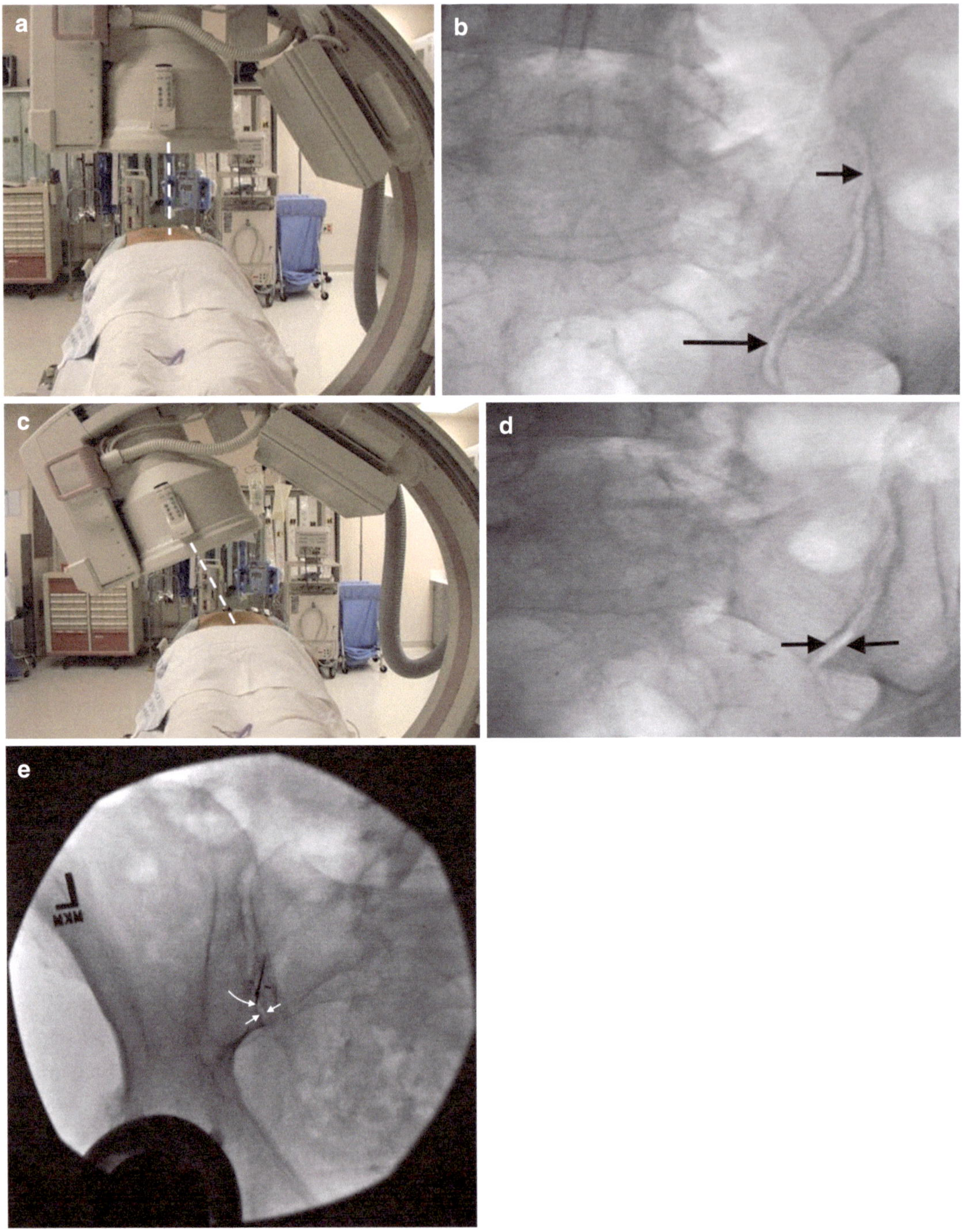

Fig. 7.7 Accessing the sacroiliac joint with fluoroscopy. Photograph of prone subject (**a**) with a fluoroscope oriented in the frontal projection (*dashed line*). Corresponding frontal projection (**b**) of the right sacroiliac joint shows "two" joints, a superior joint space (*small arrow*) and an inferior joint space (*small arrow*). Photograph (**c**) with the fluoroscope placed in the contralateral oblique projection (*dashed line*) in order to align the right sacroiliac joint. Corresponding frontal projection (**d**) of the right sacroiliac joint now shows alignment of the joint (*arrows*). Single frontal fluoroscopic image (**e**) with the patient in prone position using contralateral oblique projection to align the inferior sacroiliac joint (*small arrows*) thereby allowing down-the-barrel advancement of a 22 gauge spinal needle (*curved arrow*) into the sacroiliac joint.

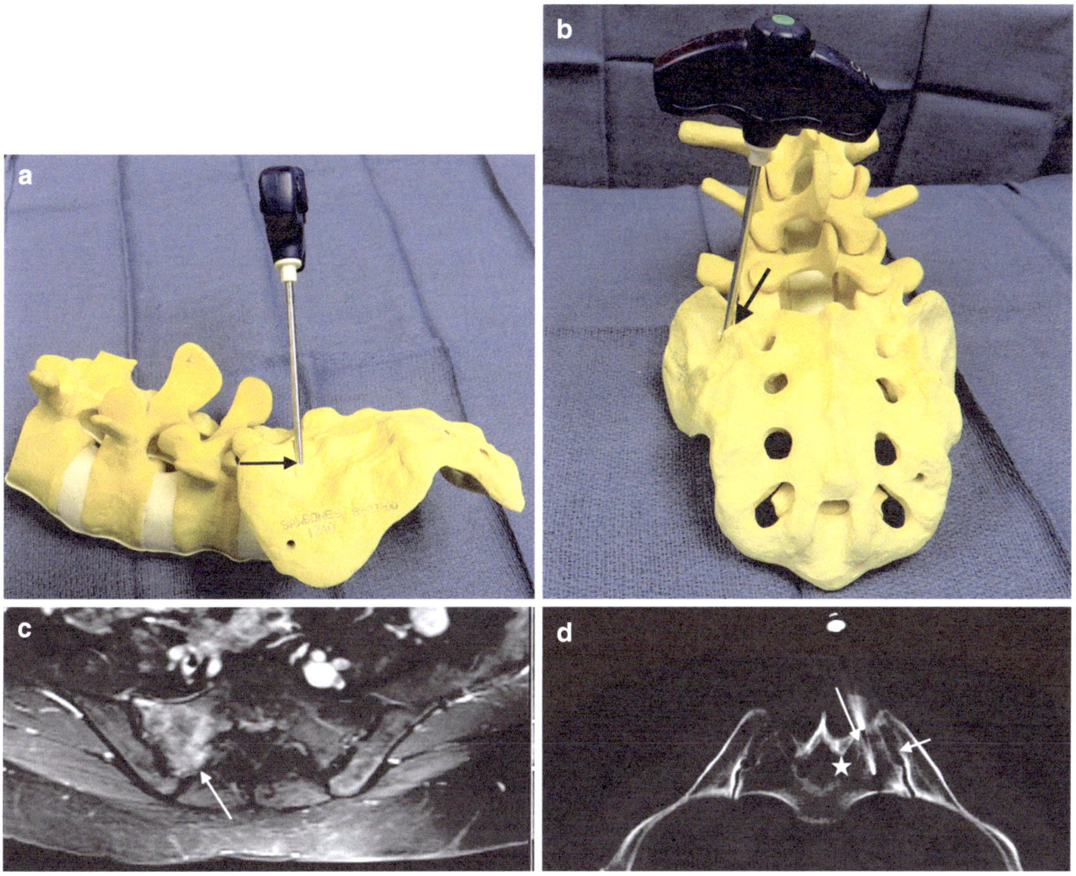

Fig. 7.8 Short-axis technique. Photograph with lateral view of sacral sawbones model (**a**) shows a relatively perpendicular orientation (*arrow*) of the biopsy needle with respect to the dorsum of the sacrum. Rearview of the same needle placement (**b**) shows an oblique orientation of the needle (*arrow*); relative to the sacrum, the needle tip is angled away from the midline in order to avoid the neural foramina. Fat-suppressed contrast-enhanced axial image (**c**) in patient with lesion (*arrow*) in the sacral ala. Axial CT image (**d**) during a biopsy of this lesion shows the angulation of the needle (*large arrow*) parallel to the sacroiliac joint (*small arrow*) that allows for sampling of the lesion while avoiding the neural foramen (*star*)

the patient's mental status and the patient's ability and willingness to undergo the sacral biopsy procedure. It also enables the operator to examine the skin overlying the sacrum for any possible wounds, scars, tattoos, and hair. Most importantly, it allows the operator to assess the patient's ability to lie in the prone position. These factors along with the lesion location and the intended approach will influence the patient position. The patient should be as comfortable as possible as this will improve their ability to cooperate throughout the biopsy procedure. By keeping the patient comfortable, you are able to help them stay relaxed.

The informed consent process affords the operator the opportunity to discuss the procedure with the patient and their family members, clarifying their expectations, and to also discuss the other diagnostic options to the procedure. The diagnostic alternative to a percutaneous biopsy procedure is an open biopsy procedure which is performed in the operating room under general anesthesia. Open biopsy procedures require a somewhat longer recovery period and are associated with greater morbidity as compared to percutaneous biopsy procedures (Mankin et al. 1996). Sacral biopsies with CT guidance are well tolerated, with rare early or delayed complica-

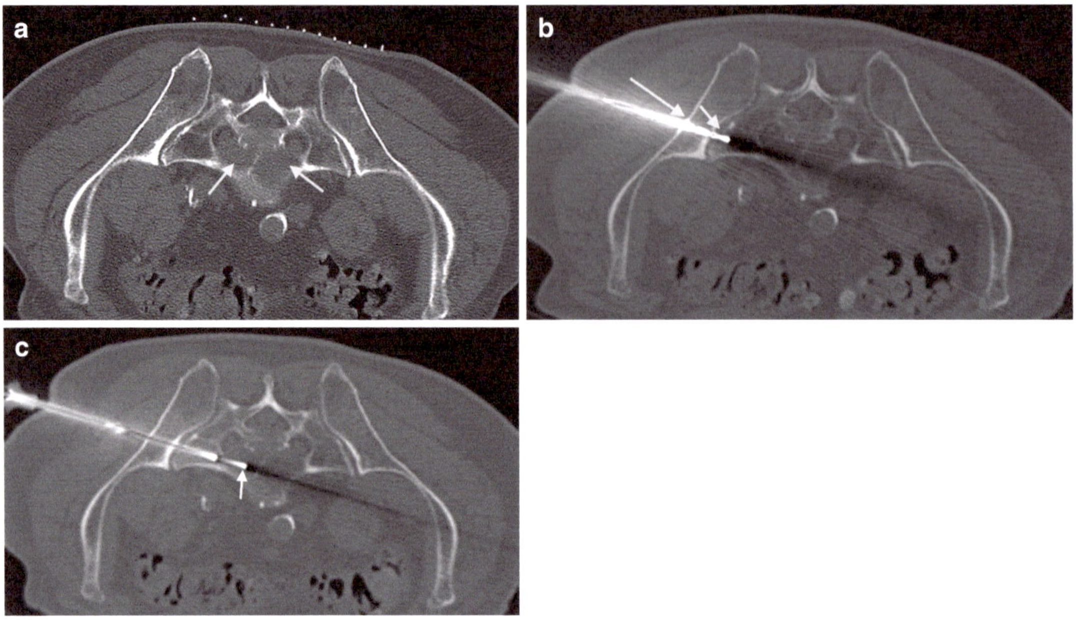

Fig. 7.9 A 79-year-old male with history of colon cancer and low back pain. Axial CT image (**a**) during biopsy procedure shows the skin grid in place and a lytic lesion within the sacral promontory (*arrows*). A posterior approach was not feasible in this case; therefore, a lateral (**b**) or trans-iliosacral approach (*large arrow*) was used to cross the fibrous portion of the sacroiliac joint (*small arrow*) with a twist drill. Axial CT image (**c**) shows a coaxial bone biopsy needle advanced anterior to the sacral foramen and into the lesion (*arrow*). The pathology showed metastatic adenocarcinoma of the colon

tions (Huang 2012). Other treatment options, though less optimal, include continued medical and imaging surveillance or empiric antibiotic therapy (if there is concern for infection). The patient should always be informed of the possibility of a nondiagnostic biopsy procedure; this rarely occurs but may require a repeat percutaneous, or an open biopsy, procedure.

For inpatients, pre-procedure orders will state that the patient is scheduled for a sacral biopsy and that they should remain NPO after midnight. Specific medications that affect blood coagulation should already be managed prior to the biopsy procedure. Intravenous access should ideally be located on the forearm, wrist, or hand as the patient's elbows are often bent during the procedure, and this adversely affects the functionality of the intravenous line. For outpatients, an instruction sheet can be reviewed with the patient. Again, it is very important to exercise an agreed upon management strategy with the patient's referring physician with respect to anticoagulant and antiplatelet medication. Outpatients should have someone available to drive them and escort them back home (*Please refer to the* Chap. 1).

7.7.1.2 Staff Factors

It is best practice for the interventional team to pause for a "time-out" communication and discuss the procedure ahead of time with all staff that are involved in the procedure. This type of communication increases the safety, efficiency, and potential success of the procedure. By facilitating specimen collection, handling, and analysis, techniques such as fine-needle aspiration become efficient procedures. The patient is ideally included in the verification phase of this process (correct patient, correct procedure, correct level, and correct side) – this will enhance the patient's trust and confidence in their healthcare team.

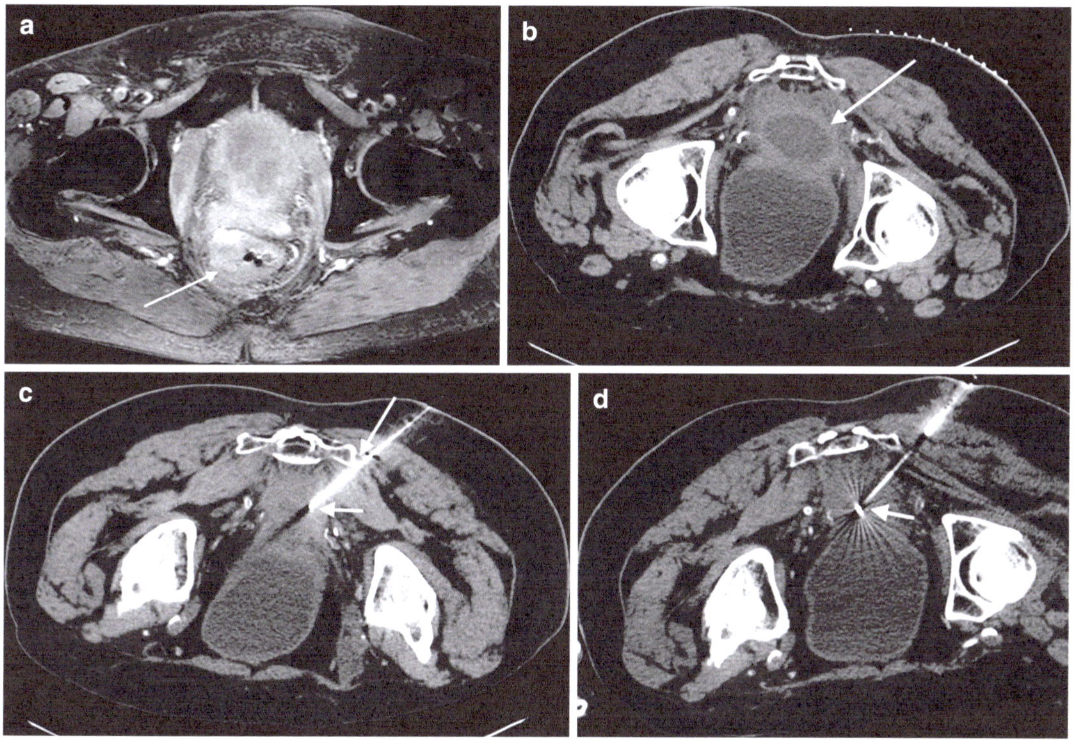

Fig. 7.10 A 73-year-old male with colorectal cancer. Fat-suppressed contrast-enhanced T1-weighted axial image (**a**) shows enhancing rectal mass (*arrow*). Axial CT image (**b**) shows skin grid in place and rectal mass (*arrow*); the arrow also indicates the trajectory for subsequent needle placement. Axial CT image (**c**) shows biopsy needle passing just lateral to the sacrum (*large arrow*) and entering the lesion (*small arrow*). Axial CT image (**d**), after coaxial fine-needle aspiration confirmed the presence of neoplastic cells, shows coaxial placement of a fiducial marker into the lesion (*arrow*). The fiducial marker is used to guide subsequent navigation with CyberKnife radiosurgery

7.7.2 Anesthesia

Sacral and sacroiliac joint biopsies are relatively quick procedures that tend to be relatively well tolerated by patients. These procedures can be performed under local anesthesia if absolutely necessary. Alternatives to this form of anesthesia include intravenous sedation and analgesia or intravenous anesthesia with propofol. The latter requires the consultation and assistance of an anesthesiologist. A major determinant of the choice of anesthesia is the patient's medical condition. Other factors that influence the choice of anesthesia include patient preference and operator preference. Patients are almost always placed in the prone position for this procedure, and all of these anesthesia options can be used as necessary.

7.7.3 Patient Preparation

The patient is placed on the procedure table in the prone position, whenever possible, and monitoring equipment including a pulse oximeter, electrocardiogram leads, and a blood pressure cuff is placed on the patient. The patient's intravenous line is examined to ascertain that the line is functional. Sacral biopsy is performed with strict aseptic technique. The skin may have to be shaved in order to remove hair from the sterile field. It is important to mention the reason and need for hair removal ahead of time with patients. Once the patient is positioned on the procedure table and the skin is shaved, then an additional time-out protocol may be exercised in order to reconfirm the level and side of the procedure (when necessary).

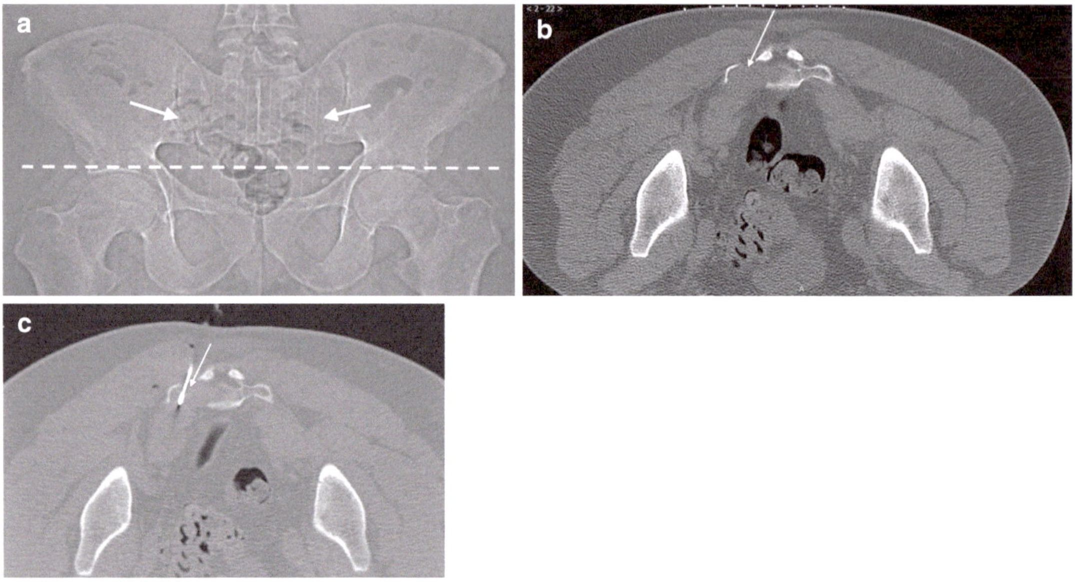

Fig. 7.11 A 47-year-old male with sacral lesion detected on an MRI examination. Scout frontal image (**a**) from CT biopsy procedure shows skin grid markers (*arrows*) oriented vertically over the sacrum. The *dashed line* indicates the level of the lower sacrum. Axial CT image (**b**) shows lytic soft tissue mass (*arrow*) within the left lateral sacrum at the level of the sacral hiatus; the arrow also indicates the optimal posterior trajectory for this lesion. Axial CT image (**c**) shows 14 gauge cutting needle (*arrow*) within the lesion, which subsequent pathologic analysis revealed to be a plasmacytoma

7.8 Technique

7.8.1 CT Guidance

Scout images are obtained in both the frontal and lateral projections with a radiopaque skin grid in place covering the side and area of the intended approach. A limited axial CT examination is performed with the skin grid in place (Fig. 7.11). The skin entry site is identified and marked with a skin marker. The skin is then prepped with a sterile solution and draped. Intravenous sedation and analgesia or anesthesia may be initiated in those patients who require it. The skin is anesthetized with a local anesthetic agent such as 1 or 2% of lidocaine using a 25 gauge needle. A small cross hair incision is made at the skin insertion site using a #11 scalpel blade. Single-needle or coaxial needle technique can be used for performing CT-guided percutaneous sacral biopsy (Geremia et al. 1992).

7.8.1.1 For Bone Biopsy

Coaxial technique can be used for larger patients with thick soft tissue overlying the planned biopsy site. With a coaxial needle technique, a 20 cm long, 20 gauge guide needle with a removable hub is slowly advanced under CT or CT fluoroscopic guidance toward the target lesion, with a trajectory that avoids the neural foramina and sacral canal (Elson, Cook Inc., Bloomington, IN). When the needle tip approaches the osseous surface of the dorsal sacrum, approximately 1 mL of local anesthetic can be administered in order to minimize patient discomfort. Once the optimal trajectory and needle position are established with CT guidance and the periosteum has been anesthetized, the needle hub of this insert or guide needle is removed. The guide needle effectively transforms into a guidewire for subsequent coaxial insertion of a guide cannula. Prior to passing the guide cannula over the guidewire, a blunt dissector is first inserted coaxially into the guide cannula (Fig. 7.12). The

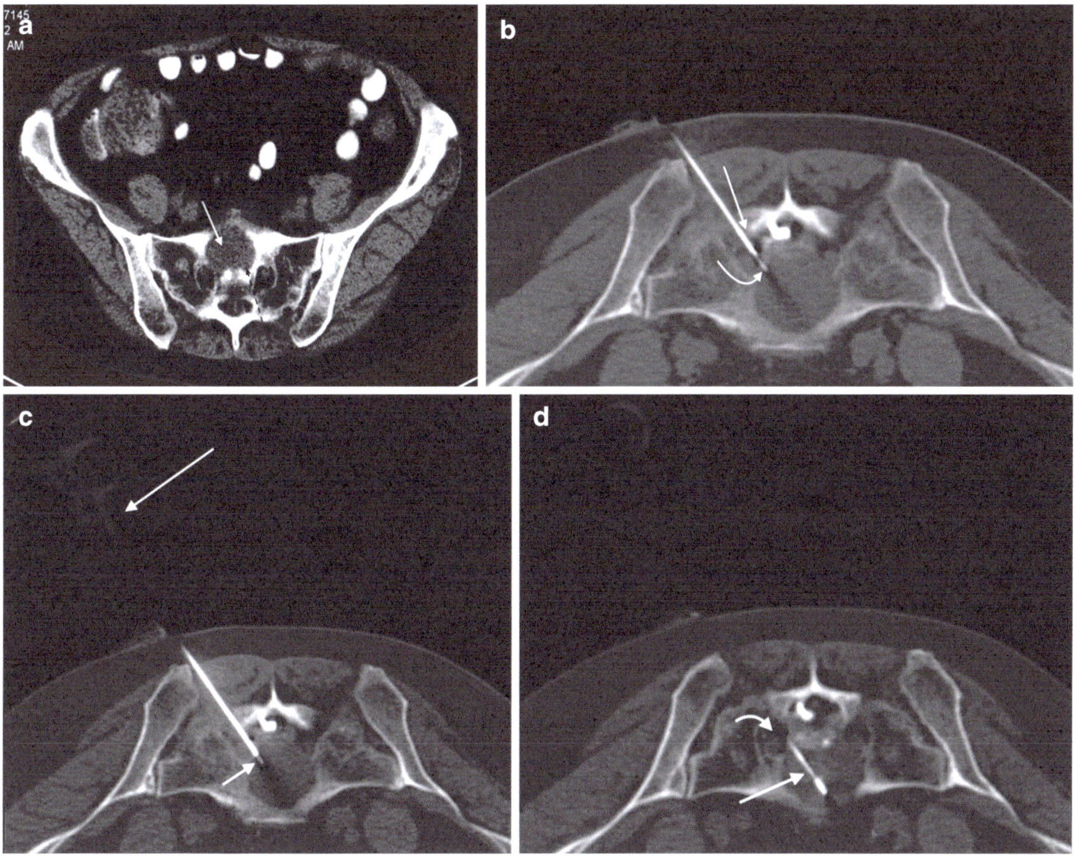

Fig. 7.12 An 81-year-old female with severe low back pain and a lung mass. Axial CT image (**a**) level of the pelvis shows a round soft tissue mass within the S1 vertebra (*arrow*); the lesion erodes the anterior aspect of the sacral promontory. This lesion is challenging to access (*dashed arrow*). Axial CT image (**b**) shows the use of coaxial technique with advancement of a guide cannula (*large arrow*) over an insert needle (curved arrow) between the neural foramen and sacral canal. Axial CT image (**c**) shows a soft tissue-cutting needle (*large arrow*) advanced coaxially to the margin of the lesion (*small arrow*). Axial CT image (**d**) shows deployment of the cutting needle (*arrow*) within the lesion; this approach just avoids the neural foramen (*curved arrow*). The pathology evaluation showed metastatic lung adenocarcinoma

blunt dissector – guide cannula ensemble – is then passed over the guidewire and advanced to the dorsal surface of the sacrum using CT imaging guidance. Once the position of this construct is confirmed with imaging, the guidewire and blunt dissector can be removed and exchanged for a trephine bone biopsy needle. Make sure to hold the guide cannula in place with one hand, in order to keep the guide cannula in position, as the exchange is performed with the other hand. The trephine bone biopsy needle can be used to "dock" the guide cannula to the dorsal sacral cortex (Fig. 7.13). The guide cannula, once in place, provides a safe access port through the soft tissues and avoids repeat needle passes which could otherwise be painful. The biopsy needle is advanced through the guide cannula and into the sacrum using CT guidance to monitor the position of the needle tip relative to the target lesion and the following critical anatomic landmarks: (1) sacral foramina, (2) sacral canal, and (3) anterior sacral cortex. The trephine bone biopsy needle is carefully advanced into the sacral cortex and marrow by rotating its handle in a quick to-and-fro, clockwise-counterclockwise motion which enables the needle tip to cut through the bone with guarded forward manual pressure on the needle. Sequential biopsy needle passes can be made through the guide cannula, always with imaging guidance, and always exchanging one bone biopsy needle for the other with one hand as the guide cannula is maintained in position with the other hand. Extreme caution should be observed in patients with osteoporosis or with very osteolytic lesions as the bone needle may advance effortlessly in these situations. With experience, the operator will also learn to be able to angle the guide cannula slightly in order to sample other areas of the target lesion, thereby effectively increasing specimen yield. Always scan and check the needle position between and during biopsy passes.

Bone biopsy specimens can usually be obtained with this coaxial needle system. At times it may be necessary to aspirate the biopsy needle with a 10 or 20 mL syringe in order to secure the tissue within the biopsy needle. Another helpful maneuver is to advance the biopsy needle a few millimeters, when possible, and this may provide the tissue. Angling the biopsy needle slightly may also dislodge the biopsy specimen. When dealing with purely lytic neoplastic processes, the biopsy sample can be obtained using fine needle (1 mm diameter or less) aspiration or core needle (diameter greater 1.5 mm) biopsy through the guiding cannula. It is important to sample as much tissue as safely as possible (Monfardini et al. 2014; Settle et al. 1990). For bone or lytic soft tissue cores, if possible obtain at least three specimens – more tissue will assist the pathologist in making the diagnosis (Ortiz et al. 2010). A single-pass bone biopsy needle can also be used to perform sacral biopsy. It may be useful to use a larger gauge system (10–8 gauge in diameter) in order to obtain one or two large cores of the bone.

7.8.1.2 For Soft Tissue Masses that are Within or Adjacent to the Sacrum (Parasacral)

A coaxial system can be used for parasacral lesions (Figs. 7.7 and 7.14). After the skin is anesthetized, a small guide needle (e.g.,18–14 gauge diameter) is advanced to the periphery of the soft tissue mass, and additional anesthetic agent is applied. Fine-needle aspiration can then be performed using CT-guided passes with a small gauge (22 gauge or smaller) needle. Fine-needle aspiration should be performed prior to core biopsy in order to minimize hemorrhage into the needle tract as this sequence decreases the likelihood of specimen contamination with the blood (Ayala et al. 1995). Sequential needle passes are made into the soft tissue mass with

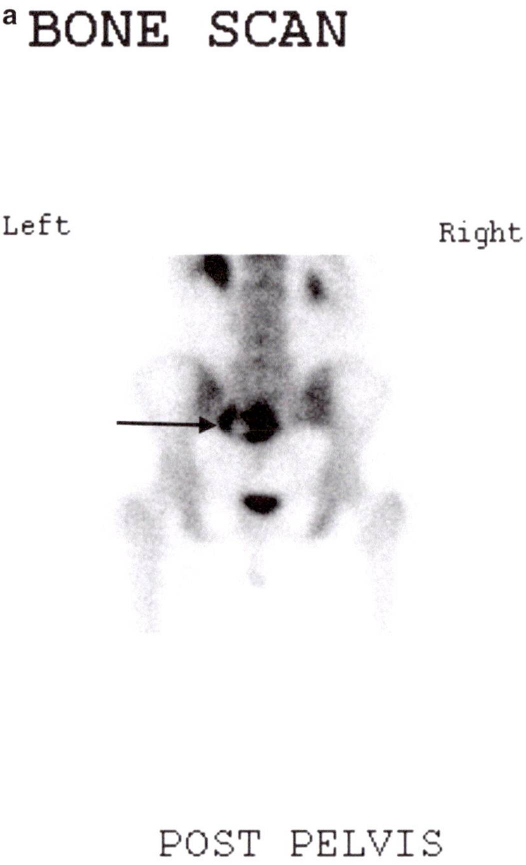

Fig. 7.13 A 62-year-old female with back pain and a prior history of carcinoma of the gall bladder. Single static posterior projection from a bone scan (**a**) shows intense radionuclide uptake within the sacrum (*arrow*). T1-weighted sagittal image (**b**) shows a hypointense expansile lesion (*arrow*) within the sacrum at S3 and S4. Fat-suppressed T2-weighted sagittal image (**c**) again shows the lesion to be relatively hypointense (*arrow*). Axial CT image in bone window algorithm (**d**) shows a sclerotic lesion predominantly involving the left side of the sacrum (*arrows*). Axial CT image (**e**) shows the use of coaxial bone biopsy needle to sample this sclerotic lesion (*arrow*) which was subsequently shown to be a metastasis

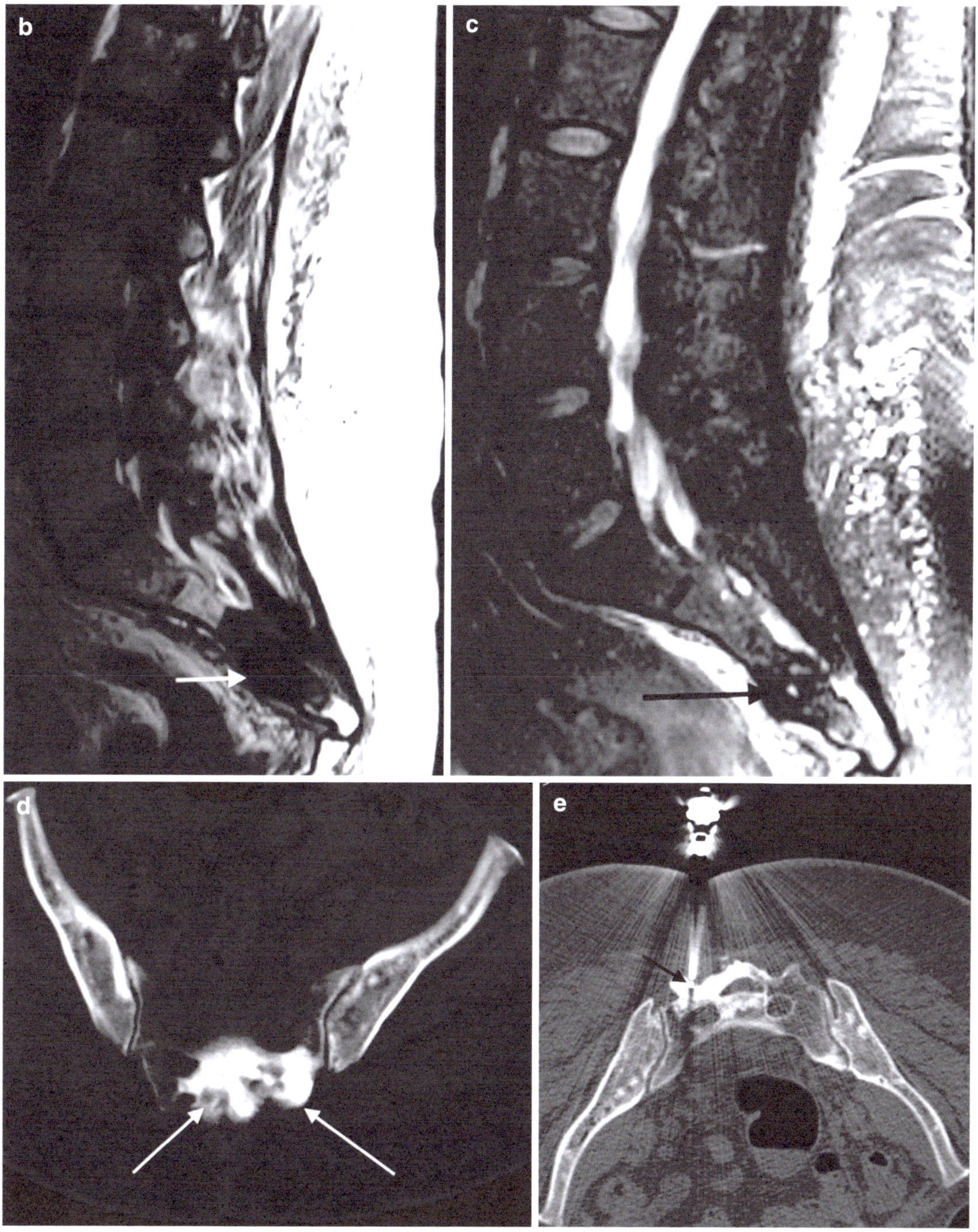

Fig. 7.13 (continued)

slight angulations in order to sample different areas of the mass. Imaging guidance is used to monitor the direction and depth of the biopsy needle and assess its relation to nearby critical structures. After the FNA passes, a core biopsy needle system can be advanced through the guide needle. Many core soft tissue biopsy needle systems contain a sampling chamber that must be exposed within the lesion. In order to perform the biopsy, this needle chamber must be exposed and

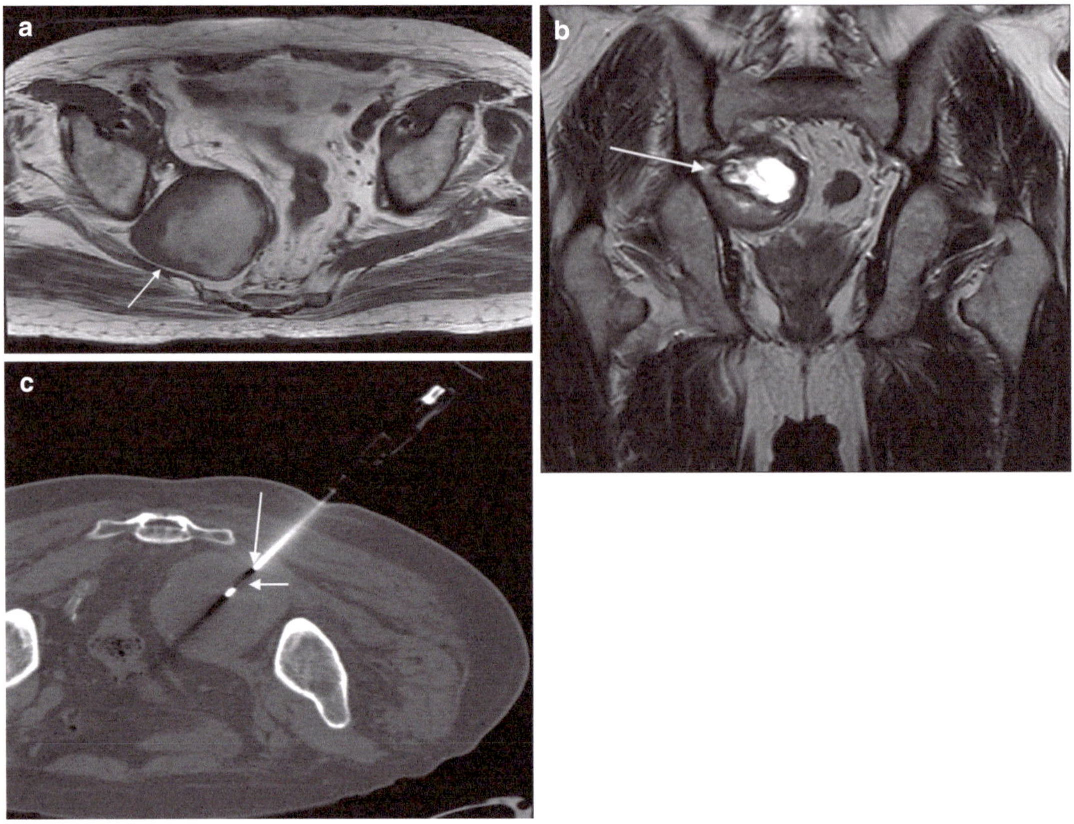

Fig. 7.14 A 77-year-old male with right leg pain. T1-weighted axial image (**a**) shows a large mass (*arrow*) anterior and lateral to the lower sacrum and anterior to the pyriformis muscle. T2-weighted coronal image (**b**) shows a solid and cystic mass (*arrow*). Axial CT image (**c**) shows coaxial (*large arrow*) insertion of cutting needle (*small arrow*) used to obtain three soft tissue cores from this neurofibroma

travel a short distance further (this often can be preset by the operator to 1 or 2 cm) within the lesion in order for the cutting mechanism to obtain the tissue within the lesion matrix. This additional distance for excursion must be accounted for when deploying the cutting needle in order to sample within the lesion and to avoid injury to a critical structure. The number of passes that can be made will be influenced by the initial success of the fine-needle aspiration passes and by the size of the lesion and its location relative to critical structures. If the fine-needle aspiration passes the yield diagnostic tissue, then it may be possible to either obtain one or more cores of the soft tissue or stop the procedure if the pathologist is certain about the diagnosis.

For soft tissue lesions or lytic lesions within the sacrum, it may be necessary to first gain access to the margin of the lesion within a bone biopsy needle system. A fine-needle aspiration and/or soft tissue core biopsy needle can then be advanced coaxially into the lesion in order to obtain the biopsy specimens (Fig. 7.12). In some cases, an expansile sacral lesion may erode the surrounding cortex; this may allow direct access to the lesion with a coaxial soft tissue biopsy system (Fig. 7.15).

7.8.1.3 For the Sacroiliac Joint

Sacroiliac joint aspiration may be performed with CT guidance (Fig. 7.16) (Lin et al. 2009). The inferior aspect of the joint, the synovial portion, is first identified on the preliminary axial images with the skin grid in place. The skin entry point is marked, the patient is prepped, and a local anesthetic agent is applied. This procedure can be performed with just local lidocaine anesthesia; some

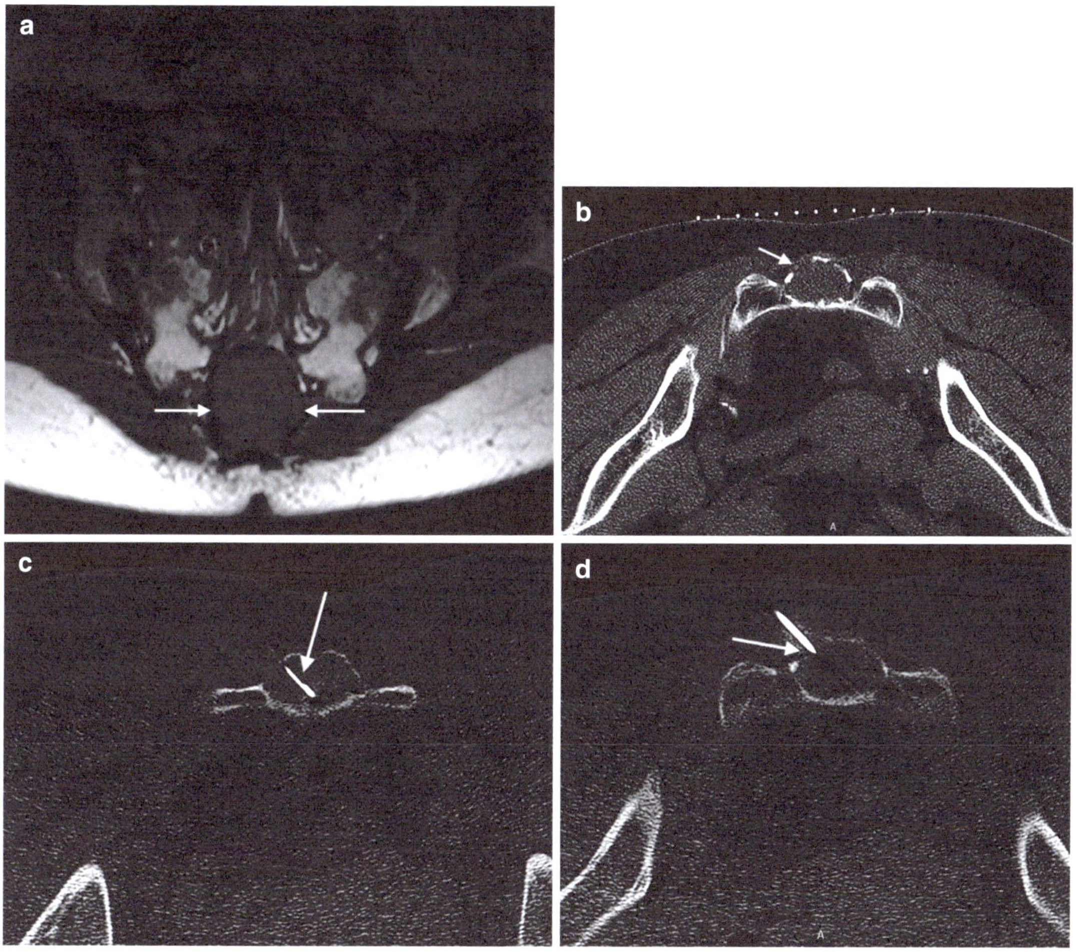

Fig. 7.15 A 66-year-old female with a sacral lesion. T1-weighted coronal image (**a**) shows a midline expansile soft tissue mass within the caudal sacrum (*arrows*). Axial CT image (**b**) with skin grid in place shows the mass partially eroding the sacrum (*arrow*). Axial CT image (**c**) shows a guide needle inserted through the eroded portion of the sacrum (*arrow*); this osseous erosion essentially provides a window for access to the lesion. Axial CT image (**d**) shows the cutting needle (*arrow*) within the substance of the lesion. Subsequent pathologic evaluation of the biopsy specimens showed the lesion to be a paraganglioma

patients, however, either prefer or may require intravenous sedation and analgesia or intravenous anesthesia. Since sacroiliac joint biopsy is almost always performed to assess for infection, a single needle, such as a 20 gauge or 18 gauge spinal needle, can be used to access the joint space. A syringe is attached to the needle hub after the stylet is removed and the joint is aspirated. Any aspirated material is placed in a sterile container for subsequent microbiologic analysis. If it is not possible to aspirate fluid, then a small volume of anesthetic can be used to infiltrate the joint – this is then aspirated and submitted for microbiologic analysis. Alternatively, a bone biopsy needle can be used to extract a small amount of the periarticular bone, and a few specimens can be obtained. Some of the specimen should be sent for microbiologic analysis, and the remainder should be sent for pathologic analysis. When switching to this latter technique, it is helpful to anesthetize the posterior aspect of the joint. It may also be necessary to give the patient intravenous medication for sedation and analgesia. Regardless of which needles are used, imaging guidance is required to monitor needle position at all times throughout the biopsy procedure.

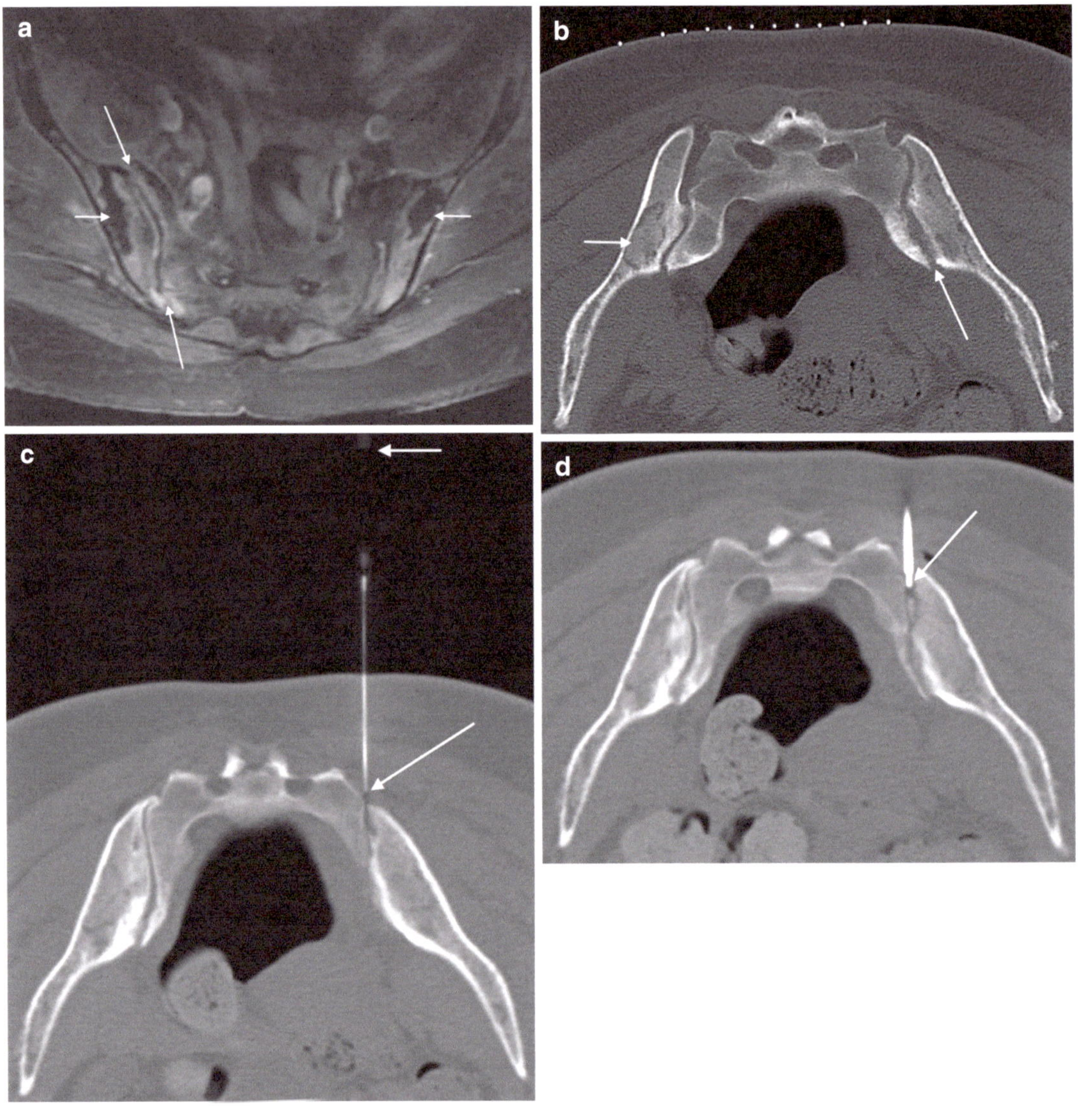

Fig. 7.16 A 51-year-old female with lower low back pain. Fat-suppressed contrast-enhanced T1-weighted axial image (**a**) shows focal enhancement surrounding the right sacroiliac joint (*large arrows*) as well as iliac crest enhancement surrounding non-enhancing hypointense lesions (*small arrows*). Axial CT image (**b**) with skin grid in place shows an expanded sacroiliac joint with focal surrounding erosion (*large arrow*) and a sclerotic focus within the iliac bone (*small arrow*). Axial CT image (**c**) shows an 18 gauge spinal needle being advanced into the posterior aspect of the sacroiliac joint (*large arrow*). After several aspirations with the 18 gauge needle, a 20 gauge needle (*large arrow*) is then used to exchange for a coaxial bone biopsy system. Axial CT image (**d**) shows the use of a coaxial bone biopsy needle (*arrow*) to obtain specimens from the sacroiliac joint.

7.8.1.4 Fluoroscopic Guidance

Fluoroscopic guidance can be used to provide prompt access to the sacroiliac joint space using a posterior-oblique approach (Hansford and Stacy 2012). With the patient prone, a contralateral oblique approach aligns the inferior joint space (Fig. 7.7). The joint is accessed taking care not to traverse the anterior border which would place the adjacent neurovascular structures in jeopardy. The extent and depth of needle insertion are monitored with frontal, lateral, and contralateral oblique projections. Single-needle or coaxial approaches with a guide needle/cannula and smaller gauge aspiration needles can be used to attempt to obtain fluid from the joint. As the majority of these biopsy procedures are being performed to evaluate for infection, additional coaxial passes with bone biopsy needles, angling them toward the osseous borders, may help to yield tissue. The number of passes that can be made with these approaches will be limited by the final location of the biopsy needle tip, which should be kept away from the anterior aspect of the joint space. Usually, sufficient aspirated material or tissue can be obtained from the posterior aspect of the joint. As with disk biopsy, performing joint aspiration biopsies prior to the initiation of antibiotic therapy will help to increase the likelihood of identifying the offending microorganism.

Image-guided percutaneous sacral biopsy: step by step

- Request for biopsy
  - Images reviewed
  - History and labs reviewed
  - Assess for coagulopathy, anticoagulants
  - Anesthesia required?
- Speak to the requesting clinician
- Speak to the patient
- Informed consent
- Position patient on scanner table
- Scout and preliminary imaging with skin grid
- Mark, prep, and drape
- Local and deep/periosteal anesthesia with spinal needle
- Small cross hair skin incision
- Biopsy needle
  - Fine-needle aspiration first for soft tissue lesions
  - Core lesion
  - Marrow aspirate
- Remove device
- Local compression for hemostasis
- Recover patient
- Follow up on biopsy results

7.9 Post-Procedure Care

All biopsy specimens are placed in the appropriate pre-labeled containers. Any special transport media, orders, or processes that are required for a given specimen would hopefully have already been discussed with the pathologist. The appropriate requisitions should be properly and thoroughly completed – good clinical history helps not only the radiologist but also the pathologist and the microbiologist. All specimens should be immediately transported to their respective destinations by individuals who understand where to bring them and to document that they were received. A significant effort has gone into your biopsy procedure, and your patient has undergone some risk in the process – do not treat the specimen handling and transport process nonchalantly. Two of the reasons for a nondiagnostic biopsy are poor specimen handling and lost specimens. Treat specimen handling and specimen transport with the same importance as every other step of the biopsy process, and you will avoid these humiliating and humbling scenarios.

Key Review Points

1. The sacrum is a complex anatomic structure.
2. Common sacral lesions include metastases and myeloma.
3. Because of its size and location, the sacrum is easy to access from a posterior approach with CT guidance.
4. Short-axis technique with or without oblique angulation is a common approach to the sacrum.
5. The sacroiliac joint may be aspirated and biopsied using fluoroscopic guidance.
6. A unilateral sacroiliac joint destructive inflammatory process may be due to infection, and an image-guided percutaneous biopsy may be required.

References

Ayala AG, Ro JY, Fanning CV, Flores JP, Yasko AW. Core needle biopsy and fine needle aspiration in the diagnosis of bone and soft tissue lesions. Hematol Oncol Clin North Am. 1995;9:633–651.

Carberry GA, Lubner MG, Wells SA, Hinshaw JL. Percutaneous biopsy in the abdomen and pelvis: a step-by-step approach. Abdom Radiol. 2016;41(4):720–42.

Carrafiello G, Fontana F, Mangini M, Ierardi AM, Cotta E, Floridi C, Piacentino F, Fugazzola C. Initial experience with percutaneous biopsies of bone lesions using

XperGuide Cone-Beam CT (CBCT): technical note. Radiol Med. 2012;117:1386–97.
Carrino JA, Campbell Jr PD, Lin DC, Morrison WB, Schweitzer ME, Flanders AE, Eng J, Vaccaro AR. Effect of spinal segment variants on numbering vertebral levels at lumbar MR imaging. Radiology. 2011;259:196–202.
Diel J, Ortiz O, Katz D, Losada R, Price DB, Hayt MW, Katz DS. The sacrum: pathologic spectrum, multimodality imaging and subspecialty approach. Radiographics. 2001;21:83–104.
Geremia GK, Charletta DA, Granato DB, Raju S. Biopsy of vertebral and paravertebral structures with a new coaxial needle system. AJNR Am J Neuroradiol. 1992;13:169–171.
Hansford B, Stacy G. Musculoskeletal aspiration procedures. Semin Intervent Radiol. 2012;29:270–85.
Huang AJ, Ambrose J, Halpern EF, Rosenthal DI. Incidence of delayed complications following percutaneous CT-guided biopsy of bone and soft tissue lesions of the spine and extremities: a 2-Year prospective study and analysis of risk factors. Skeletal Radiol. 2012;42:61–8.
Lin HM, Learch TJ, White EA, Gottsegen CJ. Emergency joint aspiration: a guide for radiologists on call. Radiographics. 2009;29:1139–58.
Mankin HJ, Mankin CJ, Simon MA. The hazards of the biopsy, revisited. Members of the Musculoskeletal Tumor Society. J Bone Joint Surg Am. 1996;78:656–663.
Monfardini L, Preda L, Aurilio G, Rizzo S, Bagnardi V, Renne G, Maccagnoni S, Vigna PD, Davide D, Bellomi M. Ct-guided bone biopsy in cancer patients with suspected bone metastases: retrospective review of 308 procedures. Radiol Med. 2014;119:852–60.
Murphy DT, Korzan JR, Quellette HA, Liu DM, Clarkson PW, Munk PL. Driven around the bend: novel use of a curved steerable needle. Cardiovasc Intervent Radiol. 2012;36:531–5.
Ortiz AO, Zoarski G, Brook A. Image-guided percutaneous spine biopsy. In Mathis JM, Golovac S, eds. Image-Guided Spine Interventions. 2nd ed. New York: Springer; 2010:75–106.
Rajeswaran G, Malik Q, Saifuddin A. Image-guided percutaneous spinal biopsy. Skeletal Radiol. 2013;42:3–18.
Sudhir G, Kalra KL, Acharya S, Chahal R. Sacral insufficiency fractures mimicking lumbar spine pathology. Asian Spine J. 2016;10:558–64.
Settle WJ, Ebraheim NA, Coombs R, Saunders RC, Jackson WT. CT-guided biopsy of metastatic sacral tumors. Orthopedics. 1990;13:753–8.

Rib Biopsy

8

A. Orlando Ortiz and Michael K. Brooks

Learning Objectives

1. To review the radiologic anatomy that is pertinent toward the safe performance of a rib biopsy
2. To review the indications and contraindications for performing a rib biopsy
3. To learn image-guided percutaneous rib biopsy approaches and techniques

8.1 Introduction

Rib biopsies are performed to identify the etiology of a rib lesion so as to determine if a lesion is malignant or benign. Metastatic disease involves the ribs in approximately 16% of patients with metastatic cancer (De Maesenner et al. 2004). The likelihood that even a solitary rib lesion is a metastasis is high; if the patient does not have a preexisting neoplasm, one series showed an incidence of metastatic foci in 28% of patients, and if the patient has a preexisting extra-skeletal malignancy, another series showed an incidence of metastatic foci in 41% (Baxter et al. 1995; De Maeseneer et al. 2004). The benign spectrum of rib lesions includes healing rib fractures and benign neoplasms such as fibrous dysplasia or hemangioma.

Image-guided percutaneous rib biopsies are infrequently performed procedures. This contributes to the challenging nature of this procedure. The procedure is made more difficult due to patient factors such as inconsistent breathing and the technical challenges related to imaging a curvilinear structure that moves in and out of the imaging plane. Furthermore, the rib is a small structure, in terms of diameter, with a small surface area and with a slick, mobile, hard cortical surface. The rib appears even more diminutive in contrast to its neighboring lung field. Image-guided percutaneous rib biopsies are performed by different radiology subspecialists; hence, an infrequently performed procedure is further diluted among these groups of operators. This creates a relative barrier to developing a consistent approach and technique for addressing this procedure when requested and when clinically indicated. Despite these challenges, given a sound appreciation of these anatomic and technical constraints, a rib biopsy can be performed, safely and efficiently, with a high diagnostic yield.

> The curved orientation of the ribs and their proximity to the lungs makes the rib a challenging structure to biopsy.

8.2 Anatomic Considerations

With a few exceptions, 12 ribs are present on each side of the thoracic cage. A minority of individuals will have either 11 or 13 ribs, and when this occurs, care should be taken in analyzing for

A.O. Ortiz, *Image-Guided Percutaneous Spine Biopsy*, DOI 10.1007/978-3-319-43326-4_8

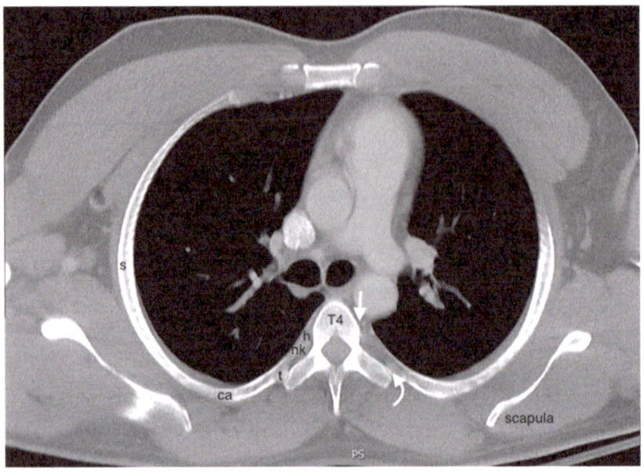

Fig. 8.1 Anatomy of a true rib. Axial CT image reconstructed in the oblique axial plane at the T4 level shows the anatomic parts of a single (fourth) rib. The rib head (*h*) articulates with the vertebral body at the costovertebral joint (*arrow*) and the rib tubercle (*r*) articulates with the vertebral transverse process at the costotransverse joint (*curved arrow*). The neck of the rib (*nk*) is located between the head of the rib and the tubercle. The shaft (*s*) or body is the longest part of the rib. The posterior curve of the rib is referred to as the costal angle (*ca*). Note that at the level of the upper thoracic spine, the scapula may limit access to the lateral rib from a posterior approach

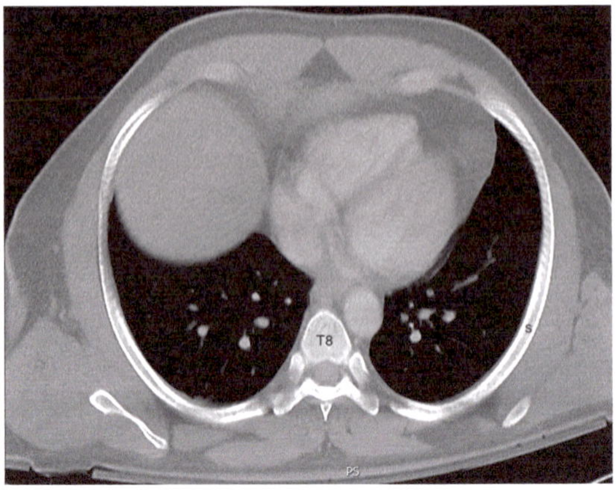

Fig. 8.2 Anatomy of a false rib. Axial CT image reconstructed in the oblique axial plane at the T8 level shows the anatomic parts of the eighth rib. These are identical to those of the true rib, but there is no direct articulation with the sternum. The shaft(*s*) is well seen

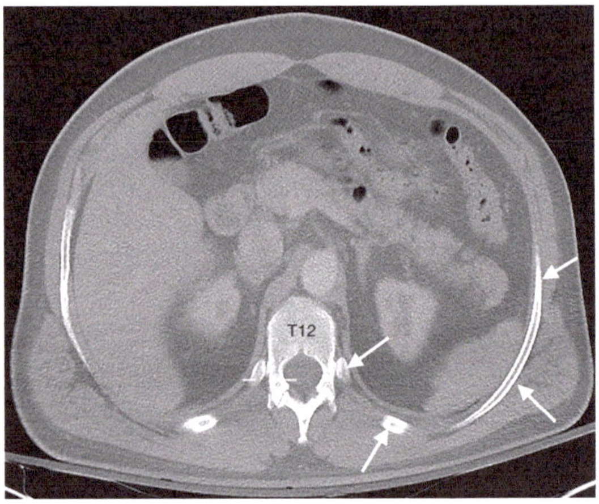

Fig. 8.3 Anatomy of a floating rib. Axial CT image reconstructed in the oblique axial plane at the T12 level shows segmental visualization of the 12th rib (*arrows*)

the presence of transitional vertebrae. The ribs form a rib cage that surrounds the thoracic cavity, including the lungs and pleural cavity. Adjoining ribs are connected by intercostal muscles and fascia. The first seven ribs are directly connected via the costal cartilages with the sternum and are referred to as true ribs (Clemente 1997). The first and second ribs are the most curved, with the second rib being longer than the first. The 8–12th ribs are indirectly connected to the sternum. Ribs number 8, 9, and 10 are continuous with costal cartilages and are referred to as false ribs. Ribs 11 and 12 terminate in the lateral soft tissues of the trunk and are referred to as floating ribs. The ribs are curvilinear tubular structures that have a downward angulation from posterior, near the spine, to anterior. Thus, on conventional axial CT images, the ribs are viewed segmentally and sequentially; the anterior portions of ribs are seen lower down on more caudal images. To study them on an axial data set requires significant scrolling through the images. An alternative technique that can be used to try to visualize a rib in its entirety is to reformat the ribs with obliquely angled images (Figs. 8.1, 8.2, and 8.3). A sagittal or coronal cross section of a rib will show that the rib consists of a semiround cortical surface which surrounds a narrow marrow containing cavity (Fig. 8.4).

A typical rib consists of a rib head, neck, tubercle, and body or shaft (Figs. 8.1, 8.2, and 8.3). The 10–12th ribs possess only a single articular facet on the rib head as compared to the remaining ribs which have two articular facets on the rib head. The rib head articulates with the vertebral body at the costovertebral junction or joint.

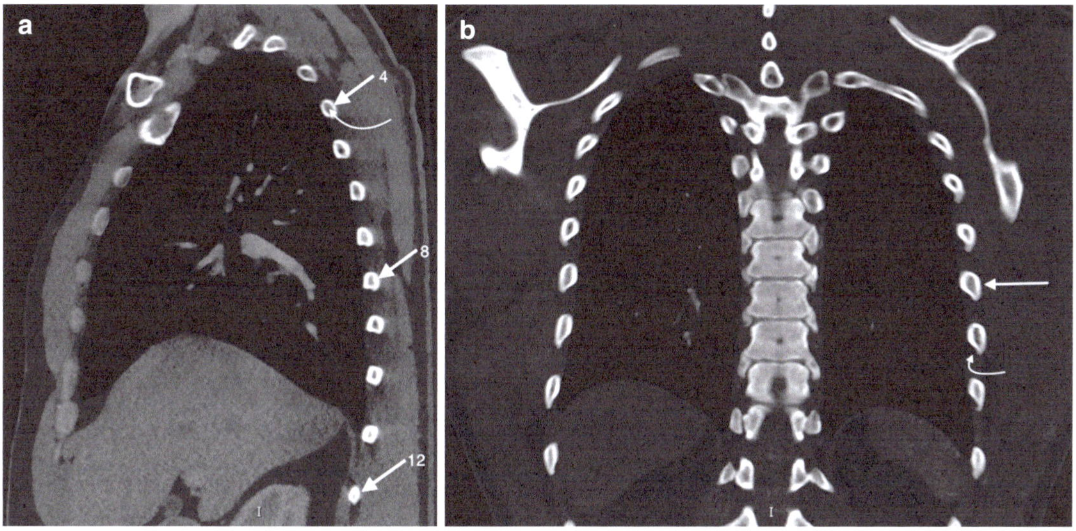

Fig. 8.4 CT cross-sectional appearance of the rib shaft. Reformatted sagittal CT image (**a**) shows sagittal cross sections of the ribs (*arrows*). The margin of the rib is comprised of an oval-shaped thick cortical layer of bone that surrounds a small marrow cavity (*curved arrow*). Coronal reformatted CT image (**b**) shows the small cross-sectional area (*arrow*) of each rib and the costal groove (*curved arrow*) of the rib

The rib tubercle, which also has an articular facet, articulates with the vertebral transverse process at the costotransverse junction or joint. The neck or crest of the rib is located between the head of the rib and the tubercle. The shaft or body of the rib commences at the tubercle just beyond the neck and curves around the lateral margin of the thoracic cavity to terminate in the sternal extremity. The initial angle of curvature of the rib is called the costal angle. The undersurface of the rib contains the costal groove. The intercostal vein, artery, and nerve are found underneath the costal groove.

The critical structures that must be considered when performing a rib biopsy are the lungs and the intercostal arteries and veins (Fig. 8.5). The lungs are mostly surrounded by the intercostal muscles. A needle that deflects off of the rounded surface of the rib could readily pass through the very short distance between the muscle and the pleural surface of the lung. Lytic rib lesions can also expose the lung to potential injury during a biopsy procedure. Care must also be exercised when advancing a needle near the inferior or costal groove of the rib as the intercostal neurovascular structures are found in this location. When

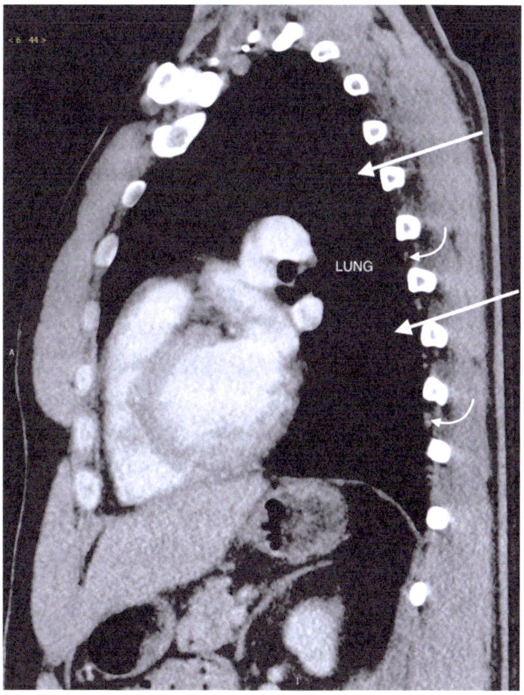

Fig. 8.5 Critical structures to consider when performing a rib biopsy. Sagittal reformation in soft tissue algorithm from a contrast-enhanced chest CT study shows the paired intercostal artery and vein (*curved arrows*) traveling underneath each respective rib. The ribs only protect a small area of lung (*arrows*)

deciding upon the feasibility of an image-guided percutaneous rib biopsy procedure, the operator must always factor these critical structures into their approach.

Critical Structures: Rib Biopsy

Lung
Intercostal vessels

8.3 Indications

Image-guided percutaneous rib biopsy is indicated for the evaluation of pathologic lesions that are located within one or more ribs (Table 8.1) (Edelstein et al. 1985; Faro et al. 1993). The most common indication for performing a rib biopsy is the evaluation of a suspected neoplastic process (Guttentag and Salwen 1999; De Maeseneer et al. 2004). Neoplastic processes within the ribs are usually secondary lesions associated with metastatic disease (Jakanani and Saifuddin 2013; Cronin et al. 2009). Direct extension from a pulmonary malignancy is another possible etiology for a rib lesion. Primary tumors within a rib, though extremely rare, may also require a biopsy procedure (Kim et al. 2008). It is very important to review all of the patient's imaging studies prior to performing a rib biopsy. The remainder of the body should be studied in order to assess for the presence of other lesions which can be more safely sampled. Since the majority of patients with metastatic disease often have lesions located elsewhere within their bodies, it is more likely than not that these other sites are in better locations for sampling. This accounts for the relatively low frequency of rib biopsy procedures. Rib biopsy procedures are performed when one or more rib lesions are detected on radiologic imaging studies in a patient with either one or more known primary tumors or with no prior history of cancer. The patient's prior imaging studies (chest radiograph, chest CT, or skeletal scintigraphy) may show only rib lesions, hence the impetus to perform a biopsy procedure in order to determine subsequent patient management, especially in patients with preexisting cancer.

Table 8.1 Indications for image-guided percutaneous rib biopsy

Neoplasm
1. Solitary rib lesion
Metastatic disease
Adult: Lung, breast, thyroid, kidney, prostate, liver Child: Ewing's sarcoma, neuroblastoma
Contiguous spread of lung or pleural-based tumor
Primary osseous neoplasm
Adult: Chondrosarcoma, myeloma, giant cell tumor Child: Ewing's sarcoma, osteosarcoma
Primary benign tumor
Fibrous dysplasia, hemangioma, Langerhans cell histiocytosis, osteoid osteoma, osteoblastoma, osteochondroma, enchondroma, chondromyxoid fibroma, aneurysmal bone cyst
2. Multiple rib lesions
Metastatic disease
Multiple myeloma
3. Other
Pathologic rib fracture vs. benign rib fracture
Infection: tuberculosis, actinomycosis, bacterial infection

Table 8.2 Contraindications to image-guided percutaneous rib biopsy

Absolute
Uncorrected coagulopathy
Relative
Patient factors
Combative or uncooperative patient
Clinically unstable patient
Factors related to the lesion in question
Probable benign lesion
Very small lesions (<5 mm in diameter)
Lesion in other location that is safer to biopsy

8.3.1 Contraindications

The major contraindication to performing a rib biopsy is uncorrected coagulopathy (Table 8.2). Because of the challenging nature of rib biopsy procedures, they should not be performed on

Table 8.3 Percutaneous rib biopsy – potential risks and complications

Tissue injury
Pneumothorax
Vascular injury
Hemorrhage
Infection
Inappropriate needle placement
Wrong level
Inadequate tissue sampling
Technical failure – biopsy system failure, lost specimen
Radiation exposure
Anesthesia complications
Aspiration, airway compromise, respiratory depression

uncooperative or unstable patients. For lesions that show a benign radiographic appearance, then it might be reasonable to delay if not avoid the rib biopsy procedure. A nondiagnostic biopsy result may be observed when performing biopsies on benign lesions (Omura et al. 2011). In this situation, the patient's prior radiologic studies should be reviewed to determine if the lesion has always been within the rib and if it is stable in appearance. Alternatively, the rib lesion can be followed at predetermined intervals with imaging surveillance.

8.4 Risks and Complications Associated with Rib Biopsy and How to Minimize Them

The risks and complications that are associated with image-guided percutaneous rib biopsy are related to potential injury to nearby critical structures (Table 8.3). The proximity of the rib to the lung puts the latter organ at risk for pneumothorax during the biopsy procedure. Fortunately, the occurrence of this complication is rare, and the likelihood of pneumothorax is further decreased by using CT-guidance and tangential coaxial biopsy techniques. The other complication that may occur is vascular injury, particularly to the intercostal vessels. This can result in hemorrhage with hematoma formation.

The risks of image-guided percutaneous rib biopsy can be decreased by using CT-guidance and coaxial biopsy techniques which utilize tangential approaches.

8.5 Imaging Guidance

CT is the most common modality that is used to perform image-guided percutaneous rib biopsy (Jelinek et al. 2002; Hwang et al. 2011). The addition of CT fluoroscopy further improves the efficiency of the rib biopsy procedure. The ability of CT to delineate osseous structures such as the rib makes CT an ideal modality for this procedure. CT provides optimal contrast resolution and is able to readily define the lung fields and intercostal soft tissues. The use of thin section acquisition techniques with immediate reconstruction also contributes to the usefulness of this modality for the purposes of performing a rib biopsy.

Large rib lesions with extraosseous soft tissue components have also been biopsied using ultrasound guidance, in a minority of cases (Jakanani and Saifuddin 2013). The probability of a neoplastic rib lesion increases when there is cortical destruction associated with an extraosseous soft tissue mass though infection may also account for these imaging findings (Lee et al. 1993). Additionally, the diagnostic yield of the biopsy procedure increases when there is an extraosseous soft tissue component and decreases with the presence of only an intramedullary rib lesion (Jakanani and Saifuddin 2013). Lesion access and tissue sampling can be challenging in the latter clinical scenario and are not feasible with ultrasound guidance.

8.6 Approaches

Biopsy approaches to the rib are determined by the lesion location and size. It is, therefore, imperative for the operator to review all pertinent pre-procedure imaging examinations in

Table 8.4 Approaches for rib biopsy

Tangential
Needle tip advanced along the long axis of the rib segment
Advantages: The inner and outer rib cortical bone (1) serves as a channel for guiding the biopsy needle's advancement, (2) reduces chances of injuring the lung or intercostal vessels, and (3) can obtain more sample from smaller, non-expansile lesions
Disadvantages: (1) Requires patient cooperation and precise needle placements
Perpendicular
Needle tip advanced vertically into the lesion, perpendicular to short axis of the rib segment
Advantages: (1) Can enter the lesion at its largest diameter and (2) can access lesion at a point of outer rib cortical breakthrough
Disadvantages: (1) Needle tip points directly at the lung – proceed with extreme caution

order to plan the most optimal approach to a rib lesion. The two principle trajectories for rib access are tangential, along the long axis of the rib, and perpendicular (to the rib outer surface – so called short axis) (Table 8.4). The tangential trajectory attempts to obtain a sample without compromising the lung or the vascular pedicle of the rib. This trajectory enables a longer throw of the biopsy needle through the marrow space of the rib. The perpendicular trajectory is direct and has the theoretical potential to puncture the lung or injure the intercostal vessels. This perpendicular trajectory is best reserved for bulky rib lesions or for directly infiltrating lesions from the adjacent pleura or lung (Fig. 8.6). In both of these clinical scenarios, the diameter of the lesion should be large enough to safely accommodate a biopsy needle without injuring the lungs or intercostal vessels.

When considering a rib lesion for biopsy, it is best to think of a single complete rib as a "C"-shaped curvilinear structure that can be divided into three segments or compartments (Fig. 8.7). The anterior portion of the rib comprises the anterior compartment. The side or lateral portion of the rib is the lateral compartment, and the posterior portion of the rib comprises the posterior compartment. The anterior and posterior compartments include curved components, with the anterior component gradually curved (second curve) and the posterior component more steeply curved (first or costal angle). These compartments and the orientations of the individual rib are important because they influence the patient position, the approach, and the direction of the needle trajectory for tangential rib biopsies (Table 8.5).

1. A patient with an anterior compartment rib lesion can be placed in the supine position (Figs. 8.8 and 8.9). The approach to the lesion is anterior. The tangential direction of the needle tip is lateral (away from the sternum) for the more medial anterior rib lesions and vertical and downward for the lateral anterior lesions that lie within the gentle second curve of the anterior compartment.
2. A patient with a lateral compartment rib lesion can be placed in the supine position with the arms up and away from the sides of the rib cage. The approach with the patient in the supine position is anterior (Fig. 8.10). For lower, infrascapular, lateral rib lesions, the patient can also be placed in the prone or prone oblique position (the scapula may limit posterior approaches to a lateral rib compartment lesion within the upper thoracic rib cage). The approach with the patient prone is posterior. The vector for the direction of the tangential needle trajectory is vertical and downward.
3. A patient with a posterior compartment rib lesion is placed in the prone position (Figs. 8.11, 8.12, 8.13, and 8.14). If the patient's condition does not permit this position, then they can be placed in the prone oblique or lateral decubitus position. The approach is posterior. The direction of the tangential needle trajectory depends upon whether the lesion is posterior and medial (within the upward portion (relative to the back) of the steep first curvature or costal angle of the rib) or posterior and lateral (within the downward portion (relative to the back) of the first or costal angle of the rib). Posterior medial rib lesions can be biopsied with a medially directed (toward

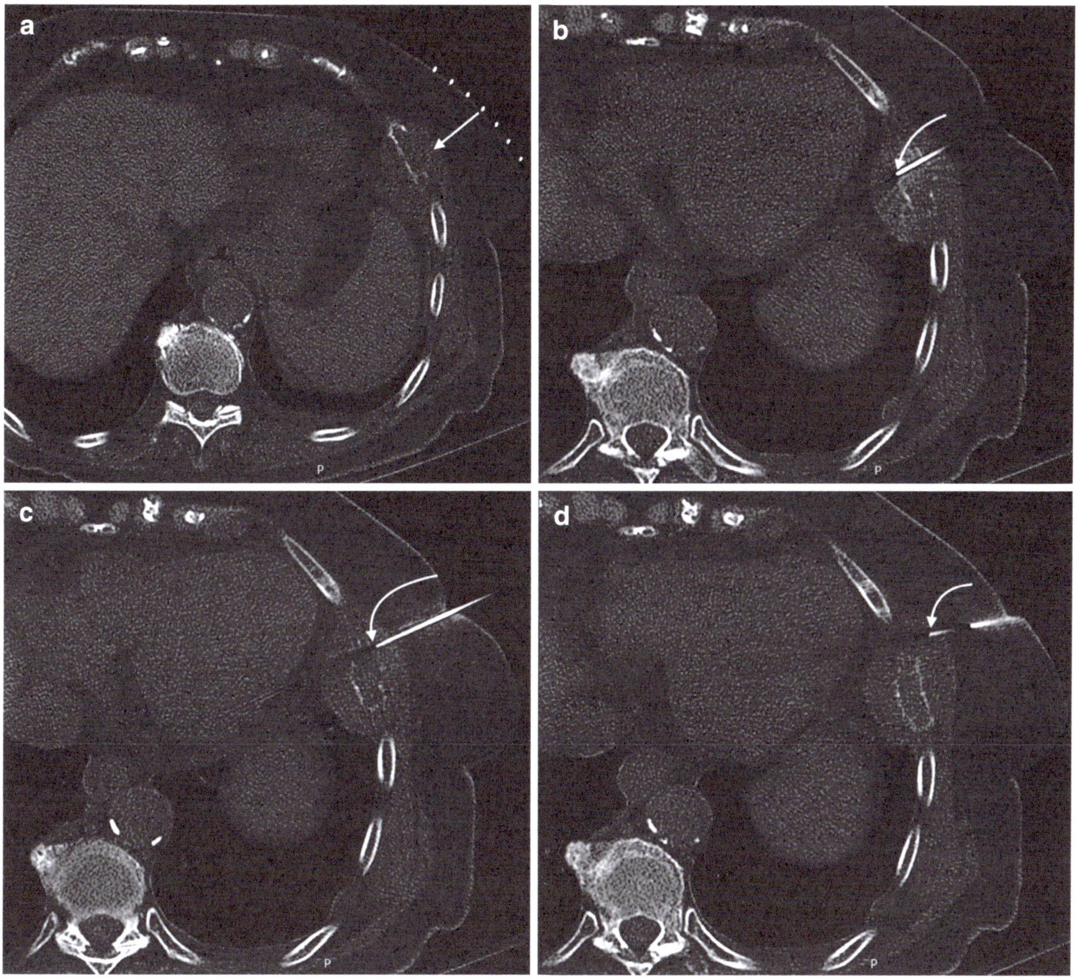

Fig. 8.6 A 76-year-old female with a history of adenoid cystic carcinoma of the submandibular gland; chest CT shows anterior sixth rib mass. Axial CT image (**a**) from a biopsy procedure shows a skin grid in place and a large expansile anterior rib lesion (*arrow*) with cortical expansion and destruction and a prominent extraosseous soft tissue component. Axial CT image (**b**) shows tip of 19 gauge guide needle (*arrow*) within the lesion; this was inserted using a perpendicular approach. An FNA procedure (not shown) was performed. Axial CT image (**c**) shows coaxial use of a 20 gauge cutting needle (*arrow*) used to sample the lesion. Axial CT image (**d**) shows coaxial use of the 20 gauge cutting needle to obtain another sample

the spine) needle trajectory. Posterior lateral rib lesions can be biopsied with a laterally directed (away from the spine) needle trajectory.

It is imperative for the operator to review all pertinent pre-procedure imaging examinations in order to plan the most optimal approach to a rib lesion.

8.7 The Rib Biopsy Procedure

8.7.1 General Considerations

8.7.1.1 Patient Factors

Image-guided percutaneous rib biopsy procedures should only be performed on cooperative patients. Image-guided percutaneous rib biopsy can be performed with the patient in the prone, prone oblique, or supine position. Some patients are

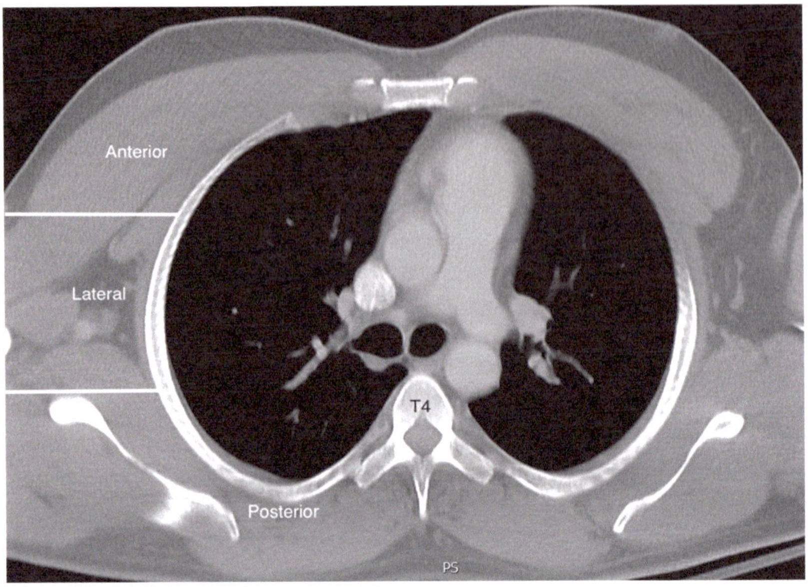

Fig. 8.7 The rib compartments or sections (anterior, lateral, posterior) as shown on reformatted oblique axial CT image at the T4 level. The location of a lesion within one of these compartments will have a significant influence on the procedure

Table 8.5 Compartment approach to rib biopsy

Compartment	Patient position	Approach	Specific lesion location	Tangential direction
Anterior	Supine	Anterior	Medial	Lateral
			Lateral	Downward
Lateral	Supine	Anterior	–	Downward
	Prone/oblique	Posterior	–	Downward
Posterior	Prone	Posterior	Medial	Medial/downward
			Lateral	Lateral/downward

unable to maintain certain positions due to pain or breathing issues. The patient should be evaluated to ascertain what position they can maintain for the anticipated procedure. The patient's medical and medication history, pertinent laboratory values, allergies, imaging studies, and NPO status should be reviewed. An informed consent is obtained from the patient. The risks and benefits of the rib biopsy procedure, and alternatives to this procedure including open biopsy and continued medical surveillance, should be discussed with the patient (Ray-Coquard et al. 2003). The patient will want to know what to expect during and after the procedure, and this should be explained to them. Additionally, let the patient know that the post-procedure recovery instructions will be reviewed with them after the procedure just prior to discharge.

8.7.1.2 Staff Factors

Since a fair number of rib biopsies are performed with fine needle aspiration techniques, it is important to prearrange the procedure so that a pathologist or cytotechnologist is present at the time of the procedure, especially when sampling a rib lesion with an extraosseous soft tissue component. Strict patient and procedure verification protocols are adhered to. The qualified and trained staff should be made aware that a rib biopsy procedure will be performed and of the intended side and location of the biopsy procedure. The patient position should be determined before the procedure; this helps the CT technologist program the patient position correctly into the CT protocol, such that the right and left side of the patient are correctly labeled on all acquired images. Careful patient transport and positioning on to the procedure table needs to be emphasized with the procedure team,

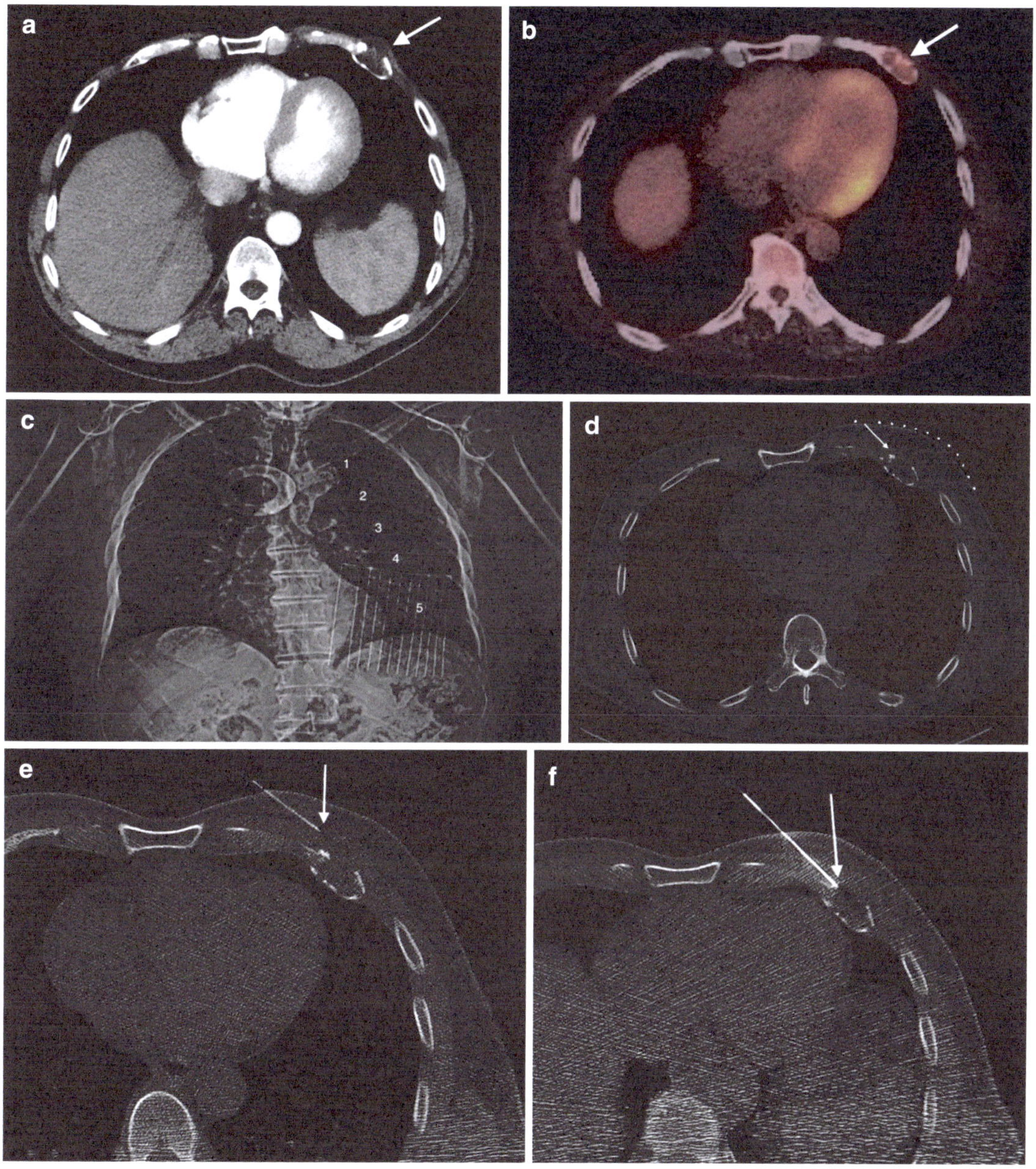

Fig. 8.8 A 70-year-old male with a palpable chest wall mass. Contrast-enhanced axial image (**a**) from chest CT study shows an expansile left anterior fifth rib lesion with anterior cortical breakthrough and a small extraosseous soft tissue component. Fused axial image (**b**) from a PET CT study shows avid FDG uptake within the lesion (*arrow*). Scout frontal CT image (**c**) with skin grid in place shows the relative location of the left anterior sixth rib (anterior ribs #1 through #5 are numbered). Axial CT image (**d**) with skin grid in place shows the lateral and downward trajectory (*arrow*) that can be used with an anterior approach to an anterior rib lesion with the patient in the supine position. Axial CT image (**e**) shows use of a 22 gauge needle (*arrow*) used to administer local anesthesia. Axial CT image (**f**) shows the insertion of a 17 gauge introducer or guide needle (*arrow*) into the margin of the lesion using a medial tangential approach. Axial CT image (**g**) shows the coaxial insertion of an 18 gauge cutting needle (*arrow*) for soft tissue core biopsy (*curved arrow*). Axial CT image (**h**) shows angulation of the guide needle with entry of the core biopsy needle (*arrow*) into the greatest span or diameter of the lesion; this case demonstrates the value of a tangential approach in this case for maximizing specimen yield. Six soft tissue cores were obtained in this pathology-proven case of chondrosarcoma

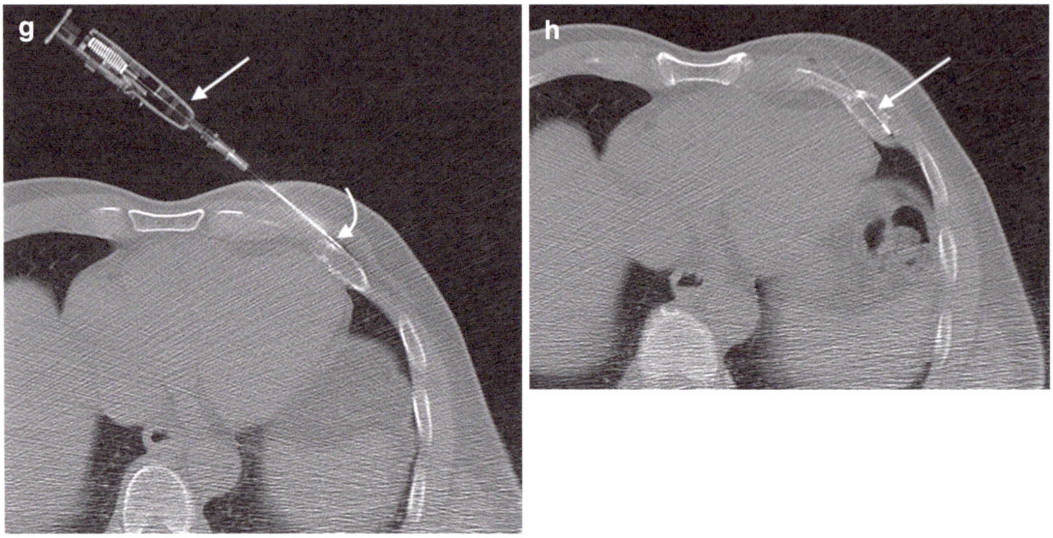

Fig. 8.8 (continued)

especially in patients who are already in severe pain due to pathologic rib fractures. Monitoring equipment can be expeditiously placed on the patient so that they can be given intravenous pain medication if necessary. Remind the staff to place the electrocardiogram leads away from the biopsy area in order to maintain a sterile field and to avoid distracting CT image artifacts during the biopsy procedure.

8.7.1.3 Anesthesia

Rib biopsies can be performed with a local anesthetic agent only, with intravenous sedation and analgesia, or with intravenous or general anesthesia. Consultation with an anesthesiologist is necessary and helpful when using deeper forms of sedation. The level of anesthesia will be primarily driven by the patient and their medical condition. The patient is actively monitored throughout the procedure with respect to vital signs, oxygen saturation, and comfort level.

8.7.2 Patient Preparation

After the patient is positioned, a time-out protocol should be exercised with the staff and the patient prior to initiating the procedure. This will decrease the likelihood of right-left confusion that sometimes occurs when patients are placed in positions other than the supine position. It confirms with all present in the procedure suite that the skin grid is being placed on the correct side of the body. After placement of the skin grid, a preliminary axial CT study is obtained through the area of interest. The image data set is usually acquired with bone window algorithm, but this is up to the operator's discretion based upon the type of lesion that is being biopsied. For example, the operator may choose to use soft tissue algorithm for a large invasive pleural-parenchymal process. It is best to perform the procedure without specific patient breathing instructions; in other words, the procedure should be performed with the patient breathing quietly. Once the images are reviewed and the approach and trajectory determined, the skin entry site is marked using the skin grid. The grid is removed and the skin is prepped and draped. The patient can start to receive intravenous sedation and/or analgesia as necessary.

8.7.3 Technique

8.7.3.1 CT Guidance

There are two types of rib lesions that tend to present for biopsy: (1) expansile rib lesions with cortical erosion or destruction and an associated soft tissue mass and (2) focal rib lesions with rib cortex intact.

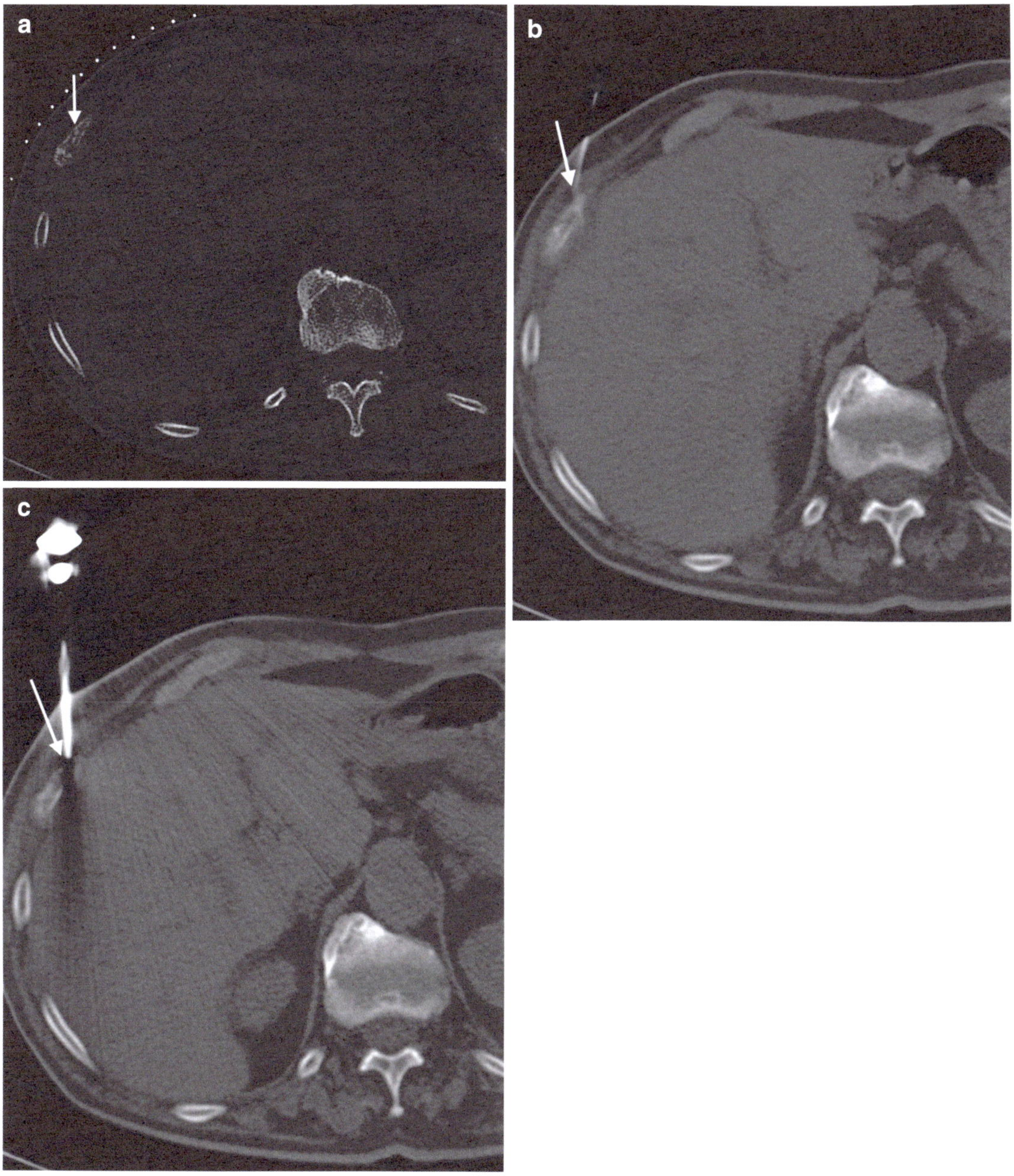

Fig. 8.9 An 81-year-old male with a lung lesion and anterior eighth rib lesion on chest CT. Axial CT image (**a**) with skin grid in place shows small mixed sclerotic lesion (*arrow*) within the anterior rib. Axial CT image (**b**) shows use of a 22 gauge needle (*arrow*) to administer a local anesthetic agent. Axial CT image (**c**) shows coaxial insertion of a 12 gauge bone biopsy needle, with a downward trajectory (*arrow*) into the lesion. Only one bone core was obtained, but this showed the presence of poorly differentiated carcinoma from a primary lung tumor

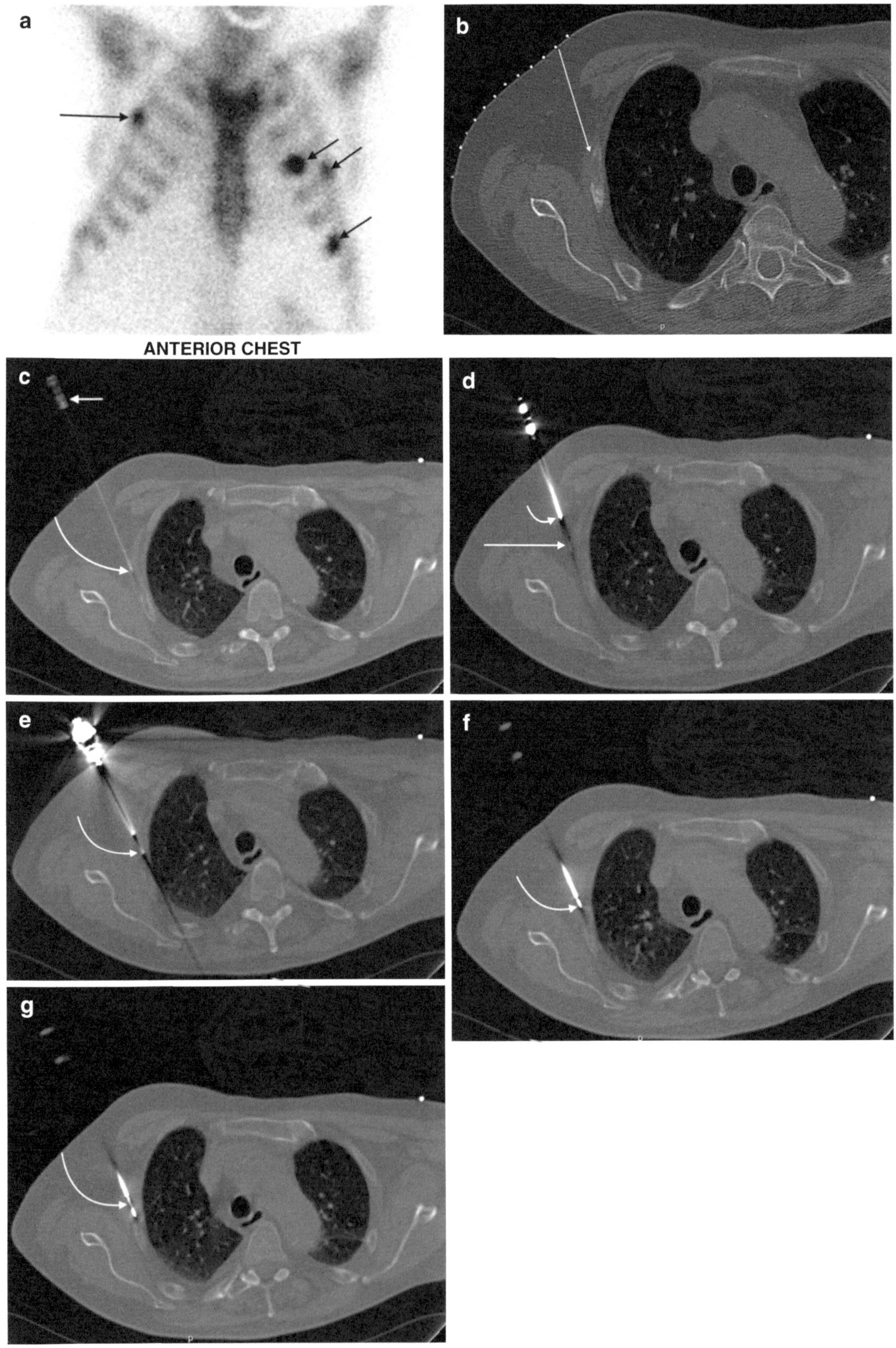
a
b
ANTERIOR CHEST
c
d
e
f
g

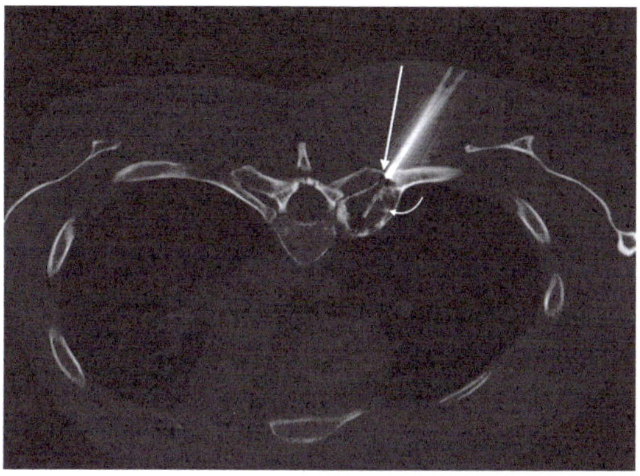

Fig. 8.11 A 34-year-old male with upper back pain. Axial CT image from a rib biopsy procedure, with the patient in the prone position, shows coaxial placement of a guide needle (*arrow*) at the notch between the transverse process and rib; this is a posterior approach with a medial trajectory for this medial lesion. A trephine bone biopsy needle is advanced into this expansile lytic lesion within the rib head and neck that contains small calcific foci (*curved arrow*). The pathologic diagnosis was chondrosarcoma

Coaxial technique is used with active imaging surveillance for all needle exchanges, placements, and advancements (Table 8.6) (Geremia et al. 1992). The skin entry site should be adequately anesthetized. Additionally, deeper administration of the anesthetic agent should be performed with imaging guidance down to the level of the lesion or rib margin. In some patients, this may be all that is necessary in order to maintain patient comfort for the biopsy procedure, especially if sampling a large soft tissue rib lesion. A guide needle, anywhere from 10 to 19 gauge size depending upon the lesion that is to be sampled, is advanced under imaging guidance to the margin of the lesion or rib, using a tangential needle orientation, whenever possible. The operator may elect to use a perpendicular needle orientation for a large expansile rib lesion with a large soft tissue component or for a pulmonary or pleural neoplasm that directly invades the rib. There are two types of rib lesions that tend to present for biopsy: (1) expansile rib lesions with cortical erosion or destruction and an associated soft tissue mass and (2) focal rib lesions with cortical bone intact.

For expansile rib lesions, the guide needle is advanced to the margin of the lesion. If there is a discrete soft tissue mass, then a fine needle aspiration (FNA) can be performed in an attempt to obtain cellular tissue. Several FNA passes can be made based upon the size of the lesion, the volume of the soft tissue abnormality, and the location of the needle tip relative to the critical structures. The FNA needle can then be exchanged for a soft tissue core biopsy needle. The cutting needle can be advanced into the lesion with imaging guidance. The biopsy chamber of the needle is exposed within the lesion. This may require 1 or 2 cm of exposure of the biopsy chamber within the lesion; the tip of the needle should be monitored as the biopsy chamber is exposed within the lesion. The cutting needle is used to obtain soft tissue cores, three or more if possible, from the lesion. The guide needle can be angled slightly to allow the cutting needle to access additional biopsy tracts within the lesion. The reason for attempting to obtain as much tissue as possible is to improve the likeli-

Fig. 8.10 A 72-year-old male with a history of transitional cell carcinoma of the bladder. Frontal projection (**a**) from a bone scan shows multiple foci of radionuclide uptake with the left ribs (*small arrows*) and the right rib (*large arrow*). Axial CT image (**b**) with a skin grid in place shows a lytic lesion within the right lateral rib compartment as well as an anterior approach with a downward needle trajectory (*arrow*) to the lesion. Axial CT image (**c**) shows the dual use of a 20 gauge guide needle to first administer a local anesthetic agent adjacent to the lesion (*curved arrow*) and then to serve as a guide wire (after removal of the hub (*small arrow*)). Axial CT image (**d**) shows coaxial advancement of a 12 gauge guide cannula and introducer (curved arrow) over the 20 gauge, now hub-less, guide needle (*arrow*). Axial CT image (**e**) shows coaxial insertion of a trephine bone biopsy needle (*arrow*) through the guide cannula and into the lesion. Axial CT image (**f**) shows exchange of the bone biopsy needle, which was used to obtain a bone core and obtain access to the medullary cavity of the rib, for a soft tissue cutting needle (*arrow*). Axial CT image (**g**) shows placement of the cutting chamber of the needle (*arrow*) within the lesion. The pathology showed poorly differentiated carcinoma of urothelial origin

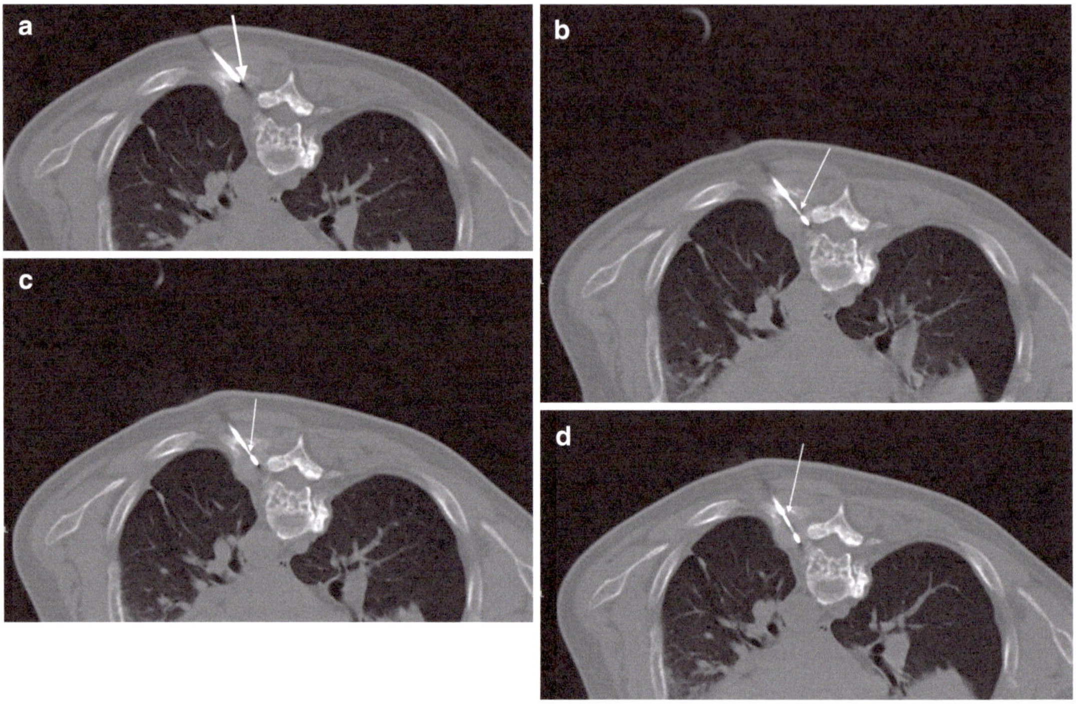

Fig. 8.12 A 66-year-old male with a history of multiple myeloma and new posterior left T6 rib lesion. Axial CT image (**a**) shows placement of a guide needle (*arrow*) at the margin of a large lytic soft tissue mass within the head of the rib. A medial trajectory is used for this posterior approach. Axial CT image (**b**) shows chamber of cutting needle (*arrow*) advanced into the soft tissue mass. Axial CT image (**c**) shows exposure of the cutting chamber (*arrow*) within the lesion. Axial CT image (**d**) shows use of different biopsy trajectory within the lesion (*arrow*). A total of two soft tissue cores were obtained, and the histopathology confirmed the presence of plasma cells and myeloma

hood of a diagnostic biopsy (Puri et al. 2006; Wu et al. 2008).

For intramedullary rib lesions with intact surrounding cortical bone, it is first necessary to access the medullary cavity with the bone needle. Either a bone needle is directly inserted into the cortical bone and this cannula serves as a guide cannula for other biopsy needles or a coaxial system is used to gain entry by advancing a trephine bone needle through a guide cannula (Geremia et al. 1992). Once inside the medullary space of the rib, it may be possible to perform an FNA, depending on the lesion matrix, prior to sequential bone biopsies. FNA will probably not be successful with sclerotic or mixed sclerotic rib lesions, but may yield cellular tissue with lytic rib lesions.

With the use of these biopsy approaches and techniques as well as careful patient selection, it is possible to optimize the diagnostic yield of the procedure. In one series involving 51 patients undergoing rib biopsy, the diagnostic yield was 88% with a diagnostic accuracy of 96%; the 12% rate of nondiagnostic biopsies occurred in rib lesions with no extraosseous component, and these lesions were subsequently demonstrated to be benign (Jakanani and Saifuddin 2013). There were no complications reported in this series of patients. In a smaller series with 11 patients, 10 of the 11 rib biopsies were diagnostic, and an open biopsy was subsequently required in one patient (Hardy et al. 1987). There were no complications in this small group of patients. There are other studies in the literature that include rib biopsies as part of their data on the diagnostic efficacy of musculoskeletal biopsies. One such study included 63 rib lesions within a large series of 800 CT-guided biopsies (Hwang et al. 2011).

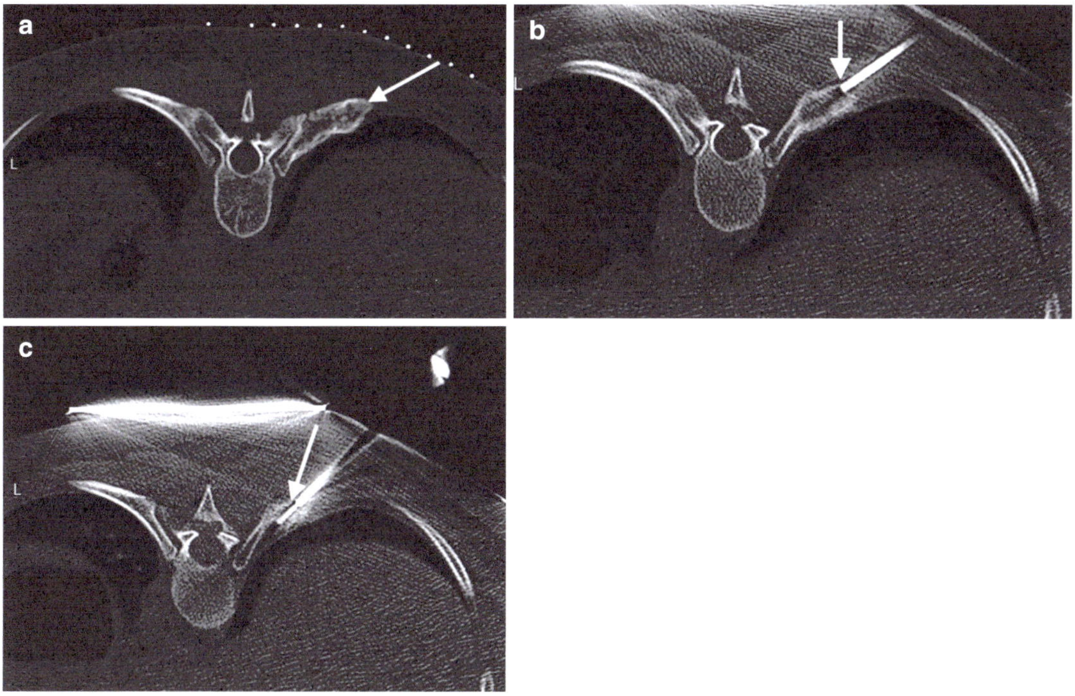

Fig. 8.13 A 34-year-old female with diabetes insipidus, an infiltrative hypothalamic lesion, and a posterior right rib lesion. Axial CT image (**a**) with a skin grid in place shows a posterior approach and medial trajectory (*arrow*) for a slightly expansile right posterior rib lesion; deformity of the posterior rib is noted. Axial CT image (**b**) shows the placement of a guide needle at the margin of the lesion (*arrow*). Axial CT image (**c**) shows coaxial placement of a trephine bone biopsy needle into the lesion. The biopsy showed nonspecific woven bone with remodeling and mild marrow fibrosis. The patient was lost to follow-up; the working differential diagnosis prior to the biopsy included Langerhans cell histiocytosis and sarcoid

The biopsies were diagnostic in 69% and indeterminate in 31% of the overall group of patients. Subsequent clinical follow-up in the indeterminate biopsies showed an eventual diagnosis of malignancy in 39% of this subgroup of cases. Another CT-guided needle biopsy study included 20 cases that were labeled as rib/scapula; the authors gave an overall diagnostic accuracy rate of 90% for the 207 musculoskeletal lesions that were biopsied and reported no complications (Tsukushi et al. 2010).

8.8 Post-procedure Care

In many ways, the post-procedure care for a rib biopsy patient in terms of recovery and pain management is similar to that of a spine biopsy patient with a couple of exceptions. First, given the concern for the possibility of a pneumothorax, a heightened clinical awareness and possible imaging surveillance may be required. Vigilance with respect to respiratory parameters, including respiratory rate, oxygen saturation, or new or increased pain with breathing must be exercised by the recovery room staff (Table 8.7). If there is a clinical concern for a possible breach of the pleural surface at the time of the biopsy, it is possible to obtain a limited CT scan of the chest to determine if there is a small pneumothorax (Fig. 8.14). If there is a pneumothorax, the subsequent clinical management depends on the size and behavior of the pneumothorax. A small pneumothorax can be followed, usually with a chest radiograph at 1 h post-procedure. If the pneumothorax is small and has not increased and the patient is stable, then the patient can be discharged with specific

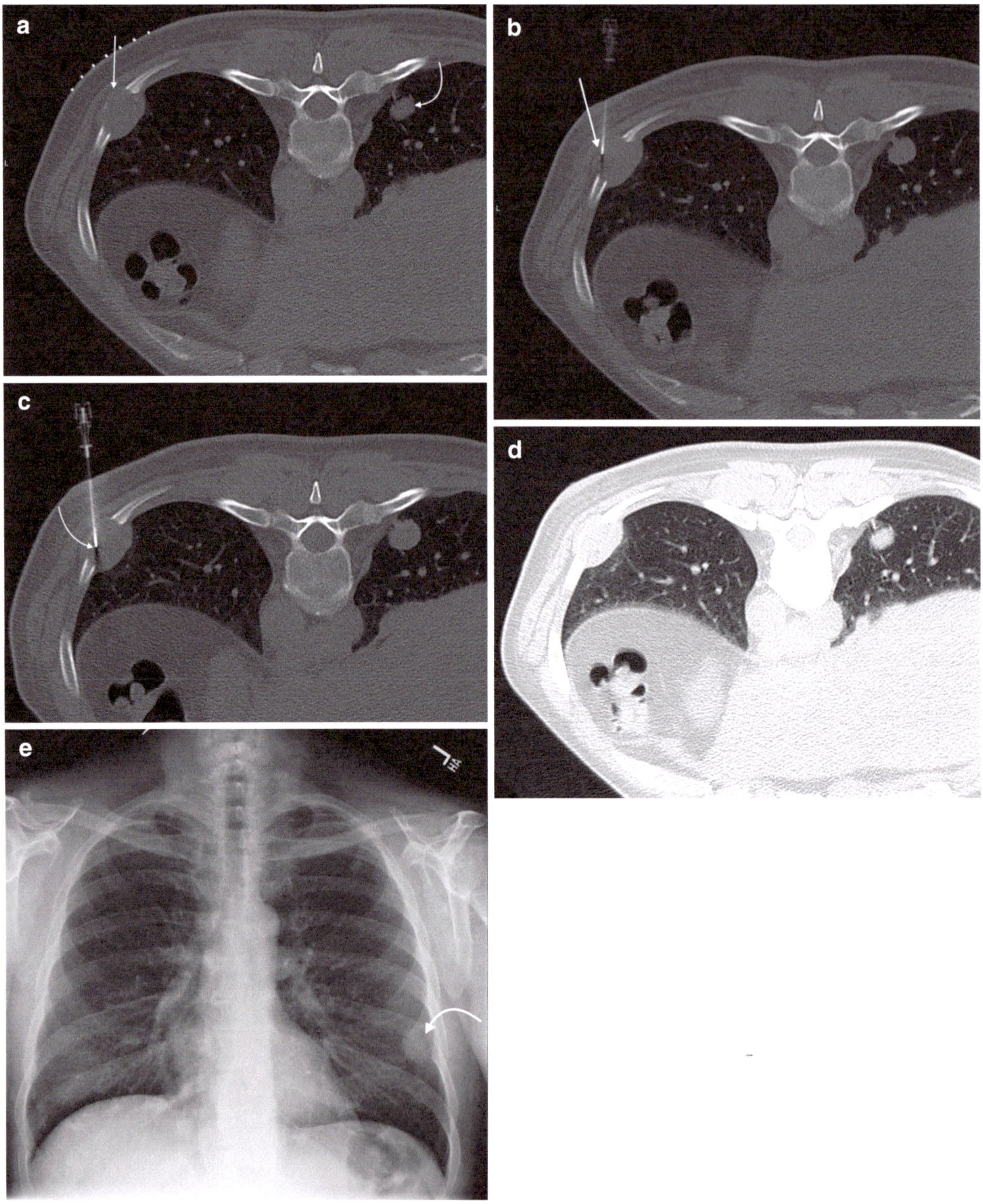

Fig. 8.14 A 53-year-old male with multiple pulmonary nodules and a rib lesion seen on a chest CT. Axial CT image (**a**) with a skin grid in place, and patient in prone position, shows a large expansile soft tissue mass within the left posterior ninth rib (*arrow*). Note the pulmonary mass (*curved arrow*). Since this lesion is located within the lateral aspect of the posterior rib, a lateral and downward needle trajectory is used to sample the lesion with this posterior approach (*arrow*). Axial CT image (**b**) shows placement of a 19-gauge guide needle at the margin of the lesion (*arrow*). Axial CT image (**c**) shows repositioning of the guide needle within the lesion (*arrow*). Axial CT image (**d**) with a lung window, performed due to patient complaints of sudden pain, shows no evidence of pneumothorax. A chest radiograph (**e**) was performed one hour after the rib biopsy procedure and shows no evidence of pneumothorax; the left rib lesion (*curved arrow*) is also seen. Four soft tissue cores were obtained; the histopathology showed small cell lung carcinoma

Table 8.6 CT-guided rib biopsy technique

Anesthetize the skin entry site up to the margin of the lesion or rib
Place the guide needle using its stylet or use coaxial technique
1. Advance guide needle to the margin of the soft tissue lesion
Perform FNA if possible
Perform soft tissue core biopsy
Or
2. Advance guide needle to the margin of the rib
Access rib with bone needle
Perform FNA of medullary compartment if possible
Perform bone biopsy

Table 8.7 Post-procedure care orders

1. Status post (anterior, lateral, or posterior) (right or left) rib biopsy (*circle correct site and side*)
2. Recover patient × 2 h
3. Bedrest × 2 h; may elevate head of bed as tolerated
4. Vital signs every 15 min until discharge
5. Continuous electrocardiogram and pulse oximetry monitoring
6. Check biopsy site for signs of active bleeding, or increasing swelling, with vital signs
7. Notify the doctor immediately for bleeding or swelling at the biopsy site, for increased patient pain, or for patient respiratory distress
8. Encourage oral intake of fluids
9. Patient may eat when recovered from anesthesia or sedation
10. Discontinue intravenous line prior to patient discharge
11. [Portable frontal chest radiograph 1 h after procedure] (*optional order as per operator*)
12. *Optional pain medication orders as per operator*

instructions to return immediately to the hospital if they experience respiratory distress. The presence of an enlarging pneumothorax will require the placement of a chest tube and admission of the patient for continued observation and care. The second difference between rib biopsy and spine biopsy patients with respect to post-procedure care is that the patients who have had anterior or lateral compartment rib biopsies do not have the secondary benefit of a "tamponade effect" that comes with lying down on their biopsy site after the procedure. Therefore, extra attention to the immediate post-biopsy hand compression and wound surveillance for signs and symptoms of bleeding or hematoma formation is highly recommended.

Key Review Points

1. Critical anatomic structures to be aware of during an image-guided percutaneous rib biopsy include the lungs and the intercostal arteries.
2. A frequent indication for performing a rib biopsy is to assess the etiology of a rib lesion.
3. The approaches for rib biopsy are either anterior or posterior, and these are determined by the location of the lesion within a specific rib compartment.
4. The use of coaxial technique with rib biopsies facilitates procedure efficiency and safety.
5. Major determinants of specimen yield in rib biopsy procedures include lesion location relative to critical structures, lesion size, and lesion type (lytic, sclerotic, or mixed).

References

Baxter AD, Coakley FV, Finlay DB, West C. The aetiology of solitary hot spots in the ribs on planar bone scans. Nucl Med Commun. 1995;16:834–7.

ClementeCD. Anatomy: a regional atlas of the human body. 4thth ed. Baltimore, Williams & Wilkins Baltimore 1997:155–158.

Cronin CG, Cashell T, Mhuircheartaigh JN, Swords R, Murray M, O'Sullivan GJ, O'Keeffe D. Bone biopsy of new suspicious bone lesions in patients with primary carcinoma: prevalence and probability of an alternative diagnosis. AJR Am J Roentgenol. 2009;193:W407–W410.

De Maeseneer M, De Mey J, Lenchik L, Everaert H, Osteaux M. Helical CT of rib lesions: a pattern-based approach. AJR Am J Roentgenol. 2004;182:173–9.

Edelstein G, Levitt RG, Slaker DP, Murphy WA. CT observation of rib abnormalities: spectrum of findings. J Comput Assist Tomogr. 1985;9:65–72.

Faro SH, Mahboubi S, Ortega W. CT diagnosis of rib anomalies, tumors, and infection in children. Clin Imaging. 1993;17:1–7.

Geremia GK, Charletta DA, Granato DB, Raju S. Biopsy of vertebral and paravertebral structures with a new coaxial needle system. AJNR Am J Neuroradiol. 1992;13:169–71.

Guttentag AR, Salwen JK. Keep your eyes on the ribs: the spectrum of normal variants and diseases that involve the ribs. Radiographics. 1999;19:1125–42.

Hardy DC, Totty WG, Funk KC. CT-directed rib biopsy. J Comput Assist Tomogr. 1987;11:994–7.

Hwang S, Lefkowitz RA, Landa J, Zheng J, Moskowitz CS, Maybody M, Hameed M, Panicek DM. Percutaneous CT-guided bone biopsy: diagnosis of malignancy in lesions with initially indeterminate biopsy results and CT features associated with diagnostic or indeterminate results. AJR Am J Roentgenol. 2011;197:1417–25.

Jakanani GC, Saifuddin A. Percutaneous image-guided needle biopsy of rib lesions: a retrospective study of diagnostic outcome in 51 cases. Skeletal Radiol. 2013;42:85–90.

Jelinek JS, Murphey MD, Welker JA, Henshaw RM, Kransdorf MJ, Shmookler BM, Malawer MM. Diagnosis of primary bone tumors with image-guided percutaneous biopsy: experience with 110 tumors. Radiology. 2002;223:731–7.

Kim S, Lee S, Arsenault DA, Strijbosch RA, Shamberger RC, Puder M. Pediatric rib lesions: a 13 year experience. J Pediatr Surg. 2008;43:1781–5.

Lee G, Im JG, Kim S, Kang HS, Han MC. Tuberculosis of the rib: CT appearance. J Comput Assist Tomogr. 1993;17:363–6.

Omura MC, Motamedi K, Uybico S, Nelson SD, Seeger LL. Revisiting CT-guided percutaneous core needle biopsy of musculoskeletal lesions: contributors of biopsy success. AJR Am J Roentgenol. 2011;197: 457–61.

Puri A, Shingade VU, Agarwal MG, Anchan C, Juvekar S, Desai S, Jambhekar NA. CT-guided percutaneous core needle biopsy in deep seated musculoskeletal lesions: a prospective study of 128 cases. Skeletal Radiol. 2006;35:138–43.

Ray-Coquard I, Ranchère-Vince D, Thiesse P. Evaluation of core needle biopsy as a substitute to open biopsy in the diagnosis of soft-tissue masses. Eur J Cancer. 2003;39:2021–5.

Tsukushi S, Nishida Y, Yamada Y, Yoshida M, Ishiquro N. CT-guided needle biopsy for musculoskeletal lesions. Arch Orthop Trauma Surg. 2010;130:699–703.

Wu JS, Goldsmith JD, Horwich PJ, Shetty SK, Hochman MG. Bone and soft-tissue lesions: what factors affect diagnostic yield of image-guided core needle biopsy? Radiology. 2008;248:962–70.

Biopsy for Spine Infection

9

Michael K. Brooks, Yuri Peterkin,
and A. Orlando Ortiz

Learning

1. To review the clinical evaluation of suspected spine infection
2. To learn the role of image-guided percutaneous spine biopsy during clinical management
3. To introduce specific biopsy techniques and tools for the proper performance of image-guided percutaneous spine biopsy

Infectious spondylitis	Infection of one or more of the spine compartments
Diskitis	Infection confined to the intervertebral disk
Osteomyelitis	Infection confined to the bone (vertebral body)
Spondylodiskitis	Infection of the disk and adjacent vertebral bodies
Septic arthritis	Infection within a facet joint
Epidural abscess	Epidural space infection with focal purulent collection
Meningitis	Infection involving the meninges

9.1 Introduction

The timely diagnosis and management of patients with spine infection are crucial as delays in diagnosis can cause neurologic impairment and mortality. Infectious spondylitis, or spine infection, is defined as infection of one or more spine structures. The structure or structures of the spine that might become infected include the intervertebral disk, the vertebral body including the vertebral endplate, the posterior elements including the facet joint, the epidural space with possible extension to the subarachnoid space, the spinal cord, and the paraspinal soft tissues (Fig. 9.1).

Although a relatively less common clinical entity, spine infections are increasing in incidence. Recent studies have reported an estimated increase in the incidence of spine infection from 5.3/100,000 population per year in 2007 to 7.4/100,000 population per year in 2010 (Akiyama et al. 2013). While an improved accuracy in diagnostic capabilities is hypothesized as an etiology for the increased incidence of spine infection, iatrogenic causes also play a significant role. Up to one-third of new cases of vertebral osteomyelitis are healthcare related, and one-third of those cases are secondary to catheter-related infections (Pigrau et al. 2015). Spine surgery is a major risk factor for spine infection (Fig. 9.2). Despite pre-procedure antibiotic prophylaxis, improved

A.O. Ortiz, *Image-Guided Percutaneous Spine Biopsy*, DOI 10.1007/978-3-319-43326-4_9

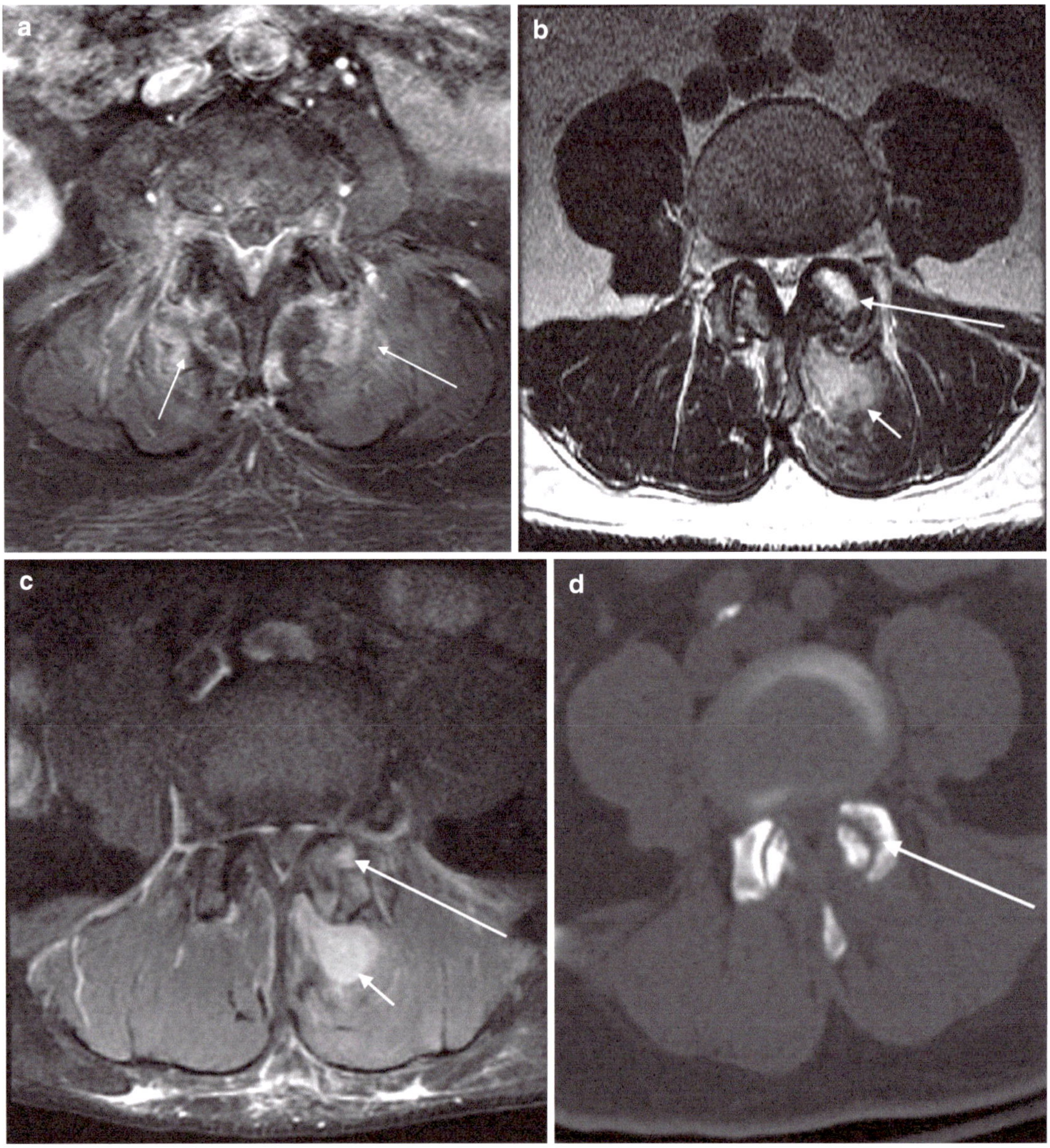

Fig. 9.1 Spectrum of spine infection. (**a**) Deep paraspinal muscle infection in an 84-year-old with low back pain and elevated ESR (90) and CRP (200) as shown on fat-suppressed contrast-enhanced T1-weighted axial image. A 56-year-old male with low back pain and fever due to septic left lumbar facet joint (*large arrow*) with edema in adjacent erector spinae and multifidus muscles (*small arrow*) as shown on T2-weighted axial image (**b**), fat-suppressed contrast-enhanced T1-weighted axial image (**c**), and axial CT image in bone window algorithm (**d**). Note the juxta-articular erosion within the infected joint (*arrow in* **d**). In this 76-year-old female with low back pain and fever, the indium-111 white blood cell study is normal (**e**), but the T1 sagittal image (**f**) shows intermediate signal soft tissue (*arrow*) posterior to the L5 vertebral body and low signal (*curved arrow*) within the sacral promontory, within hyperintense signal seen within these areas on the T2 sagittal image (**g**). The fat-suppressed contrast-enhanced T1-weighted sagittal image (**h**) shows a peripherally enhancing abscess (*large arrow*) and focal endplate enhancement (*small arrows*) as well as subtle leptomeningeal enhancement (*curved arrows*); the epidural abscess (*large arrow*) is again seen on the fat-suppressed contrast-enhanced T1-weighted axial image (**i**) as is the leptomeningeal enhancement (*curved arrow*) consistent with meningitis; deep soft tissue enhancement (*small arrow*) is also noted

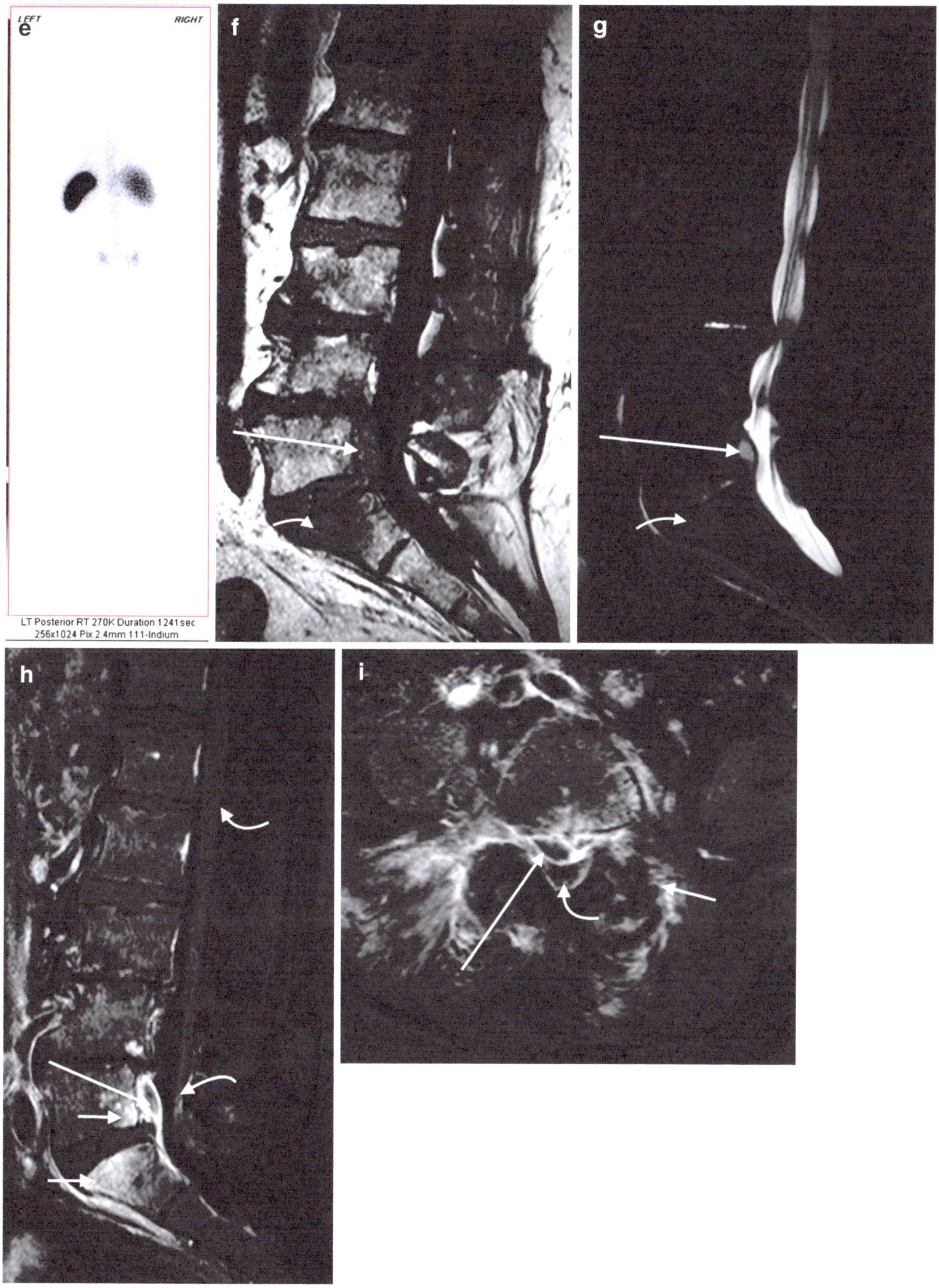

Fig. 9.1 (continued)

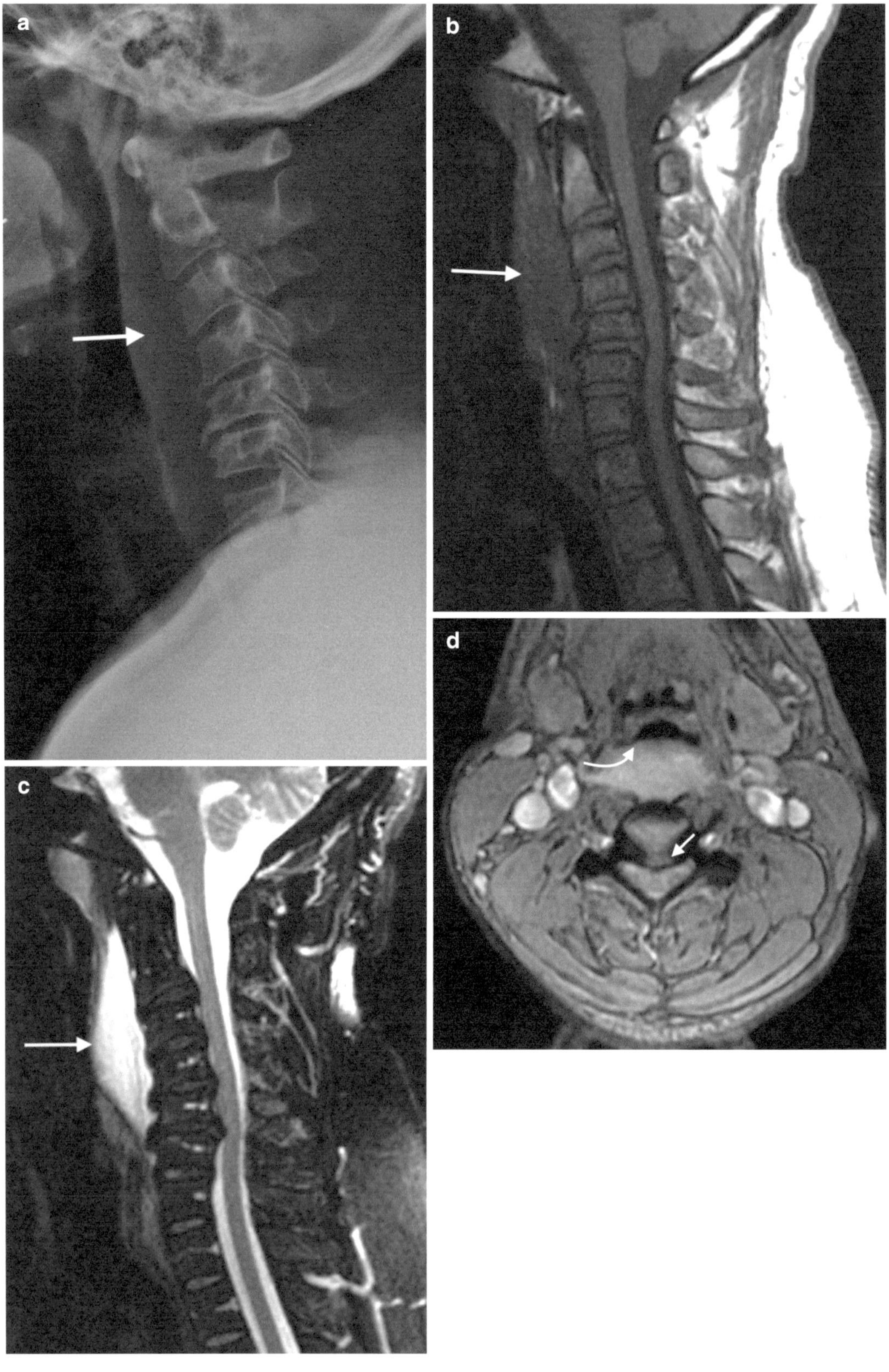
a
b
c
d

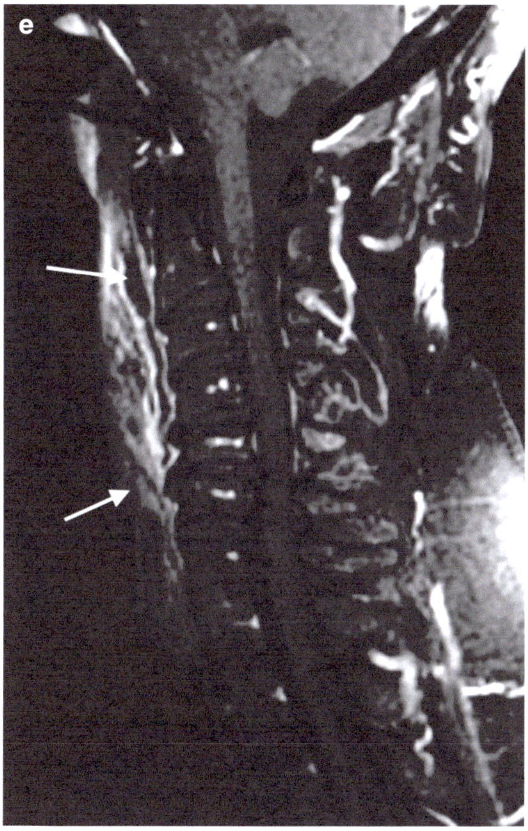

Fig. 9.2 (continued)

surgical techniques, and postoperative care, post-procedural diskitis represents up to 30% of all cases of pyogenic spondylodiskitis (Jiminez-Mejias et al. 1999). Other factors that might account for the increased incidence of spine infection include the increasing age of the overall population, advancements in medicine leading to an increased life expectancy of patients with chronic diseases, and the increased prevalence of patients on immunosuppressive medications (Bhavan et al. 2010; Duarte and Vaccaro 2013; Kim et al. 2015; Pigrau et al. 2015).

9.2 Efficacy of Image-Guided Spine Biopsy for Infection

Image-guided percutaneous spine biopsy is a safe and effective procedure with a reported overall accuracy ranging from 88 to 95% (Gupta et al. 2002; Heyer et al. 2008; Rimondi et al. 2008; Tehranzadeh et al. 2007). Although, theoretically, an adequate sample is often obtained with biopsies in patients with suspected spine infection, there is an associated lower overall success rate in identifying the causative organism (Table 9.1). The accuracy for image-guided percutaneous disk space biopsy, in patients with surgically proven spondylodiskitis, has been reported to be as low as 36–57% (Kim et al. 2012; Kim et al. 2015; Marschall et al. 2011; Michel et al. 2006). A negative spine biopsy for spine infection is operationally defined as no evidence of microbial agent growth or identification in the submitted specimen(s) and no histopathologic evidence of diskitis or osteomyelitis in the submitted specimen(s).

Operational definition of a negative biopsy for spine infection:

1. No evidence of microbial identification or growth in the submitted specimen(s)
2. No evidence of disk or vertebral end-plate inflammatory change in the submitted specimens

Fig. 9.2 A 40-year-old male with difficulty swallowing after attempted cervical disk procedure. Lateral radiograph (**a**) of the neck shows extensive prevertebral soft tissue swelling (*arrow*) with slightly hypointense signal intensity (*arrow*) on the T1-weighted sagittal image (**b**) and hyperintensity (*arrow*) on the T2-weighted sagittal image (**c**). The fat-suppressed axial image (**d**) shows mass effect (*large arrow*) upon the hypopharynx at C4-C5 with a disk herniation that impinges upon the spinal cord (*small arrow*). The fat-suppressed contrast-enhanced T1-weighted sagittal image (**e**) shows a heterogeneously enhancing (*arrows*) retropharyngeal fluid collection which was emergently drained and shown to be an infected hematoma

Table 9.1 Reasons for a negative biopsy result in patients with suspected spine infection

1. Patient
Patient is on concurrent antibiotic therapy
Incomplete patient work-up in imaging study that mimics spine infection
Incomplete imaging work-up and analysis prior to performing the biopsy procedure
2. Procedure
Unable to access the site of infection
Wrong level or wrong side is biopsied
Presence of transitional vertebra
Abnormality on MRI not well visualized with imaging guidance
Use of instruments that fail to collect an adequate amount of tissue and fluid
3. Specimen
Improper specimen handling
Insufficient specimen
Specimen not sent for both microbiologic *and* pathologic analysis

The length of pre-biopsy antibiotic therapy is inversely related to the likelihood of identifying a causative organism and is the most common reason for a false negative biopsy result (Enoch et al. 2008; Kim et al. 2012; Kim et al. 2015; Marschall et al. 2011; Mazzie et al. 2014; Wu et al. 2007). Ideally, a biopsy should be performed before the initiation of antibiotic therapy in order to maximize the probability of obtaining a positive culture result. Alternatively, if the clinical circumstances dictate, then the biopsy should be performed within 48 h of antibiotic administration. A patient who has been placed on antibiotic therapy for a period of time longer than this should have their antibiotic regimen stopped for a minimum of 2 days prior to attempting a biopsy procedure. Other common causes of a false negative biopsy in patients with suspected spine infection include insufficient specimen, improper specimen handling and processing, and obtaining disk material without adjacent subchondral bone (Michel et al. 2006). A repeat spine biopsy in patients with a negative first biopsy and negative blood cultures may yield a positive culture result, and this option, in the appropriate clinical setting, might be considered in patients who are not on antibiotic therapy (Terreaux et al. 2016).

> The length of pre-biopsy antibiotic therapy is inversely related to the likelihood of identifying a causative organism and is the most common reason for a false negative biopsy result.

9.3 Spine Infection: Mechanisms of Spread

Understanding the pathophysiologic basis of spine infection is integral to perform image-guided percutaneous spine biopsy in patients with suspected spine infection. There are three possible routes of spread that may result in spine infection: (1) hematogenous spread, (2) direct inoculation, and (3) contiguous spread from adjacent structures. Hematogenous spread from a distant site, frequently the genitourinary tract or skin, is the most common cause of spine infection (Bhavan et al. 2010; Diehn 2012; Govender 2005). In adults, hematogenous seeding of vertebral body infection occurs at the level of the end-arterioles adjacent to the subchondral endplates. End-vessel occlusion results in ischemic and necrotic bone; the formation of a bony sequestrum in turn serves as a nidus for progression of infection. Pyogenic infection subsequently spreads from the infected vertebral endplate into the adjacent intervertebral disk (Bhavan et al. 2010; Duarte and Vaccaro 2013; Govender 2005; Jimenez-Mejias et al. 1999). In children, the end-arterioles extend into the intervertebral disk; hence, spine infections in children originate within the disk proper. In adults, therefore, in the setting of suspected vertebral osteomyelitis, disk aspiration and core needle biopsy of the subjacent subchondral vertebral body endplate should both be attempted (Mazzie et al. 2014; Michel et al. 2006). Direct inoculation is frequently due to an iatrogenic etiology. It occurs secondary to spine instrumentation, including spine surgery, lumbar puncture, and percutaneous epidural or facet joint injections. A penetrating injury into or near the spine may also result in direct inoculation. Contiguous spread from an adjacent focus of infection is the least common of the three mechanisms responsible for spine infection. Skin infection (including decubitus ulcers), pulmonary infection, and kidney infection are examples of conditions that can be associated with direct contiguous spread to the adjacent segment of the spine.

9.4 Clinical Presentation

The clinical presentation depends upon two major factors, the virulence of the infectious agent and host resistance factors (Table 9.2). Potential infectious agents include bacterial, mycobacterial, fungal, or parasitic organisms depending on the clinical scenario. Clinically, spine infections are generally challenging to diagnose as patients may present with subtle and non-specific symptoms, which range in acuity. Therefore, a significant delay in clinical diagnosis may occur. A strong clinical suspicion of spine infection should be supported by correlation with pertinent imaging studies and laboratory analysis. On initial presentation, the most common reported symptom is unremitting back pain, which worsens at night and does not dissipate with rest. The lumbar spine is the spinal segment that is most frequently involved. Fever is an unreliable sign of spine infection as up to 54% of patients are afebrile at initial presentation (Bhavan et al. 2010). Neurologic deficits including lower extremity weakness, radiculopathy, and urinary incontinence have been reported in up to one-third of patients and are often associated with delays in diagnosis (Duarte and Vaccaro 2013). Spine infections are more common in males, and the incidence increases with age, most commonly affecting adults who are 50 years of age or older. Predisposing risk factors include intravenous drug abuse, chronic disease such as renal failure or diabetes, previous spinal surgery, or HIV infection or other immunocompromised state (Bhavan et al. 2010; Diehn 2012; Duarte and Vaccaro 2013; Govender 2005).

Table 9.2 Risk factors for spine infection

1. Age greater than 50 years
2. Intravenous drug use
3. Pre-existing source of infection
4. Diabetes
5. HIV infection or other immunocompromised state
6. Previous spine surgery
7. Chronic steroid use
8. Chronic medical condition (renal failure, cirrhosis)

A key initial step in diagnosing spine infection is to suspect it!

9.5 Laboratory Findings

There are several serum laboratory markers, which may be helpful in diagnosing and managing spine infection. The erythrocyte sedimentation rate (ESR) and C-reactive protein (CRP) are inflammatory markers that are commonly elevated at initial presentation. ESR is a sensitive but non-specific measure of inflammation. It is the rate at which red blood cells layer, or sediment, in 1 h (Singh 2014). ESR directly correlates with the amount of fibrinogen in the blood, increasing with any condition that elevates fibrinogen. Other causes of an increased ESR include pregnancy, anemia, autoimmune disorders, multiple myeloma, and lymphoma. CRP is an acute phase protein of hepatic origin, which rises in response to the release of interleukin-6 by macrophages and T-cells (Go et al. 2012; Singh 2014). Infections and inflammatory diseases are common causes of an increase in serum CRP levels (Heyer et al. 2012). Pregnancy, obstructive sleep apnea, and malignancy can also cause an elevated CRP. Typically in spine infection, both ESR and CRP are elevated at initial presentation. However, bone pathology, specifically in diabetics, is reported as a common factor in causing an elevated ESR with a normal CRP level (Singh 2014). ESR is the most useful marker of inflammation, with elevation reported in 70–100% of infections at presentation (Go et al. 2012). Inflammatory markers are often followed to assess the patient's response to treatment. Serum CRP returns to normal with treatment faster than ESR and is therefore a better marker for therapeutic response in patients with infection (Brigden 1999; Duarte and Vaccaro 2013; Singh 2014). The white blood cell count (WBC) is the least useful of the inflammatory markers due to its low sensitivity. In a large 2-year retrospective cohort study, 40% of patients who presented with or developed hematogenous vertebral osteomyelitis had a normal initial WBC (Bhavan et al. 2010). Positive blood cultures may be seen in approximately 24% of patients with suspected spine infection and may assist in identifying the offending microorganism and guiding subsequent treatment. In specific situations, when a coagulase-positive *Staphylococcus* infection is suspected, the use of counterimmunoelectrophoresis to detect serum anti-teichoic acid antibodies may be helpful in confirming the presence of staphylococcal infectious spondylitis (Dhale et al. 2003). Ribitol teichoic acid, found within the cell wall of *Staphylococcus aureus* species, is antigenic and a high serum titer (> 4) of anti-teichoic acid antibodies which may be detected in patients with staphylococcal spine infection.

9.6 Imaging

Due to the insidious and non-specific clinical presentation of infectious spondylitis, radiologists have an integral role in facilitating this diagnosis. Radiographs are often the initial imaging examination performed; however, plain films have an extremely low sensitivity for detection of early infection and may remain normal for several weeks (Diehn 2012; Govender 2005). Despite the low sensitivity for acute spine infection, radiographs often demonstrate findings of spine infection due to the delayed presentation that is associated with this condition. Loss of cortical definition with irregularity of the vertebral endplate is the earliest radiographic finding in spondylodiskitis (Diehn 2012; Go et al. 2012; Govender 2005). Radiographic detection of bone loss requires a 30–40% loss of the bony matrix typically occurring 2 weeks after initial symptoms (Go et al. 2012). Prevertebral or paraspinal soft tissue swelling, fullness, or bulging with loss of fat planes can also be identified on radiographs in early cases of spine infection (Diehn 2012; Go et al. 2012; Govender 2005). As the infection progresses, there is subsequent involvement of the intervertebral disk space, with loss of disk height and erosive changes of the vertebral endplates (Fig. 9.3). Radiographic findings of chronic infection include sclerosis of the vertebral endplates with variable collapse of the infected vertebral body, obliteration, and fusion across the affected disk space, leading to spinal deformities such as kyphosis and/or scoliosis (Diehn 2012; Go et al. 2012). In chronic spine infection, especially tuberculous spondylitis, calcification may be observed within the paraspinal soft tissues or within the epidural space.

Computed tomography (CT) has a higher sensitivity than plain radiography for the detection of early bony changes in spine infection due to the increased anatomic resolution. CT findings of spine infection are similar to those seen on radiographs; however, subtle endplate irregularity and erosions are better depicted (Fig. 9.4). Loss of the normal architecture of the trabecular bone is one

Fig. 9.3 An 11-year-old male with *S. aureus* proven septic spondylodiskitis. Lateral radiograph (**a**) of the lumbar spine shows L5-S1 disk space narrowing (*arrow*) with vertebral endplate erosions and subchondral sclerosis. Reformatted sagittal CT image (**b**) in bone window algorithm shows irregularity, sclerosis, and erosion of the subchondral bone (*arrow*) along the L5-S1 endplates. Sagittal T1-weighted image (**c**) shows obliteration of the disk space with loss of the cortical margins (*arrow*), while the sagittal T2-weighted image (**d**) shows hyperintense T2 signal within the disk space, as well as extensive vertebral bone marrow edema (*arrow*). Sagittal (**e**) and axial (**f**) T1-weighted fat-suppressed contrast-enhanced images show intradiskal enhancement with intradiskal abscess (*arrows*). Axial CT image acquired during biopsy at the level of the L5-S1 disk space (**g**) shows coaxial advancement of the biopsy needle through the guiding cannula (*arrow*) via a right S1 transpedicular approach utilizing cranial angulation through the pedicle (*P*) for successful sampling of the vertebral endplate and the adjacent disk

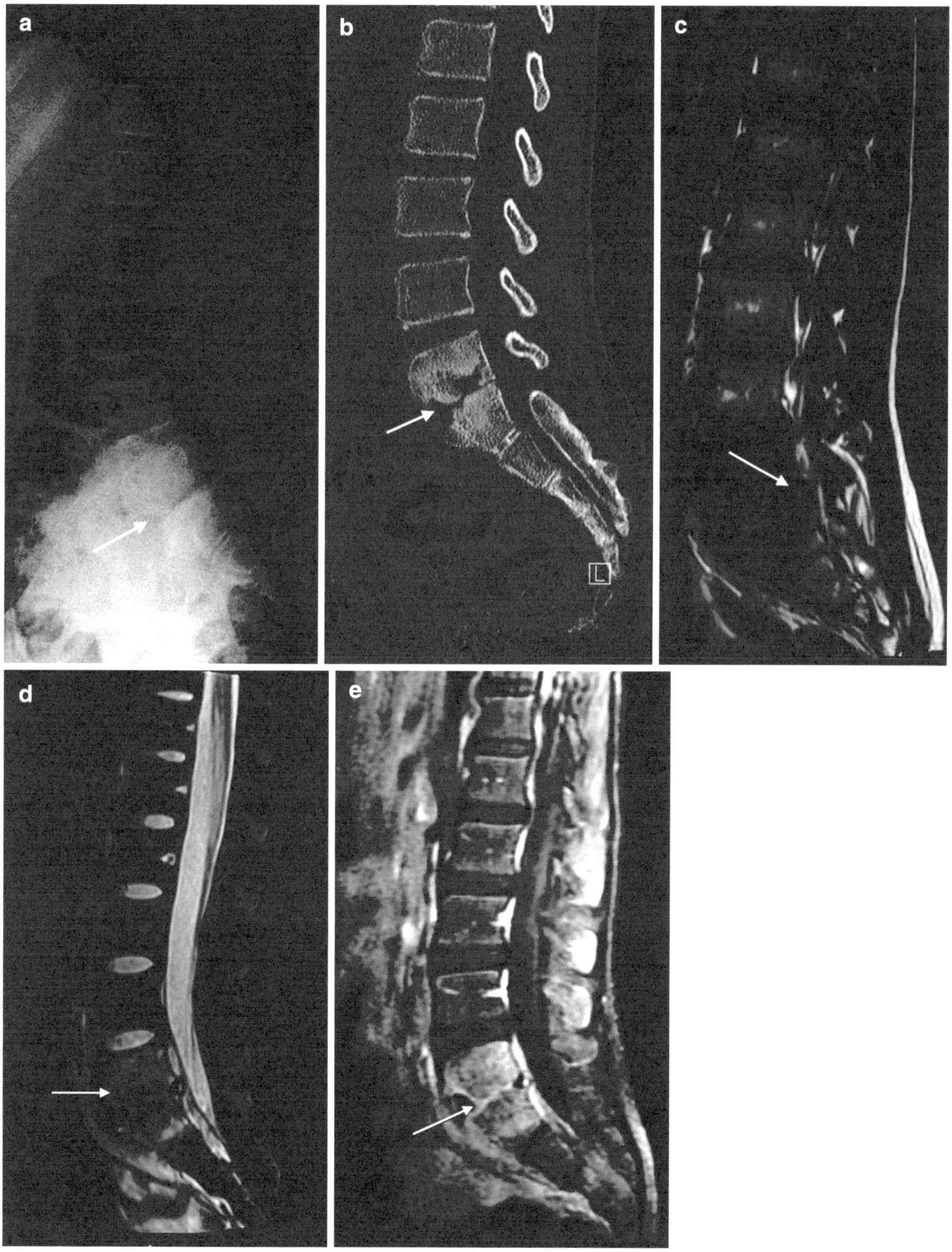
a
b
c
L
d
e

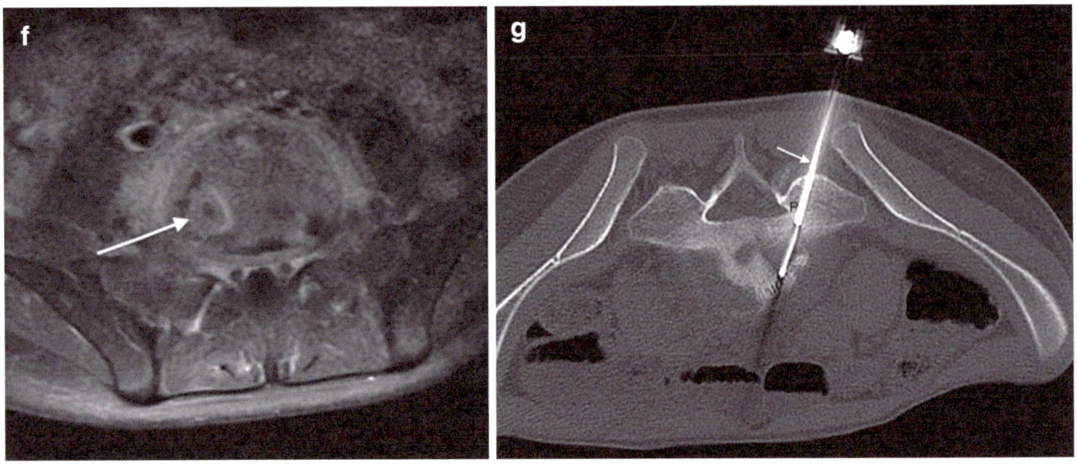

Fig. 9.3 (continued)

of the early CT findings of pyogenic vertebral osteomyelitis, which is rarely appreciated on radiographs (Go et al. 2012). CT is commonly utilized in patients with contraindications to magnetic resonance imaging (MRI) and for differentiating mimickers of spondylodiskitis, such as reactive vertebral endplate changes. CT is useful for the depiction of the spread of infection and helps to characterize prevertebral and paraspinal soft tissue involvement. Mass effect from infected paraspinal collections can compromise the neural foramen and may cause nerve root impingement. Posterior extension of infection can involve the epidural space and, in the cervical or thoracic spine, may result in spinal cord compression. In patients that cannot undergo an MRI examination, this study may need to be performed with an intravenous contrast agent or, less commonly, with an intrathecal contrast agent.

Magnetic resonance imaging is the study of choice for diagnosing spine infection, with a reported sensitivity of 96%, specificity of 92%, and accuracy of 94%. Endplate irregularity, with loss of cortical definition, and erosions are common and may later progress to vertebral body destruction. The earliest MRI finding in spine infection is altered bone marrow signal manifested as hypointense T1- and hyperintense T2-weighted signal with contrast enhancement, most prominent along the vertebral endplates (Fig. 9.4). Involvement of the adjacent intervertebral disk space may manifest with loss of intervertebral disk height, alteration of normal disk morphology including loss of the intranuclear cleft, focal T2 hyperintensity, and variable contrast enhancement patterns (Fig. 9.5). Infection may also spread posteriorly into the epidural space and laterally into the paravertebral soft tissues. Because of the initial involvement of the vertebral endplate, loss of the normal disk-endplate margin may be a helpful sign in suspecting possible infection. Psoas musculature T2 hyperintensity shows a high sensitivity and specificity (92% at a 95% confidence interval) with a high positive likelihood ratio for spondylodiskitis; this may be a helpful imaging finding especially when an unenhanced MRI study is performed and may raise a concern for possible spine infection (Ledbetter et al. 2016). A contrast-enhanced MRI examination is the study of choice to evaluate a patient with a suspected spine infection and/or epidural abscess with possible spinal cord compression (Fig. 9.6). Initially, irregular, thick paraspinal, or epidural soft tissue enhancement is seen compatible with phlegmon. Paraspinal abscesses are readily identified on MRI as T1-hypointense and T2-hyperintense fluid collections with peripheral enhancement. Spine infections however can have a variable appearance on MRI, with atypical imaging characteristics and

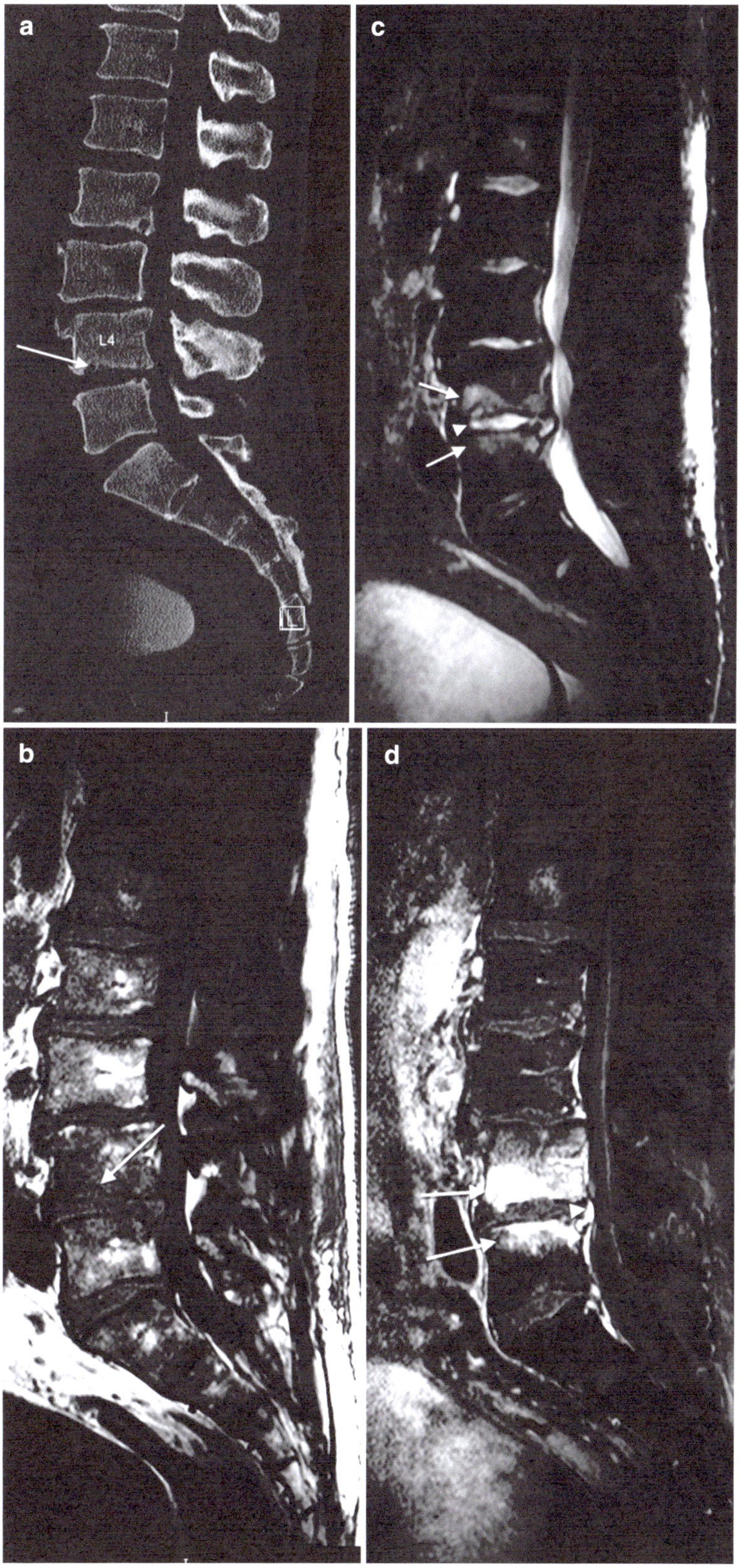

Fig. 9.4 A 53-year-old male with pathological analysis showing acute inflammation and purulent exudates and culture-positive gram-positive cocci in pairs. Reformatted sagittal CT image (**a**) in bone window algorithm shows irregularity of the inferior endplate of L4 with loss of cortical bone (*arrow*) and increased intervertebral disk height anteriorly. Sagittal T1-weighted image (**b**) also shows loss of the normal hypointense line along the inferior endplate of L4 (*arrow*) as well as hypointense T1 signal adjacent to the vertebral endplates of L4 and L5. Sagittal T2-weighted image (**c**) shows corresponding bone marrow edema (*arrows*) and hyperintense signal within the disk (*arrowhead*). Sagittal T1-weighted fat-suppressed contrast-enhanced image (**d**) shows prominent endplate enhancement (*arrows*) and focal epidural enhancement (*arrowhead*). Axial CT image (**e**) acquired during biopsy shows the biopsy needle (*small arrow*) advanced coaxially through a guide cannula (*large arrow*) via a posterolateral paravertebral approach directly into the L4-L5 disk space

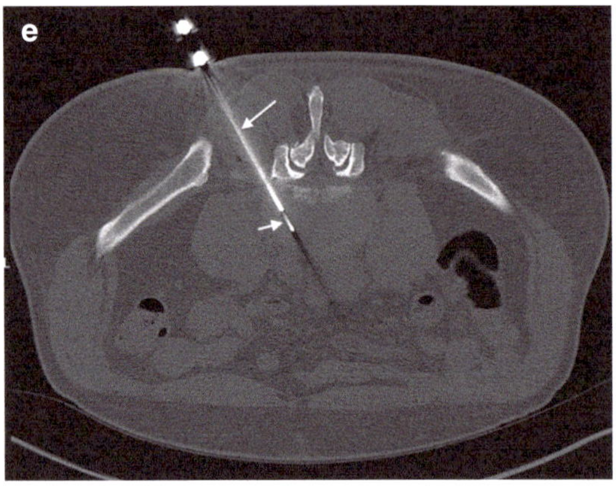

Fig. 9.4 (continued)

variable vertebral involvement with sparing of the intervening disk spaces. MRI findings with the reported highest sensitivity for the diagnosis of spine infection are vertebral body T1-hypointense signal, intervertebral disk space T2-hyperintense signal, and disk space enhancement (Diehn 2012) (Fig. 9.7). Epidural abscess formation may be associated with spondylodiskitis or, depending on the etiology (e.g., a spinal procedure), may be seen in isolation (Fig. 9.8). MRI will show a heterogeneous T1-hypointense and T2-hyperintense variable-length fluid collection within the epidural space that is associated with prominent peripheral and epidural contrast enhancement. It should be noted that, at the cervical and/or thoracic spine level, a patient's myelopathic presentation may be disproportionately greater than the severity of spinal cord compression because the associated spinal cord ischemia also reflects the presence of epidural venous plexus vascular congestion. Untreated epidural abscesses can progress rapidly and cause significant morbidity and mortality. The detection of a suspected epidural abscess should prompt immediate spine surgical consultation for consideration of emergent drainage and decompression of the epidural abscess.

> The MRI detection of a suspected spinal epidural abscess should prompt immediate spine surgical evaluation.

In patients with lumbar spondylosis and advanced degenerative disk disease, diffusion-weighted MR images (DWI) may distinguish between reactive fibrovascular vertebral endplate changes and spondylodiskitis (Patel et al. 2014). With respect to reactive endplate change, DWI will show a focal diffusion pattern referred to as the "claw" sign, whereas in infection, a diffuse DWI pattern or absent "claw" sign is noted. The abnormal MRI findings that are seen with spine infection may persist for a variable period of time despite successful treatment of the spine infection.

Nuclear medicine imaging can sometimes be useful in diagnosing spine infection. The radionuclide imaging method of choice is a combined triple phase ^{99m}technicium-methylene diphosphonate bone and ^{67}gallium-citrate scan. This dual radionuclide study has a high sensitivity and high specificity for spine infection (Diehn 2012; Duarte and Vaccaro 2013; Go et al. 2012; Mazzie et al. 2014). Discordant or increased radionuclide uptake on the gallium scan, in comparison to the technetium bone scan, is the most common finding in spondylodiskitis. Radionuclide imaging for spine infection, however, is typically reserved for certain clinical situations due to limited spatial resolution, a long examination time, and the greater availability and sensitivity of MRI (Fig. 9.9). The combined bone and gallium scan is most useful in patients with contraindications for MRI or with equivocal CT and MRI results.

9.7 Spine Infection in the Immunocompromised Patient

Due to a blunted immune response, the diagnosis of spine infection is often further delayed in immunocompromised patients. These patients often do not manifest the typical signs and symptoms of spine infection and can even be asymptomatic. The causative microorganisms also differ in immunocompromised patients, who are prone to atypical bacterial, fungal, and parasitic infections. HIV/AIDS predisposes patients to fungal infections due to neutrophil and leukocyte

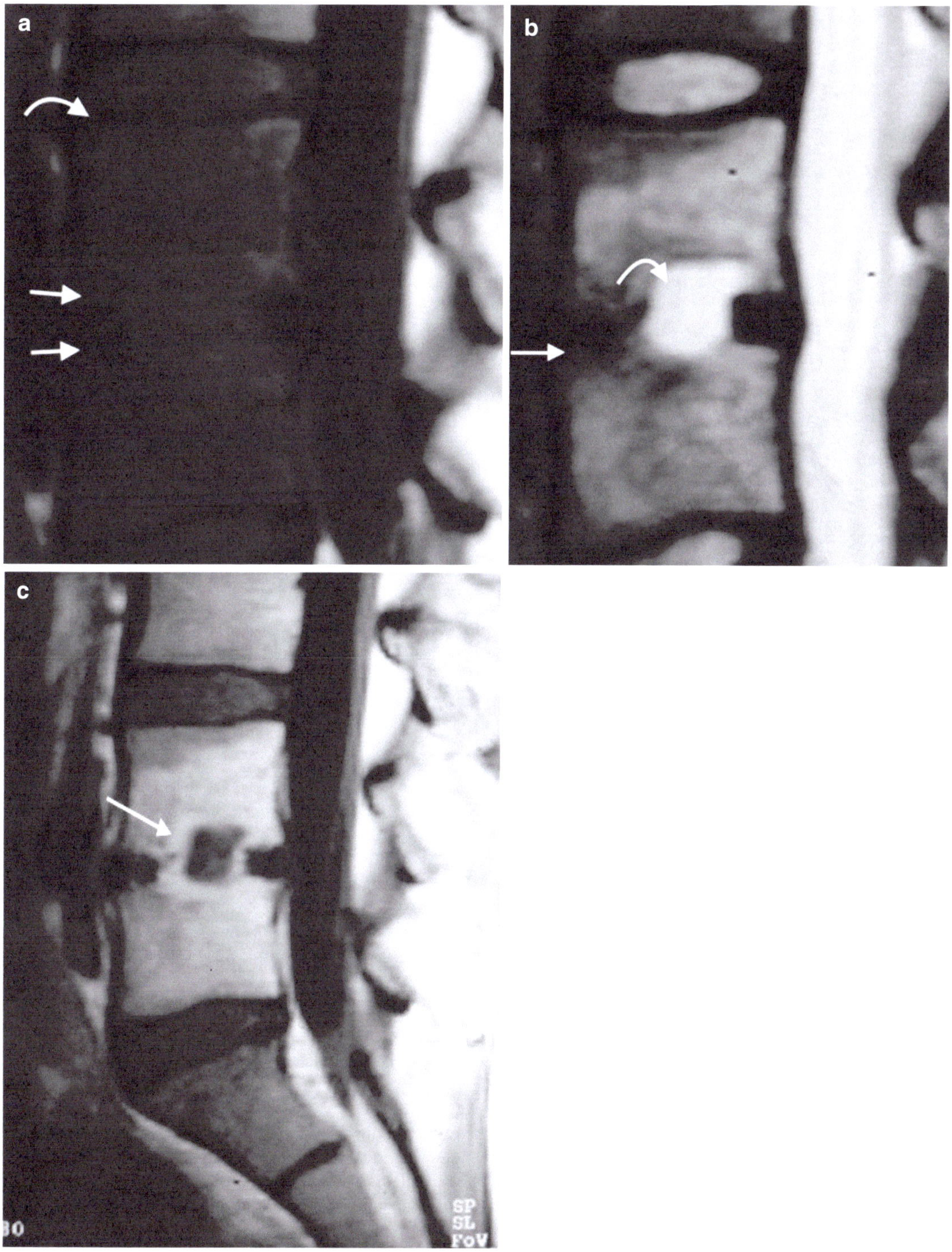

Fig. 9.5 MRI signs of early disk space infection. T1-weighted sagittal image (**a**) shows loss of the hypointense lines (*arrows*) that correspond to the vertebral endplate; compare to the normal vertebral endplate at the level above (*curved arrow*). T2-weighted sagittal image again shows vertebral endplate irregularity/erosion (*arrow*) and loss of the normal intranuclear cleft (*curved arrow*). Contrast-enhanced T1-weighted sagittal image (**c**) shows prominent marrow enhancement and ring enhancement surrounding an intradiskal abscess (*arrow*)

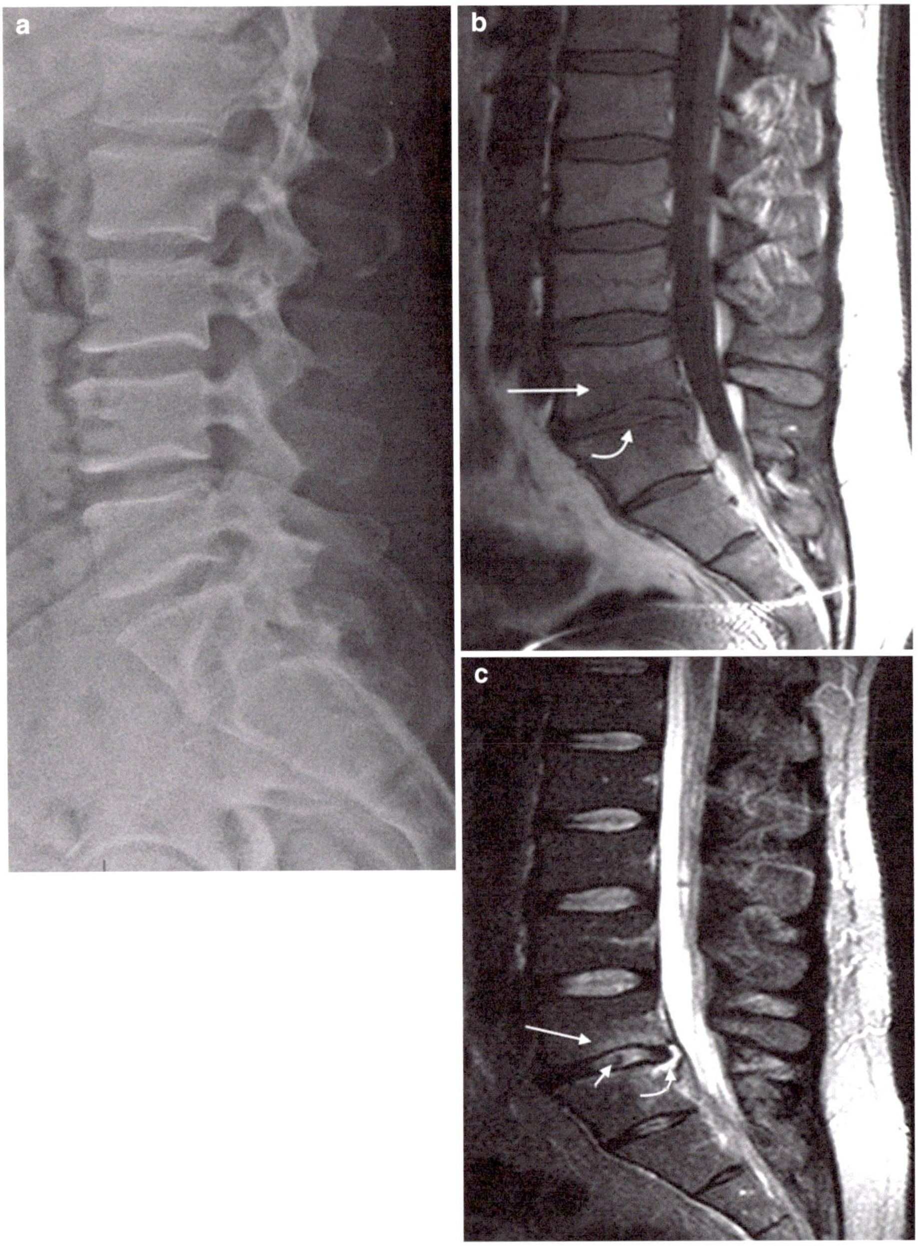

Fig. 9.6 Chronology of a case of spine infection. Lateral radiograph of the lumbar spine (**a**) in a patient with acute low back pain is normal. T1-weighted sagittal image (**b**) obtained on the same day shows hypointense endplate signal (*arrow*) which was attributed to degenerative endplate change at L5-S1; note the subtle cortical erosion of the endplate (*curved arrow*). The T2 sagittal image (**c**) shows reactive endplate edema (*large arrow*), loss of the intranuclear cleft (*small arrow*), and thick hyperintense signal (*curved arrow*) adjacent to the posterior annulus. Three weeks later, a repeat MR examination shows further loss of the normal T1 hypointense endplate signal (**d**) as compared to the level above (*curved arrow*) and prominent marrow edema. The T2-weighted sagittal image (**e**) shows progression of intradiskal signal increase (*arrow*) with contrast enhancement confined to the endplates and adjacent marrow as shown on the fat-suppressed contrast-enhanced T1-weighted image (**f**). The findings were attributed to degenerative disk disease with reactive endplate change at L5-S1, and conservative medical management was continued. The patient's back pain symptoms persisted, and lateral radiograph (**g**) obtained 10 weeks after the initial onset of the patient's symptoms shows complete loss of the cortical endplates at L5-S1 (*arrows*); compare to the normal level above (*curved arrow*). A third MRI study obtained 12 weeks from the onset of symptoms now shows extensive marrow edema and disk space height loss with disorganization and signal abnormality with extensive vertebral body and intradiskal enhancement at L5-S1 as shown on the sagittal T1(**h**), T2 (**i**), and fat-suppressed contrast-enhanced T1-weighted (**j**) images

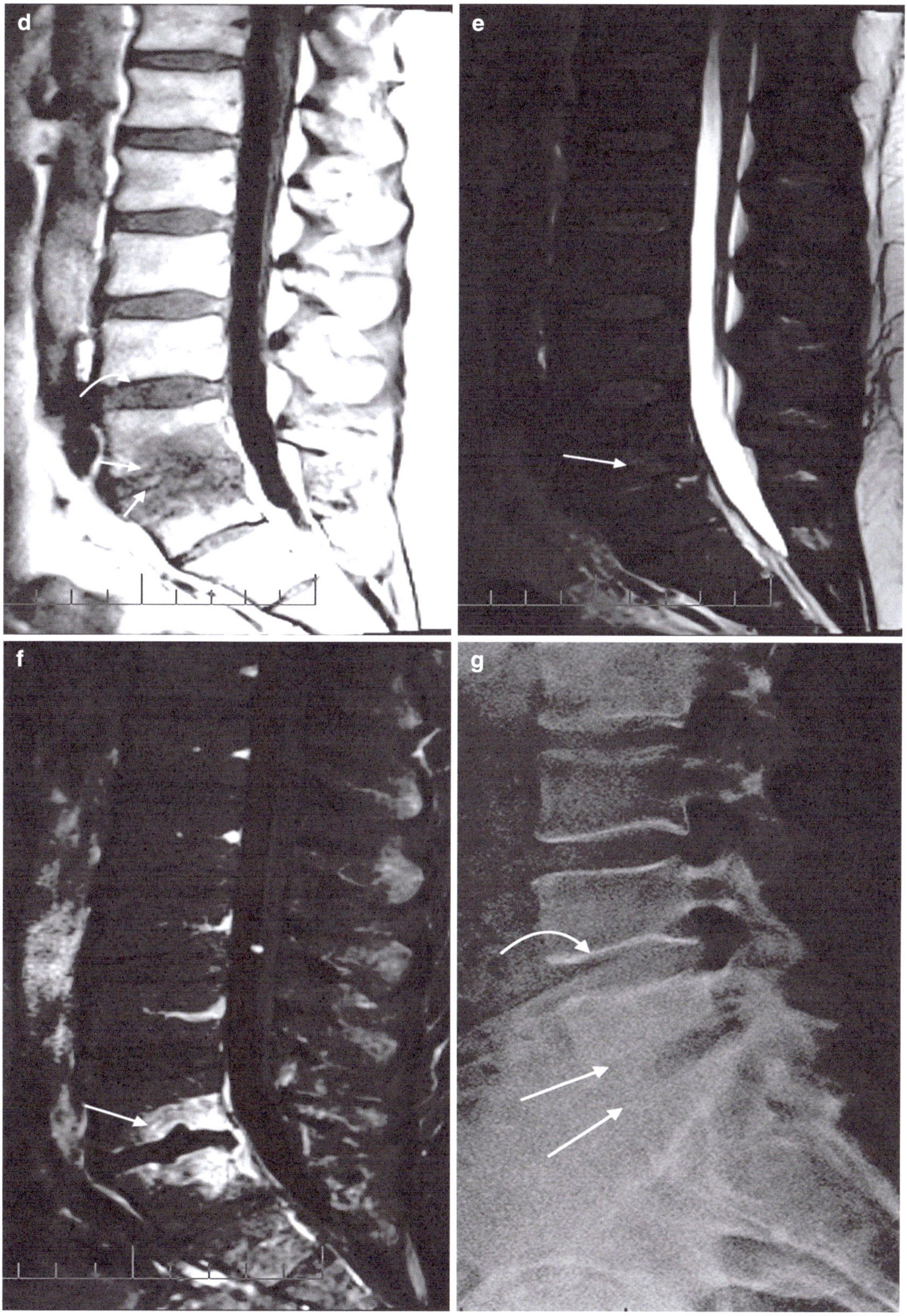

Fig. 9.6 (continued)

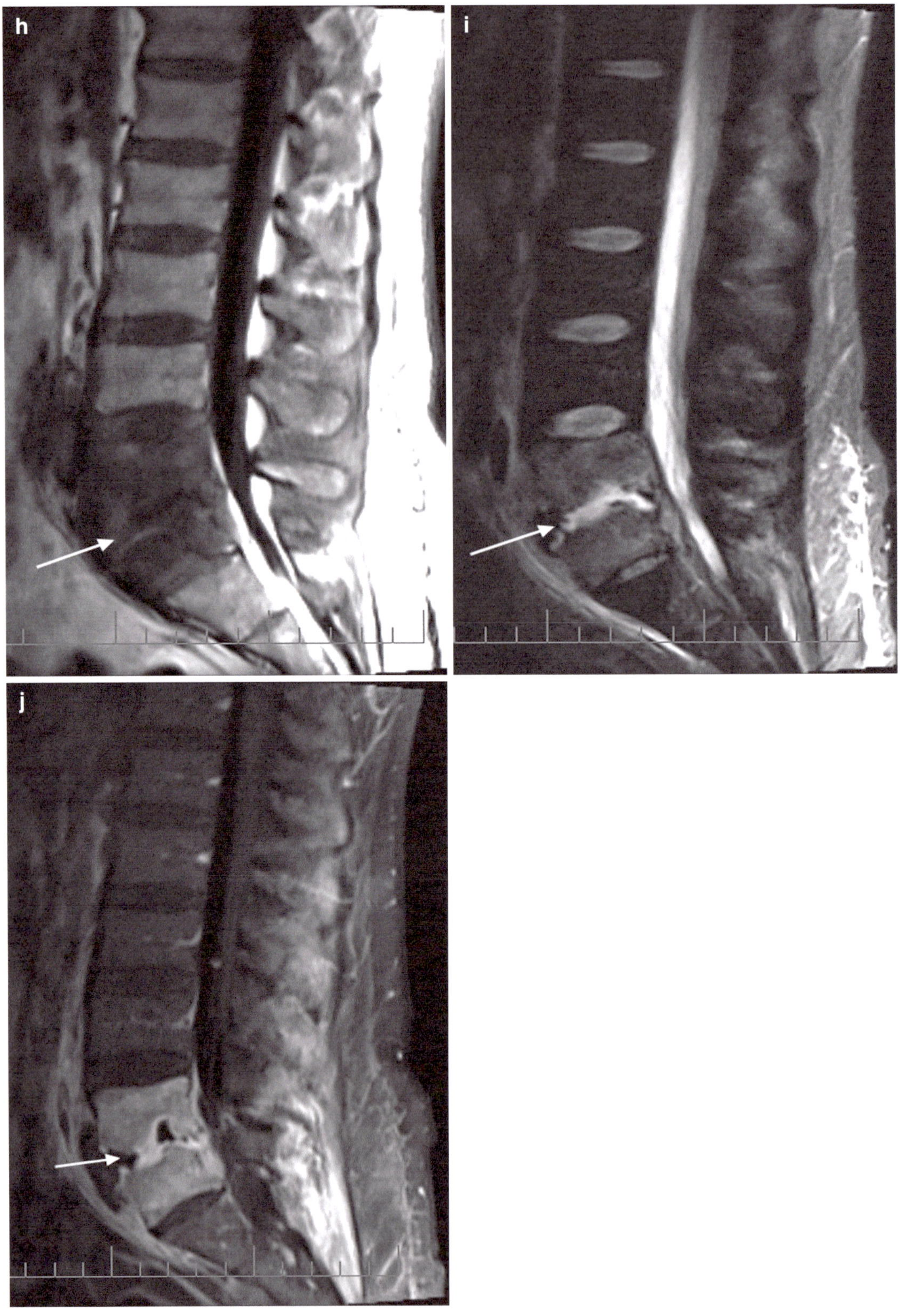

Fig. 9.6 (continued)

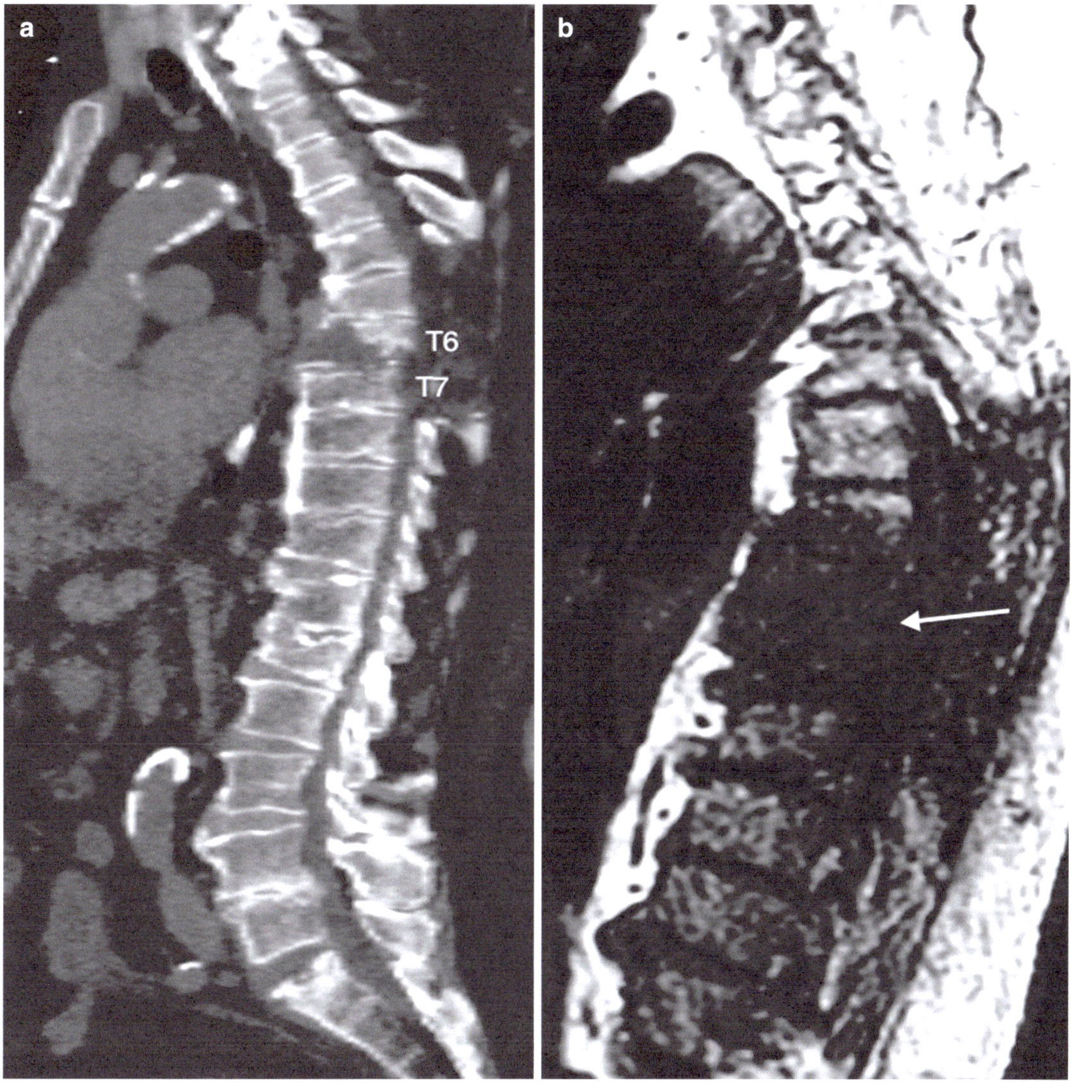

Fig. 9.7 A 65-year-old male with methicillin-resistant *Staphylococcus aureus* (*MRSA*) proven T6-T7 septic spondylodiskitis. Reformatted sagittal CT image in bone window algorithm (**a**) shows irregularity of the T6 and T7 endplates with advanced erosion and destruction of the T6 vertebral body. Sagittal T1-weighted image (**b**) shows diffuse hypointense signal (*arrow*) from T6 to T7 with loss of the normal endplate cortical margins. Sagittal T2-weighted image (**c**) shows hyperintense fluid signal within the T6-T7 disk space and T6 vertebral body (*arrow*). Sagittal T1-weighted fat-suppressed contrast-enhanced image (**d**) shows peripheral enhancement around the fluid collection (*arrow*) indicative of a large intradiskal and vertebral body abscess. Axial CT images (**e**, **f**) acquired during a spine biopsy show the biopsy needle (*arrow*) advanced between the right seventh rib (*R*) and transverse process (*TP*) (a costotransverse approach), in order to access the T6-T7 disk space

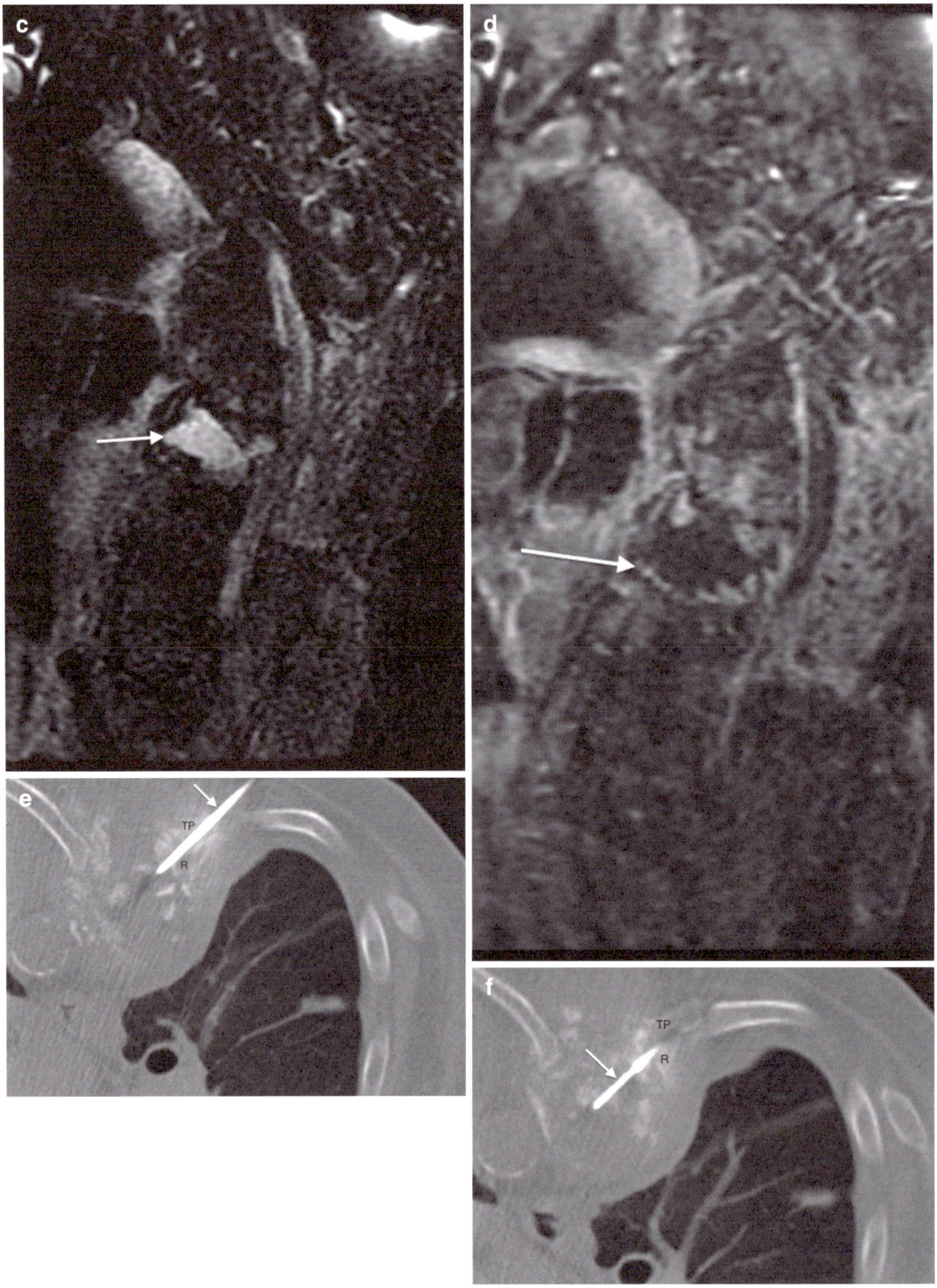

Fig. 9.7 (continued)

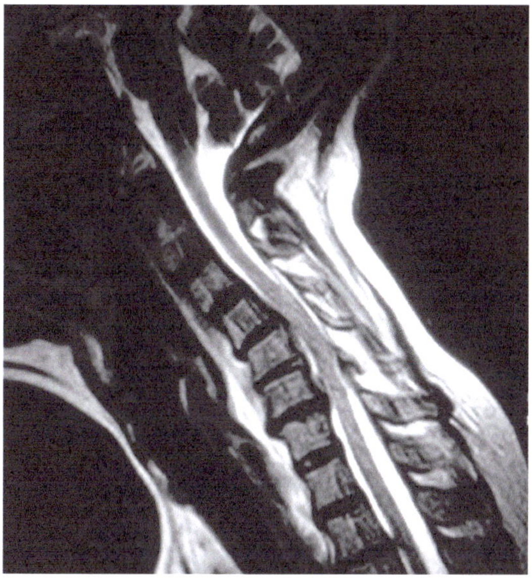

Fig. 9.8 Epidural abscess in patient with severe neck pain. T2-weighted sagittal image shows a small focal hyperintense ventral epidural fluid collection at C5-C6 that is associated with mass effect upon the spinal cord

dysfunction (Govender 2005). *Mycobacterium tuberculosis* is a particularly common cause of spine infection in HIV-positive patients, reported in up to 60% of identified pathogens (Duarte and Vaccaro 2013). On imaging, involvement of the vertebral pedicle, lamina, and spinous process is uncommon for pyogenic infection and should raise the suspicion for *Mycobacterium tuberculosis* (Duarte and Vaccaro 2013). The duration of treatment for tuberculous spondylodiskitis is also longer with recommendations of at least 12 months, to prevent multidrug resistance in the immunocompromised patient.

9.8 Spine Infection in the Postoperative Spine Patient

The diagnosis of spine infection in the postoperative spine patient is a challenging situation that requires correlation with the surgical procedure, clinical presentation, laboratory, and imaging findings. Clinically, the signs and symptoms of pain and elevated temperature are unreliable and may occur with the healing response in the postoperative patient. A persistently elevated CRP for greater than 2 weeks following spine surgery is an early indication of postoperative infection (Mazzie et al. 2014). Postsurgical change following a spine intervention and developing infection are difficult to differentiate on diagnostic imaging examinations. For example, hyperintense T2 signal is seen within the intervertebral disk space and subchondral endplates after diskectomy, with varying contrast disk enhancement (Mazzie et al. 2014). Asymptomatic post-diskectomy patients often have contrast-enhanced MR studies that show focal enhancement at the diskectomy site, linear enhancement within the intervertebral disk, and, less often, vertebral endplate enhancement (Ross et al. 1996). While initially these "normal" postsurgical changes are confined to the surgical tract and site, subsequent spread of signal change and contrast enhancement beyond the surgical bed, a so-called triad of vertebral bone marrow, and intradiskal and posterior annulus fibrosis enhancement may herald infection (Boden et al. 1992). Due to the overlap between expected inflammatory changes and infection on diagnostic imaging of the postoperative spine, image-guided percutaneous biopsy is sometimes requested in order to evaluate for possible postoperative spine infection (Fig. 9.10). When identified either via biopsy or blood culture, the most common pathogens that are encountered for postoperative spine infections are *Staphylococcus* species.

Postoperative spine paraspinal fluid collections are common and may be incidental or require further intervention, based upon the patient's clinical presentation (Fig. 9.11). These paraspinal fluid collections can be classified as seromas, hematomas, pseudomeningoceles, or abscesses. Differentiating a non-infected fluid collection from an infected collection may be difficult but is critical for appropriate patient care. Paraspinal seromas are collections of lymphatic-type fluid, which may be encapsulated. Seromas follow the imaging characteristics of fluid on CT and MRI; however, a small hematocrit level may be evident (Jain et al. 2014). Encapsulated seromas may demonstrate homogenous wall enhancement on contrast-enhanced MRI. Treatment options range

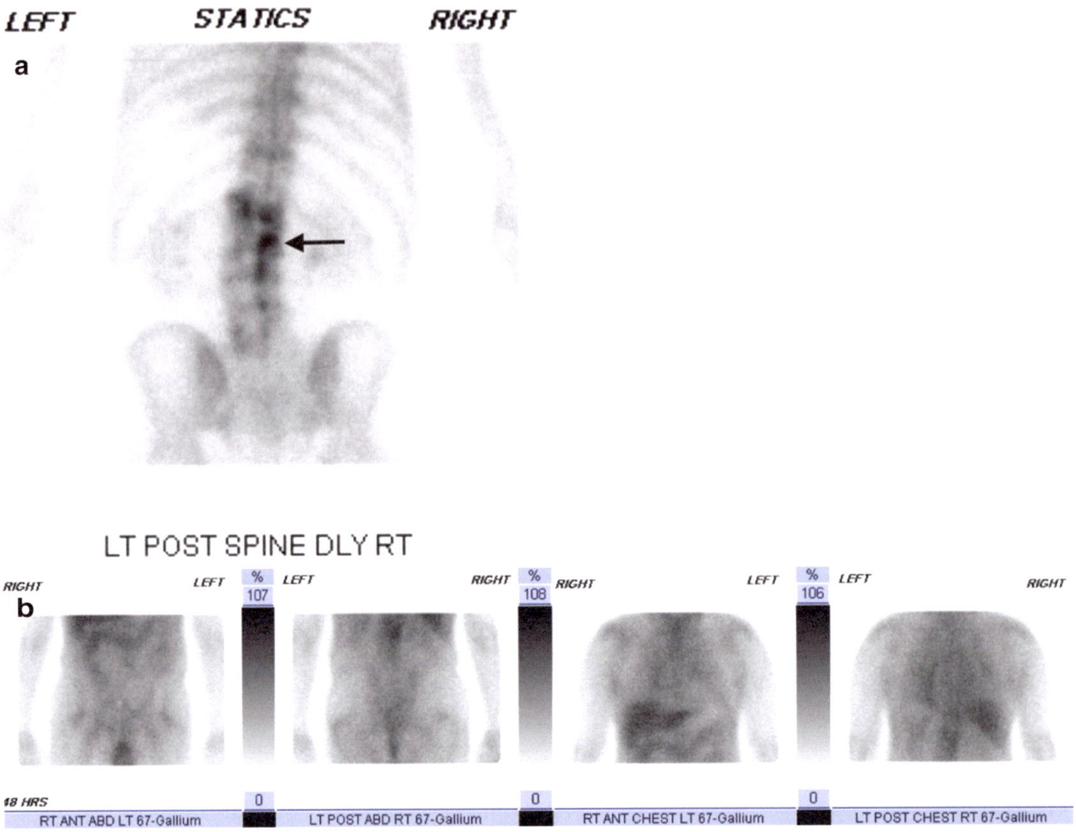

Fig. 9.9 An 85-year-old male with intermittent low back pain and abnormal gait. Static posterior image from bone scan (**a**) shows asymmetric focal radionuclide uptake (*arrow*) within the upper lumbar spine; this was attributed to osteoarthritis. Multiple static images from a negative gallium scan (**b**). Frontal radiograph (**c**) of the lumbar spine shows degenerative changes of the spine; there is focal erosive change on the right at L1-L2 (*arrow*). T1-weighted sagittal image (**d**) shows extensive hypointense signal extending from T12 to L2 (*arrows*) with loss of the vertebral endplate margins. T2-weighted sagittal image (**e**) shows patchy hyperintense signal in the same distribution (*arrows*) and focal increased signal (curved arrow) within the T12-L1 disk space. Fat-suppressed contrast-enhanced T1-weighted axial image (**f**) shows prominent patchy enhancement throughout the T12-L1 disk (*small arrow*), left peri-diskal soft tissue enhancement (*large arrow*), and left peri-facet soft tissue enhancement (*curved arrow*). Due to the relatively asymptomatic nature of the patient's clinical presentation, this was initially thought to be related to aggressive degenerative changes of the spine, and the patient was referred for spine injections. However, the MR imaging findings and their location within the upper lumbar spine suggested the possibility of an indolent spine infection; the high degree of radiologic suspicion prompted a consideration for an image-guided percutaneous biopsy

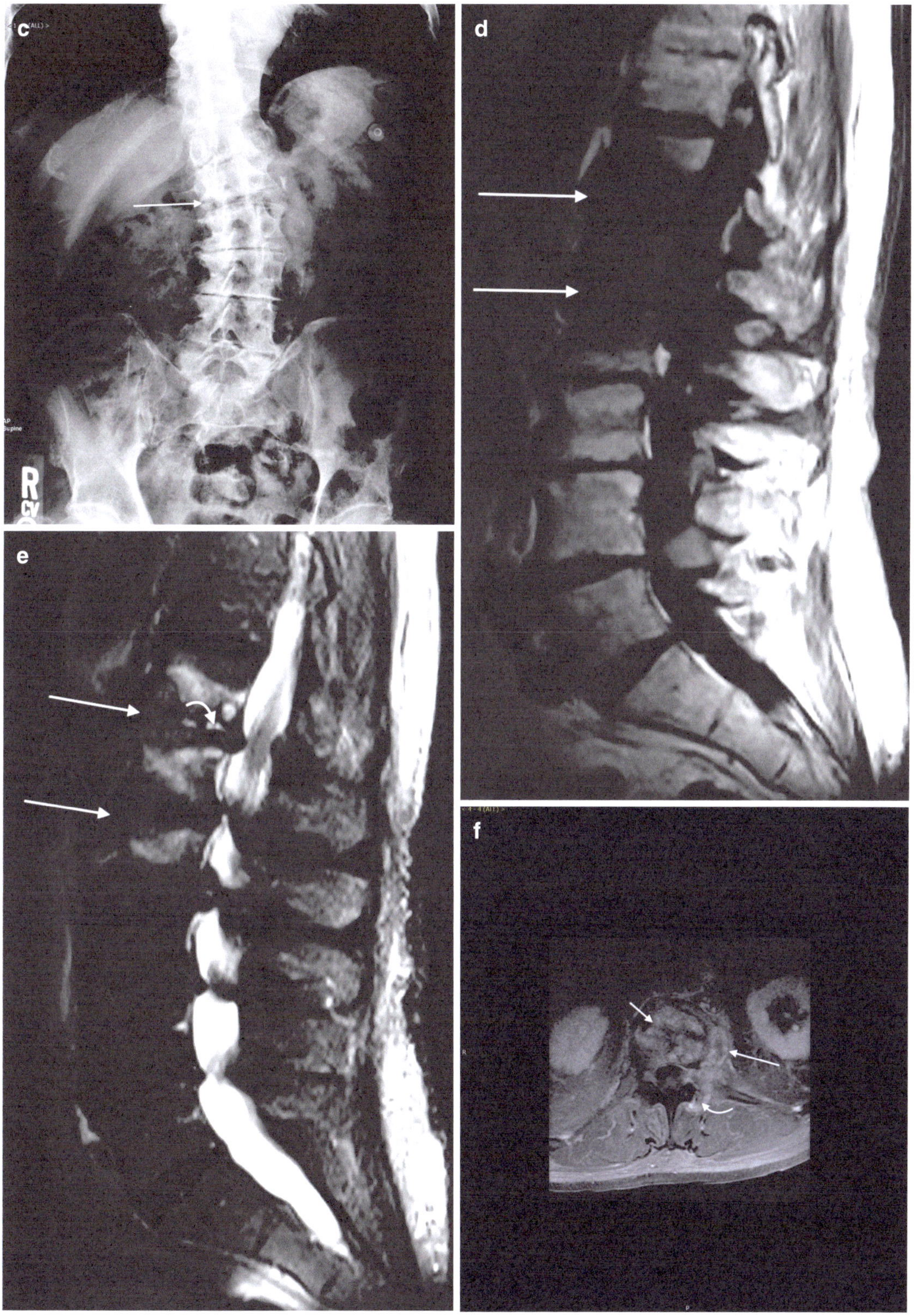

Fig. 9.9 (continued)

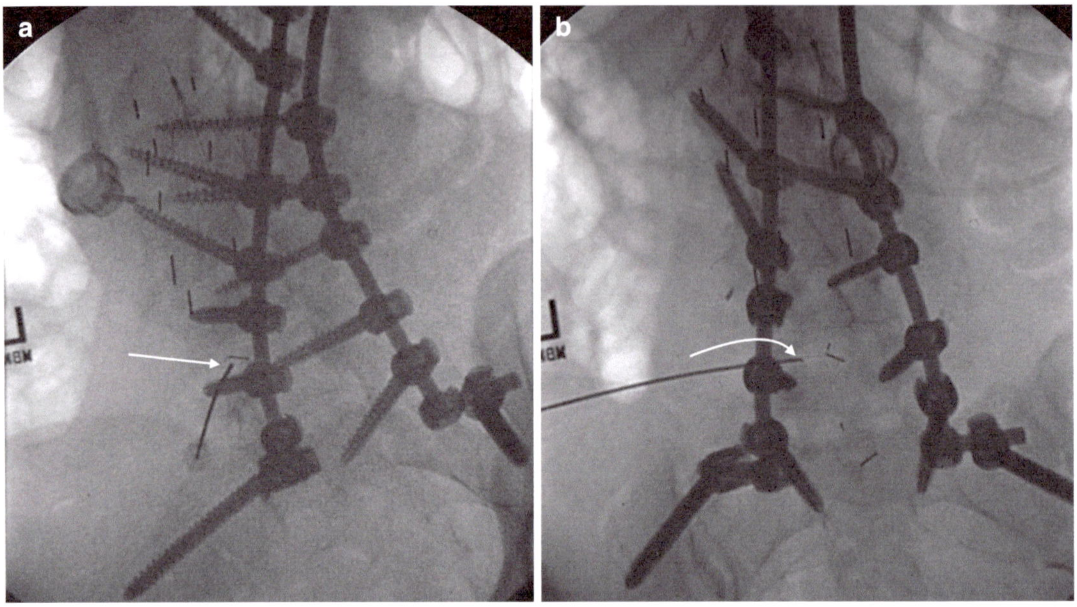

Fig. 9.10 A 53-year-old female with fever and back pain presenting for fluoroscopic-guided aspiration of the L4-L5 disk space, previously noted to be abnormal on an MRI study. The patient is status post extensive spinal fusion for scoliosis 3 months prior to presentation. Oblique and AP fluoroscopic images (**a**, **b**) of the lumbar spine show a 13-gauge needle (*arrow*) advanced into the L4-L5 disk using a left posterior oblique approach

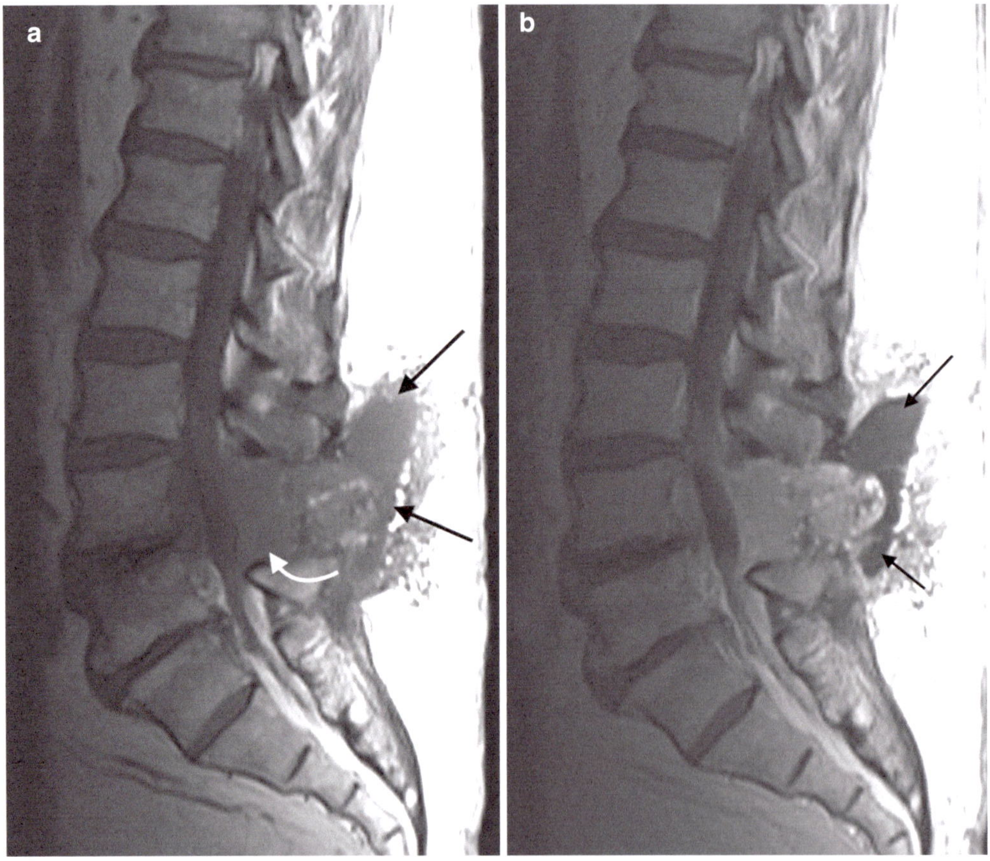

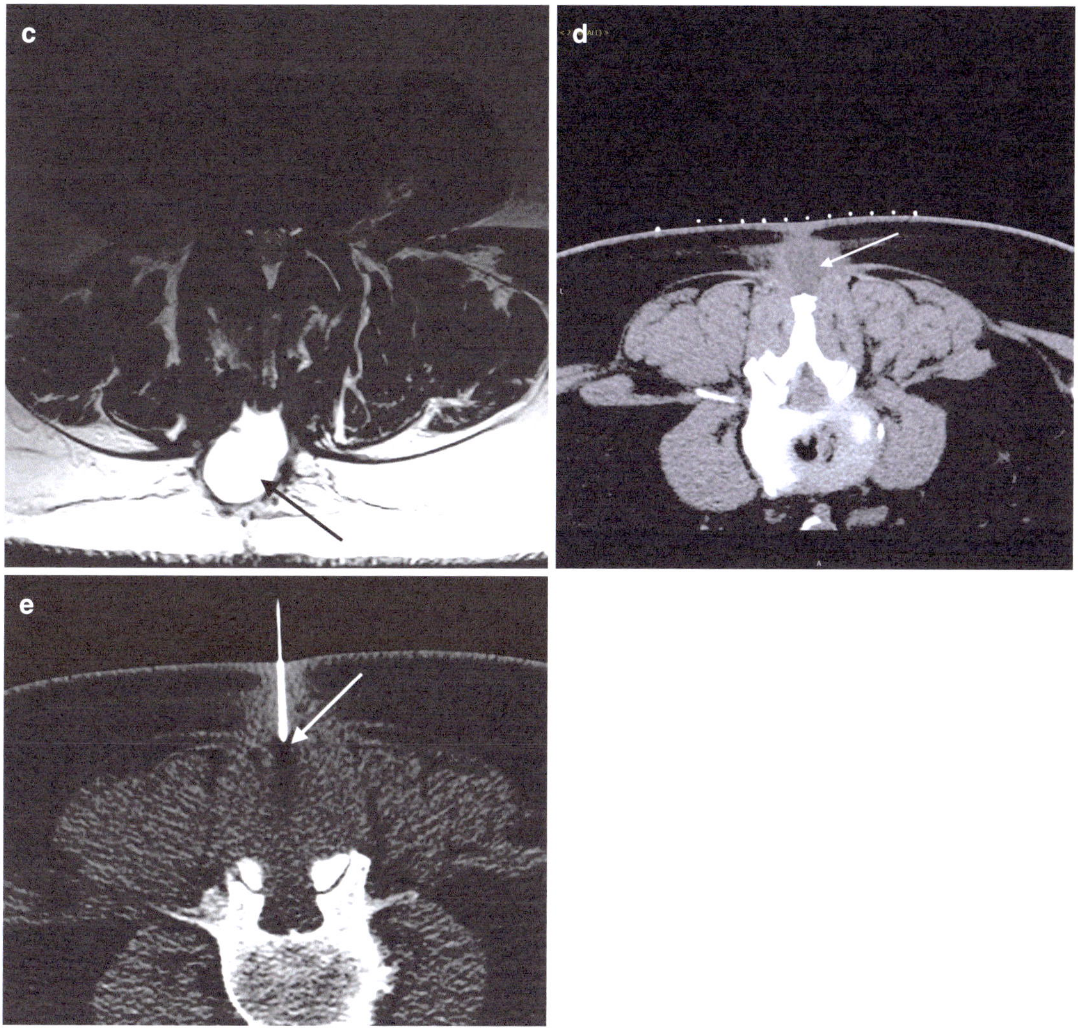

Fig. 9.11 (continued)

Fig. 9.11 A 76-year-old male with low back pain following a laminectomy and diskectomy for an L4-L5 extruded disk herniation. T1-weighted sagittal image (**a**) shows a laminectomy (*curved arrow*) and a posterior paraspinal fluid collection (*arrows*). The collection (*arrows*) does not enhance as shown on the contrast-enhanced T1 image (**b**) and is well circumscribed and hyperintense (*arrow*) as shown on the T2-weighted axial image (**c**). The patient's laboratory parameters (WBC, ESR, CRP) were all normal, and he was afebrile; nevertheless, because of his pain symptoms, the surgeon requested an aspiration drainage procedure. This was performed using strict aseptic technique and with initiation of intravenous antibiotic prophylaxis at the start of the procedure. Axial CT image in soft tissue algorithm (**d**) with skin grid in place shows the hypodense fluid collection (*arrow*) just superficial to the spinous process. A coaxial system (**e**) with a small guide cannula (*arrow*) was used to aspirate the collection – a seroma

from conservative management to percutaneous or surgical drainage depending on the nature and extent of the patient's symptoms. Hematomas are uncommon in the postoperative spine patient, occurring in less than 1% of cases (Jain et al. 2014). They are extravascular collections of blood, which result from iatrogenic manipulation and are found at or immediately adjacent to the operative site. Hematomas have variable imaging characteristics depending on the stage of hemorrhage. On CT, acute hemorrhage is hyperdense and decreases in density as time progresses. Signal changes on T1- and T2-weighted MR sequences follow the evolution of blood products within the collection. Because of their location within the epidural space, epidural hematomas may cause spinal cord compression and edema and require immediate spine surgical consultation for possible evacuation. Pseudomeningoceles are collections of cerebrospinal fluid (CSF) that extend from the spinal canal into the adjacent paraspinal soft tissues and are typically the result of a breach of the dura mater. Pseudomeningoceles follow the imaging characteristics of CSF on CT and MRI and may also contain a small hematocrit level due to hemorrhage. Variable treatment options are available and include observation with monitoring, compression bandages, epidural blood patch, percutaneous or surgical drainage, or direct surgical repair of the dural defect. An abscess is a focal collection of infected fluid. Edema of the paraspinal soft tissues or epidural space can be present and with contiguous spread of infection may progress into an abscess. Paraspinal and epidural abscesses can have a variable imaging characteristics depending on stage and water content. Classically, they appear as a thick-walled fluid collection, which demonstrates avid irregular wall enhancement following the intravenous administration of contrast agent. In many instances, it may be difficult to distinguish between an abscess, pseudomeningocele, and seroma on diagnostic imaging examinations. Positive blood cultures and persistently elevated CRP are laboratory findings suggestive of infection. Ultimately, percutaneous or open surgical drainage may be necessary for diagnostic evaluation with therapeutic implications. Because it is highly desirable to avoid superinfecting a sterile fluid collection, image-guided percutaneous aspiration procedures are best discussed with the referring clinician in order to develop the appropriate treatment plan for the patient.

> The diagnosis of spine infection in normal patients, immunocompromised patients, or postoperative spine patients requires a high index of clinical suspicion and utilizes a combination of clinical, laboratory, and imaging findings.

9.8.1 Indications

The indication for performing image-guided percutaneous spine biopsy is to diagnose or exclude the presence of spine infection and, when spine infection is indeed present, to identify the causative microorganism. Suspected spine infection is the second most common indication for spine biopsy, after suspected metastatic disease in a patient with known primary malignancy (Tehranzadeh et al. 2007). Spine infections are typically mono-microbial with *Staphylococcus aureus* accounting for the majority of cases. *Mycobacterium tuberculosis*, *Escherichia coli*, and *Brucella* are other common pathogens that have been identified as a source of spine infection. Despite a suspicious clinical picture, including imaging findings that are consistent with spine infection, a definitive causative organism can only be obtained by microscopic analysis of an infected specimen. The offending pathogen may be harvested from the infected spine segment or, less commonly in the case of sepsis, from a positive blood culture. Identifying the causative organism is important as it can change patient management by allowing clinicians to adjust the antibiotic treatment regimen and tailor other treatments specific to the patient's condition (Rankine et al. 2004). Image-guided percutaneous spine biopsy may be considered in patients with suspected spine infection, based on the clinical presentation, laboratory data, and imaging studies, when a microbiologic diagnosis for a known associated organism has not been established by blood cultures or serologic tests (Berbari et al. 2015; Garg et al. 2014).

9.8.2 Contraindications

Bleeding diathesis and uncorrected coagulopathy (INR > 1.5 or platelets < 50,000/mm^3) are the primary contraindications to performing image-guided percutaneous biopsy in patients with suspected spine infection. Discussion with the referring physician and the patient is critical to determine the appropriate actions in either temporarily discontinuing or reversing anticoagulant and antiplatelet medications prior to spine biopsy procedures to reduce the risk of bleeding or thromboembolic events (*refer to the Chap. 1 Pre- and Peri-procedural Planning and Patient Management for Spine Biopsies*). Informed consent must also be obtained from the patient or an appropriate designated individual prior to performing image-guided biopsy.

9.9 Image Guidance and Biopsy Techniques

Image-guided percutaneous sampling of vertebral lesions and the intervertebral disk for suspected infectious spondylitis is a safe procedure that offers several advantages compared to open surgical biopsy (De Lucas et al. 2009). Percutaneous image-guided spine biopsy procedures can be performed efficiently and expeditiously within an imaging suite and do not require an operating room or an overnight hospital stay, therefore resulting in overall lower healthcare costs. Furthermore, image-guided spine biopsy procedures do not require general endotracheal anesthesia and have a lower risk of procedure-related infection or bleeding resulting in lower morbidity and complication rates as compared to open biopsy. The option for an image guidance modality is ultimately determined by the preference of the operator and equipment availability. Although the use of ultrasonography and magnetic resonance imaging have been described for performing percutaneous spine biopsy, conventional fluoroscopy, CT, or CT with fluoroscopy are the most frequently used modalities for performing image-guided spine biopsy. Conventional fluoroscopy with a multidirectional fluoroscope enables prompt access to the vertebral body or intervertebral disk with real-time monitoring of the biopsy needle relative to the level of interest. Coaxial exchanges are quickly performed with fluoroscopic guidance. Nevertheless, subtle or small lesions may not be visible or accessible with this form of imaging guidance (Kim et al. 2013). Furthermore, many critical structures such as the aorta are not well visualized with fluoroscopy. CT is advantageous in that it provides a comprehensive view of all anatomic and critical structures within the biopsy field. The biopsy needle tip location and trajectory relative to the target lesion and/or disk can be readily and precisely monitored with CT, lessening the likelihood of injury to adjacent neurovascular structures. CT fluoroscopy increases the efficiency and safety of percutaneous CT-guided spine procedures, combining the real-time benefits of fluoroscopy and the axial resolution of CT (Wu et al. 2014).

9.10 General Considerations

Communication and discussion between the operator and the referring clinician regarding the patient and the intended biopsy procedure is very important prior to performing the spine biopsy procedure. Although percutaneous image-guided spine biopsy procedures are regarded as safe and effective procedures, both the performing radiologist and referring clinician should agree that the biopsy results will affect the patient's clinical management and that this benefit firmly outweighs the risks of this interventional procedure. Additionally, if there is concern that the site to be sampled may be a malignant bone lesion, a multidisciplinary team approach with discussion between the radiologist, surgeon, oncologist, infectious disease specialist, and pathologist can be essential for patient management. Before proceeding with biopsy, the operator must review the patient's clinical data, including medical and surgical history and laboratory results, as well as perform a thorough review of all imaging studies. Adherence to these basic principles will ensure that a biopsy is indeed indicated while avoiding unnecessary procedures. It will also help to determine the optimal location and spine level to sample. Written informed consent including the risks and benefits of the procedure should be explained to the patient and/or patient's family, as well as the alternatives to percutaneous sampling including open surgical biopsy or continued medical monitoring with imaging surveillance.

Helpful steps when considering a biopsy for spine infection:

1. Obtain all pertinent clinical information (history, past medical history, past surgical history, current and recent medications, medical allergies).
2. Review all pertinent recent and prior imaging studies.
3. Consult with the referring clinician when possible.
4. Obtain and/or order laboratory studies (white blood cell count with differential, ESR, CRP; coagulation profile if necessary).

9.11 Preparation

Pre-procedural laboratory parameters including hematocrit, hemoglobin, platelet count, and coagulation profile (prothrombin time [PT], partial thromboplastin time [PTT], and international normalized ratio [INR]) should be acquired. The operator should be aware of concurrent patient medications that may be contraindicated or perhaps alter the biopsy results. Patients on antiplatelet and/or anticoagulant therapies should have these medications temporarily discontinued prior to biopsy to minimize bleeding. In the setting of suspected vertebral spondylodiskitis, a white blood cell count with differential, an erythrocyte sedimentation rate (ESR), and a C-reactive protein (CRP) should also be obtained. It should be noted if the patient has recently been placed on or is currently on antibiotic therapy. If the patient is indeed already receiving antibiotics, then the biopsy procedure should be performed within 48 h of commencing antibiotic therapy, or antibiotics should be discontinued for at least 48 h prior to performing the biopsy. The operator must be aware of any potential patient drug allergies, especially reactions to anesthetic agents and intravenous radiographic contrast media. Ideally, patients should not eat or drink (NPO status) for a minimum of 8 h prior to the procedure. A majority of image-guided spine procedures can be performed utilizing local anesthetic administration and intravenous sedation and analgesia. Intravenous sedation usually consists of a combination of a short-acting benzodiazepine (Versed) for anxiety relief, as well as an analgesic agent such as fentanyl (Sublimaze). It is best to obtain intravenous access via the forearm or hand, as the patient's arms are often bent during the procedure, a position that often compromises the functionality of antecubital venous access. Automated patient monitoring equipment, including a pulse oximeter, an electrocardiogram, and a blood pressure monitor, adds yet another level of safety to these procedures.

Patient positioning is dependent upon the anatomic region of interest and lesion location. The prone position is preferred for accessing the thoracic and lumbosacral spine, as well as the posterior elements of the cervical spine. Accessing cervical intervertebral disk spaces and vertebral body lesions is performed with the patient in the supine position in order to facilitate an anterior approach. All patients, regardless of the spine biopsy location, are prepared for the procedure using a standard protocol. Once written informed consent and intravenous access are obtained, the patient is placed on the CT or fluoroscopy table in a position to facilitate a safe and successful biopsy, without causing discomfort to the patient. A "time-out" is then initiated by the operator to verify the correct patient and procedure to be performed. Intravenous sedation and analgesia can also be administered at this time.

9.12 CT Guidance

A radiopaque grid is placed on the skin over the anticipated skin entrance site, followed by acquisition of scout images in the frontal and lateral projections. After review of the preliminary images through the spine level of interest, an entrance site is selected and marked with a skin marker. The skin is then prepped via standard sterile technique and draped. The skin entrance site is then anesthetized utilizing a local anesthetic agent (e.g., 2% lidocaine) utilizing a 25-gauge needle, which is advanced deeper along the expected needle path and trajectory. For deeper local anesthesia, additional anesthetic agent may be administered using a 22-gauge needle. Utilizing a #11 scalpel blade, a small crosshair skin incision is made to facilitate placement of larger caliber needles through the skin and superficial fascia. A coaxial bone biopsy needle system utilizing a single needle pass to access the target is our preferred method for biopsy of vertebral osteomyelitis, minimizing the possibility of injuring normal tissues and critical structures. The biopsy needles can be advanced through a guide cannula that is "parked" at the level of interest. Disk aspiration is facilitated by utilizing a 20-mL syringe connected to the biopsy needle so as to create negative pressure while performing needle excursions within the area of suspected infection. Once the needle is confirmed to be within the desired disk space, craniocaudal and mediolateral angulation of the needle can also be performed with each sample to increase specimen yield. The location of the biopsy needle should be monitored with CT for each attempted needle pass, to confirm the location of the needle relative to the area of interest and relative to adjacent critical anatomic structures. The aspirated intradiskal material and/or subchondral bone are placed into sterile containers and submitted for microbiological analysis. Aspirated blood can also be submitted for microbiologic analysis.

9.13 Biopsy Technique: The Cervical Spine

An anterior approach (*as described in Chap. 4 Cervical Spine Biopsy*) is used to access the cervical intervertebral disk space. These are not frequently performed as cervical spine infections are less common than thoracic or lumbar spine infections. The general principles in terms of using coaxial technique to minimize needle insertions adjacent to critical anatomic structures, optimal visualization and avoidance of these critical structures, and optimal lesion targeting to maximize specimen yield are particularly important in this region of the spinal axis, where the spine structures are smaller and surrounded by several important vascular and nonvascular structures. CT aids in optimal visualization of critical structures and their anatomic relation to the suspected site of infection within the cervical spine. In some cases, however, fluoroscopic techniques with manual retraction of the carotid space structures can yield quick and safe access to the intervertebral disk.

9.14 Biopsy Technique: The Thoracic Spine

When sampling the intervertebral disk space of the thoracic spine, care must be taken to avoid the lung and pleura, the thoracic aorta, and the spinal cord. The thoracic spine can be accessed via transpedicular or extrapedicular posterolateral approaches. Transpedicular approaches in the thoracic spine are employed when sampling suspected foci of osteomyelitis that occupy an accessible portion of the vertebral body. The margins of the pedicle, especially the medial margin, should be visualized, while the needle traverses the pedicle into the vertebral body. There are three extrapedicular posterolateral approaches including the costotransverse, transcostovertebral, and intercostal routes of access (Figs. 9.7 and 9.12).

The costotransverse approach is a well-established approach to sample thoracic vertebral body lesions (Fig. 9.7). This approach requires needle placement between the vertebral transverse process and the tubercle of the corresponding rib. The head of the rib articulates with superior vertebral costal facet, which is located in the posterolateral superior aspect of the vertebra immediately caudal to the superior endplate, thus allowing access to lesions in the upper portion of

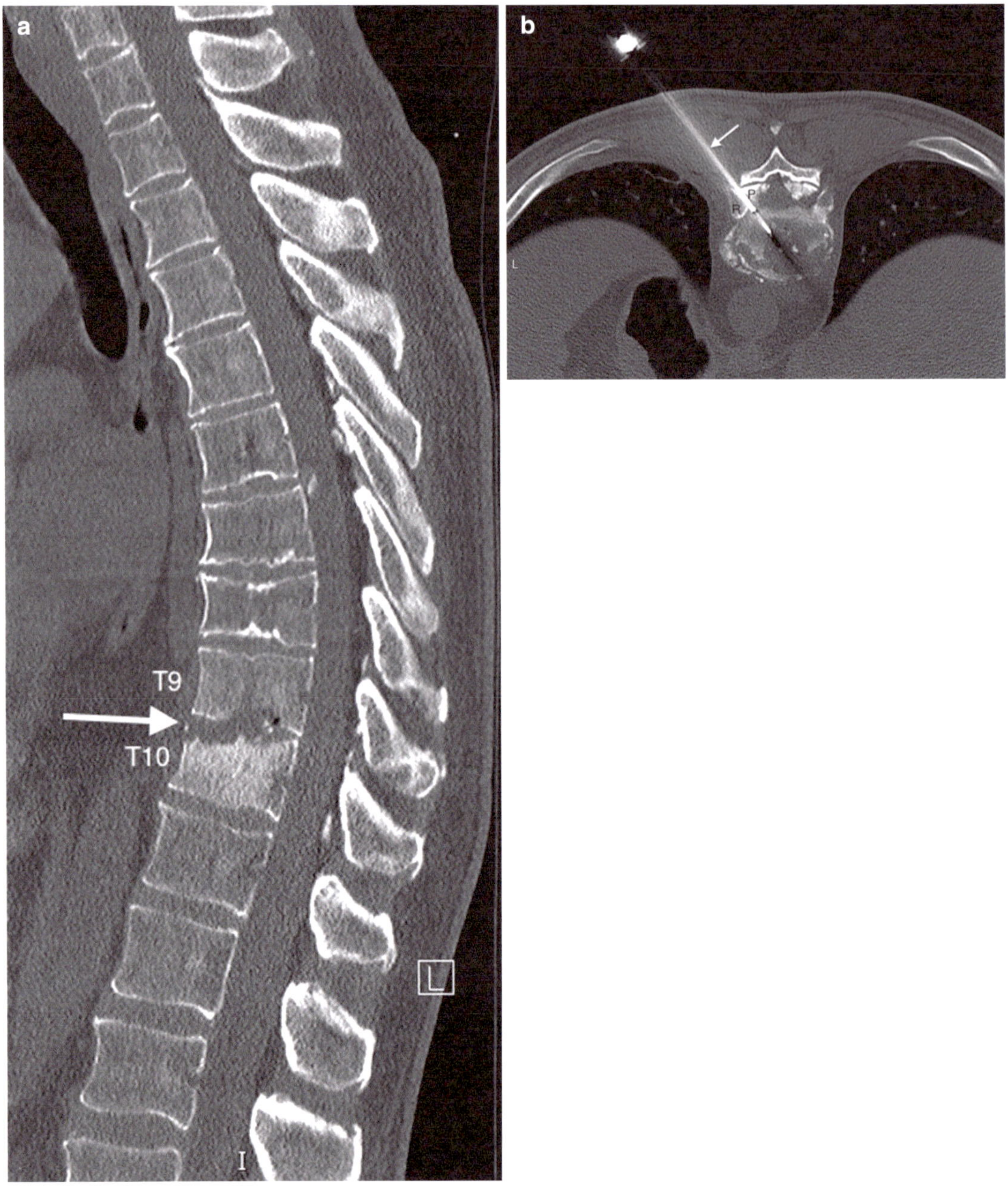

Fig. 9.12 A 65-year-old male with clinically proven acute osteomyelitis, culture positive for *S. aureus*. Reformatted sagittal CT image in bone window algorithm (**a**) shows irregularity, sclerosis, and erosion of the T9-T10 vertebral endplates (*arrow*). Axial CT image (**b**) acquired during biopsy shows the biopsy needle (*arrow*) advanced in an anatomical groove between the head of the left tenth rib (*R*) and the pedicle (*P*), a transcostovertebral approach, and safely entering the T9-T10 disk space

the vertebral body, as well as entry into the intervertebral disk space along the superior endplate of the corresponding accessed vertebra. The posteromedial margin of the rib prevents the needle from puncturing the pleura, and the transverse process prevents entrance into the spinal canal. Damaging the costotransverse articulation is a theoretical risk with the costotransverse approach.

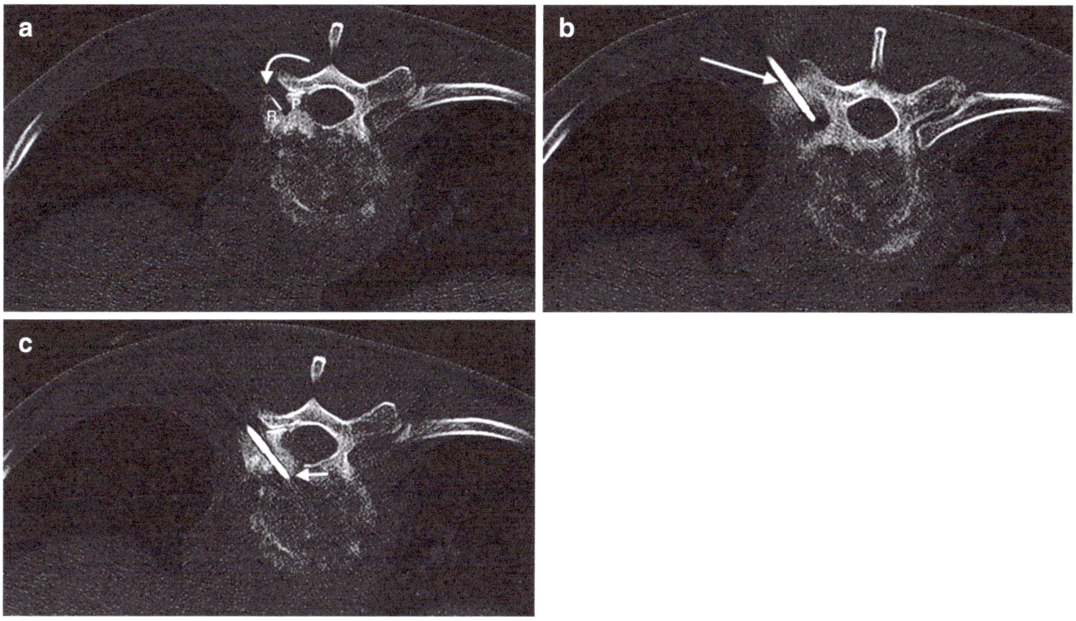

Fig. 9.13 A 59-year-old male with a history of previously treated *Streptococcus anginosus* infectious spondylitis at T9-T10 presents with back pain and elevated ESR and CRP. Axial CT image (**a**) acquired during biopsy shows a spinal needle (*curved arrow*) entering the groove between the pedicle (*P*) and rib (*R*), a transcostovertebral approach. Axial CT images (**b**, **c**) acquired during biopsy show advancement of a bone biopsy needle (*small arrow in* **c**) through a guide needle (*large arrow in b*) into the T9-T10 disk space for successful sampling of the T9-T10 disk and adjacent vertebral endplate

The transcostovertebral approach is a modification of the costotransverse approach (Fig. 9.12). This is an excellent approach for sampling the intervertebral disk space and adjacent vertebral endplate when osteomyelitis is suspected (Fig. 9.13). The needle trajectory is located slightly superior to the costotransverse joint, and the biopsy needle system is advanced in a groove formed between the pedicle and head of the corresponding rib, preventing inadvertent lung puncture and injury to the exiting nerve root. This anatomical groove is located just above the transverse process, which allows more freedom for needle angulation and, as with the costotransverse approach, allows access to lesions within the superior aspect of the vertebral body and the adjacent intervertebral disk space, facilitating both vertebral endplate and disk sampling.

The posteromedial intercostal approach is infrequently performed, but it is a reported technique that is used to access paravertebral thoracic soft tissue masses that extend from the vertebral body into the adjacent paravertebral soft tissues. Needle placement is located within the posteromedial intercostal space, anterior to the head of the rib and the costovertebral joint. Given the more tangential needle trajectory, sampling vertebral body lesions with intact cortex via the intercostal approach assumes a higher risk of inadvertent lung puncture because the needle has a tendency to be deflected anteriorly. This approach also has the added risk of causing intercostal vascular injury. When using this approach to sample a paravertebral soft tissue mass, it might be helpful to infiltrate a few milliliters of sterile normal saline into the paravertebral soft tissues so as to create more space for needle manipulation by pushing the parietal pleura and lung anteriorly.

9.15 Biopsy Technique: The Lumbar Spine

In lumbar spine biopsy, the critical anatomic structures of interest include the abdominal aorta, inferior vena cava, kidneys, bowel, and exiting spinal nerves. Accessing the lumbar intervertebral disk spaces and the adjacent subchondral vertebral endplates for evaluation of vertebral osteomyelitis is performed via the transpedicular or the extrapedicular posterolateral approach. The transpedicular approach is often utilized for lesions that are located within the pedicle or are centrally located within the vertebral body. Access to the intervertebral disk can also be obtained by utilizing the transpedicular approach (Michel et al. 2006). For this approach, the biopsy needle is placed in the groove between the superior articular process and the transverse process, thereby directly entering the ipsilateral pedicle. The upper lumbar vertebral disk spaces and vertebral endplates are often oriented either parallel or angled superiorly relative to the needle trajectory; therefore, once the needle passes through the pedicle, cranial angulation is performed to sample both the superior endplate and the disk space with a single biopsy pass (Fig. 9.3). Care must always be taken not to penetrate the medial cortex of the pedicle as this would constitute a breach into the spinal canal and its contents. The transpedicular approach is preferred by some operators as compared to the posterolateral approach due to the shorter and more direct path of the former. Nevertheless, efficient and successful biopsy of the intervertebral disk and vertebral endplate can be performed by utilizing the posterolateral approach (Fig. 9.4). The entry site and trajectory are through the soft tissues just lateral to the superior articular process before entering the disk space or the lateral vertebral cortex. The exiting lumbar nerve roots pass through the upper portion of the neural foramen, just posterior to the disk-endplate complex. The posterolateral route allows access to the disk space by traversing the inferior margin lateral to the neural foramen. Careful attention to the patient's anatomy and imaging guidance will help to avoid injury to the exiting nerve root. In the lumbar spine, this can be achieved with CT guidance or with fluoroscopic guidance. While the advantages of CT have already been described, lumbar disk biopsy can be quickly and safely performed using fluoroscopic guidance. This requires craniocaudal angulation of the fluoroscope in order to align the vertebral endplates at the level of interest. Next, the fluoroscope is rotated ipsilateral oblique in a mediolateral direction depending on the side of percutaneous access (toward the right on the patient's right side and toward the left on the patient's left side). This maneuver effectively creates a "scotty dog" configuration on the fluoroscopic image such that superior articular process projects over the disk space of interest anywhere from 30 to 50% along the visualized width of the disk space. A steeper oblique angulation allows for access of the more median and posterior aspect of the disk. The biopsy needle system will "ride" along the lateral aspect of the superior articular process in order to access the disk space (Fig. 9.14). The biopsy needle system can also be angled cephalad to sample the inferior cortical endplate or caudal to sample the superior cortical endplate.

A lateral access route (Garces and Hidalgo 2000) which places the patient in a lateral decubitus position displaces the abdominal viscera forward and allows for direct access to the lumbar vertebral body, intervertebral disks, and paravertebral masses while avoiding the nerve roots, bowel, kidneys, and vessels. The transforaminodiskal method (Sucu et al. 2003) is an alternative to the posterolateral approach.

9.16 Challenging Disk Biopsies

L5-S1 disk space biopsy can pose a challenge. With fluoroscopic guidance and a steep oblique lateral-to-medial approach, along with craniocaudal angulation to align the L5 inferior vertebral endplate and S1 superior vertebral endplate, the fluoroscope is used to create a radiolucent triangular portal of entry to the

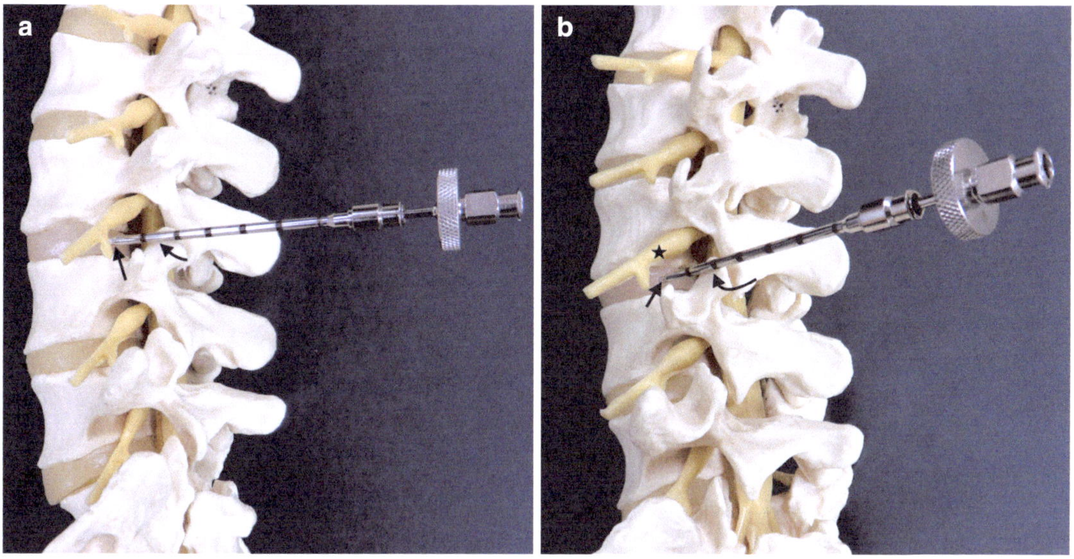

Fig. 9.14 Photographs of a lumbar spine model with a coaxial needle biopsy system inserted via posterolateral approach. Lateral view (**a**) shows guide needle overlying the superior articular process (*curved arrow*) and then passing underneath the exiting nerve root (*arrow*) to enter the disk space. Oblique view (**b**) again shows the close proximity of the guide needle as it passes over the superior articular process (*curved arrow*) to then enter the disk (*arrow*) beneath the exiting nerve root (*star*)

disk (Fig. 9.15). The anatomic relations of this radiographic inverted triangle include the iliac crest laterally, the S1 superior articular process medially, and the L5 inferior vertebral endplate superiorly. This approach helps to avoid the exiting L5 nerve root. Sometimes, due to the patient's intrinsic spinal axis geometry, it is not possible to access the L5-S1 disk despite maximal angulation maneuvers. In this situation, it is often helpful to use abdominal and pelvic bolsters to correct for steeply oriented disk spaces or, alternatively, place the patient in a prone oblique position. Bolsters can also be utilized when performing L5-S1 disk biopsy with CT guidance. Alternatively, angulation of the CT gantry parallel to the L5-S1 disk space can be helpful in gaining access for disk sampling. As previously mentioned, a transpedicular approach with appropriate angulation of the needle, depending on which pedicle is entered (L5, angle caudally, or S1, angle cranially), can be used to access the L5-S1 disk and vertebral endplate (Fig. 9.3).

9.17 Disk Aspiration Techniques

Obtaining a satisfactory specimen from a disk biopsy is not an easy task. The conventional method for attempting to biopsy the disk is to place a small gauge needle within the disk and to aspirate using continuous suction with a syringe that is attached to the needle as the needle is moved back and forth within the disk. This is often followed by the injection of a small amount of sterile saline into the disk and aspiration of the saline lavage. Neither of these techniques is particularly suited to obtaining disk material due to the small caliber of the aspiration needle (often 18–22-gauge), the connective tissue characteristics of the disk annulus, and the high viscosity of disk material. An alternative to this approach is to perform a mixed vertebral endplate disk biopsy by angling the bone biopsy needle into the vertebral endplate.

Another technique that can be used to perform a disk biopsy is to utilize a percutaneous

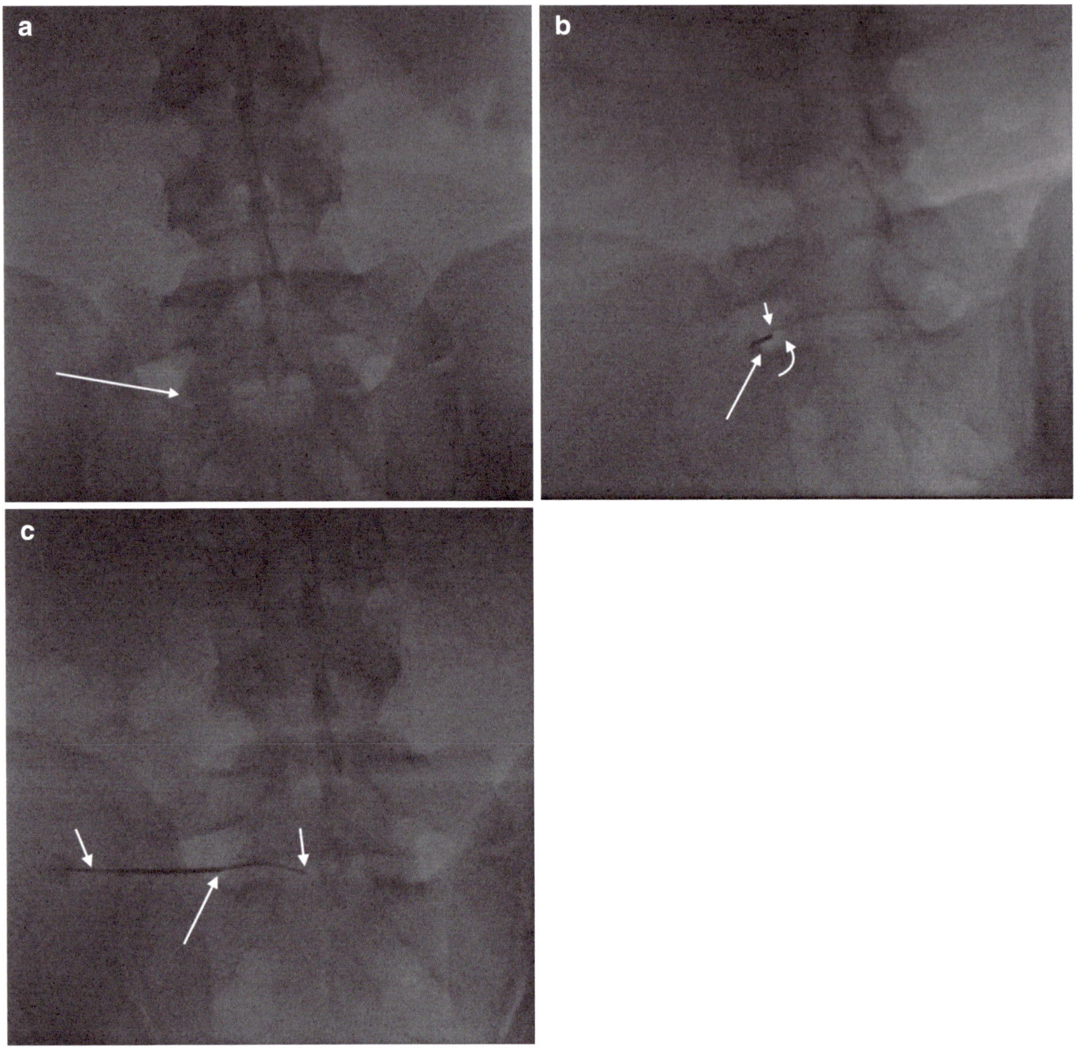

Fig. 9.15 Fluoroscopic approach to the L5-S1 disk space. Frontal radiograph (**a**) shows L5-S1 disk (*arrow*). In order to access this disk space, the fluoroscope is angled both in the craniocaudal direction, so as to align the vertebral endplates at L5-S1, and in an ipsilateral mediolateral orientation so as to keep the iliac crest from obscuring and preventing access to the disk space. The result of these fluoroscopic maneuvers should result in an image (**b**) that projects the superior articular process of S1 (*curved arrow*) over the L5-S1 disk space. A radiolucent inverted triangle is formed by the inferior endplate of L5 (*small arrow*), the iliac crest (*large arrow*), and the superior articular process of S1 (*curved arrow*) as shown on the oblique radiograph (**b**). A needle can then be advanced with a "down-the-barrel" approach toward the disk. In this case, an insert needle (*small arrows*) has been advanced into the disk through a guide needle (*large arrow*) as shown on the frontal radiographic projection (**c**)

diskectomy device (Wattamwar and Ortiz 2010). A 13- or 17-gauge guide needle is advanced into the margin of the disk (Fig. 9.16). A 6-in. automated percutaneous device is then inserted coaxially via the guide needle into the disk. The device is then activated, and its excursions to and fro within the disk are actively monitored with fluoroscopy. This device is able to aspirate infected purulent fluid material within the disk as well as disk tissue. Coaxial technique allows for multiple passes with this device in order to obtain adequate amounts of disk specimen for subsequent microbiologic and histopathologic analysis. The initial experience with this type of device has been extremely favorable in terms of obtaining an adequate specimen yield. In addition, the guide needle can then be exchanged over a removable hub insert needle, with subsequent placement of a bone biopsy system that can then be used to obtain specimens from the adjacent vertebral endplates.

9.18 Specimen Handling

The operator should obtain as much specimen as reasonably possible, be given the location and extent of the suspected infectious process, and be given the limitations of the biopsy tools that the operator is using. Specimen handling and transfer are important steps in the biopsy process for spine infection. Under optimal conditions, specimens should be submitted for both microbiologic and pathologic analysis. All microbiology specimens should be placed in sterile containers and transported as soon as reasonably possible to the microbiology laboratory. The clinical, including whether or not the patient is already on antibiotic therapy, and imaging information should be communicated with the request for microbiologic analysis. If a specific pathogen, for example, *Mycobacterium tuberculosis*, is suspected, then this information should also be communicated to the laboratory personnel. Most specimens are submitted for bacterial, fungal, and mycobacterial stains and cultures. The specimens (e.g., mycobacterial) may be kept for a long period of time, and the operator should periodically check for the final results of each specific test. For pathology, the specimens can be placed in a container with 10% formalin and then transported to the pathology department. Bone specimens will require additional processing time in order to allow for appropriate decalcification prior to histopathologic analysis.

Key Review Points

1. The incidence of spine infection appears to be increasing.
2. The imaging diagnosis of spine infection is improved by not only being aware of the early imaging findings in spine infection but also by suspecting this diagnosis.
3. MRI is the imaging modality of choice for helping to diagnose spine infection.
4. Spine biopsy, whenever possible, is best performed before the initiation of antibiotic therapy.
5. A persistently elevated CRP for greater than 2 weeks following spine surgery is an early indication of postoperative spine infection.
6. Postoperative paraspinal fluid collections are common and include seroma, hematoma, pseudomeningocele, and abscess. Percutaneous image-guided biopsy is sometimes requested to exclude an infected collection.
7. Coaxial techniques with sampling of the intervertebral disk and the adjacent vertebral endplates maximize specimen yield.

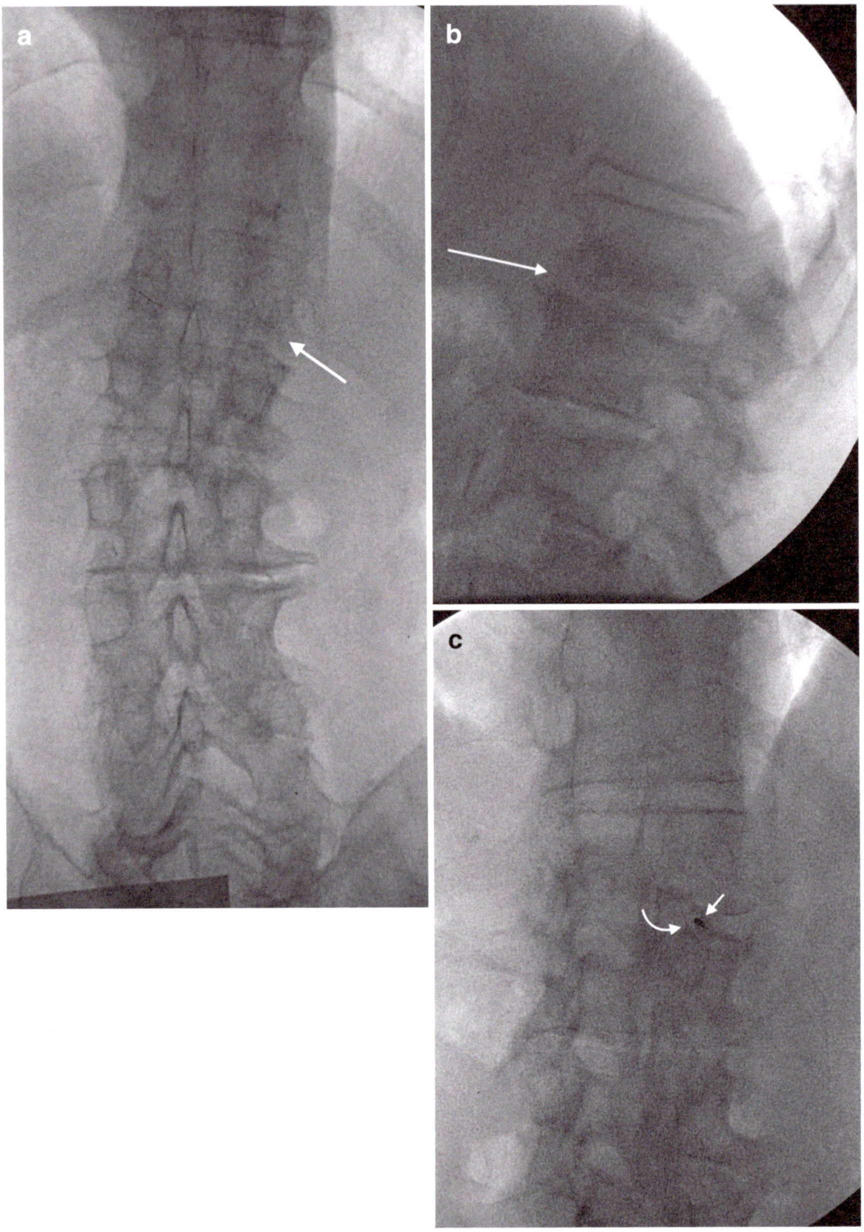

Fig. 9.16 An 85-year-old male with intermittent low back pain and abnormal gait. Frontal projection of the lumbar spine (**a**) shows vertebral endplate erosion at T12-L1 (*arrow*). Lateral radiograph of lumbar spine (**b**) shows disk space narrowing and reactive sclerosis at T12-L1 (*arrow*). Oblique fluoroscopic image (**c**) of lumbar during the spine biopsy shows advancement of a 17-gauge spinal needle (*arrow*) adjacent to the superior articular process of L1 (*curved arrow*). Note that this mediolateral angulation of the fluoroscope places the superior articular process (*curve arrow*) or ear of the "scotty dog" at least 30–40% of the width of the vertebral body as seen on this projection. A lateral fluoroscopic image (**d**) shows the needle tip (*arrow*) at the posterior aspect of the T12-L1 disk with subsequent advancement into the disk (*arrow in* **e**). The stylet of the needle is removed, and an aspiration of the disk is performed with the needle left in place. A percutaneous diskectomy device is then coaxially inserted into this guide needle (*arrow*) as shown on this lateral fluoroscopic image (**f**), and disk material is obtained. The diskectomy device is removed, and the guide needle is left in place such that a 20-gauge insert needle with a removal hub is then inserted into this guide needle. The 20-gauge insert needle (*small arrow*) serves as a guide pin for a coaxial exchange for a bone biopsy guide cannula (*large arrow*) and introducer (*curved arrow*) as shown in the lateral fluoroscopic image (**g**) and frontal fluoroscopic image (**h**). Lateral (**i**) and frontal (**j**) fluoroscopic images show a trephine biopsy needle that is inserted coaxially through the guide needle and angled cephalad in order to sample the inferior endplate of T12 (*arrows*)

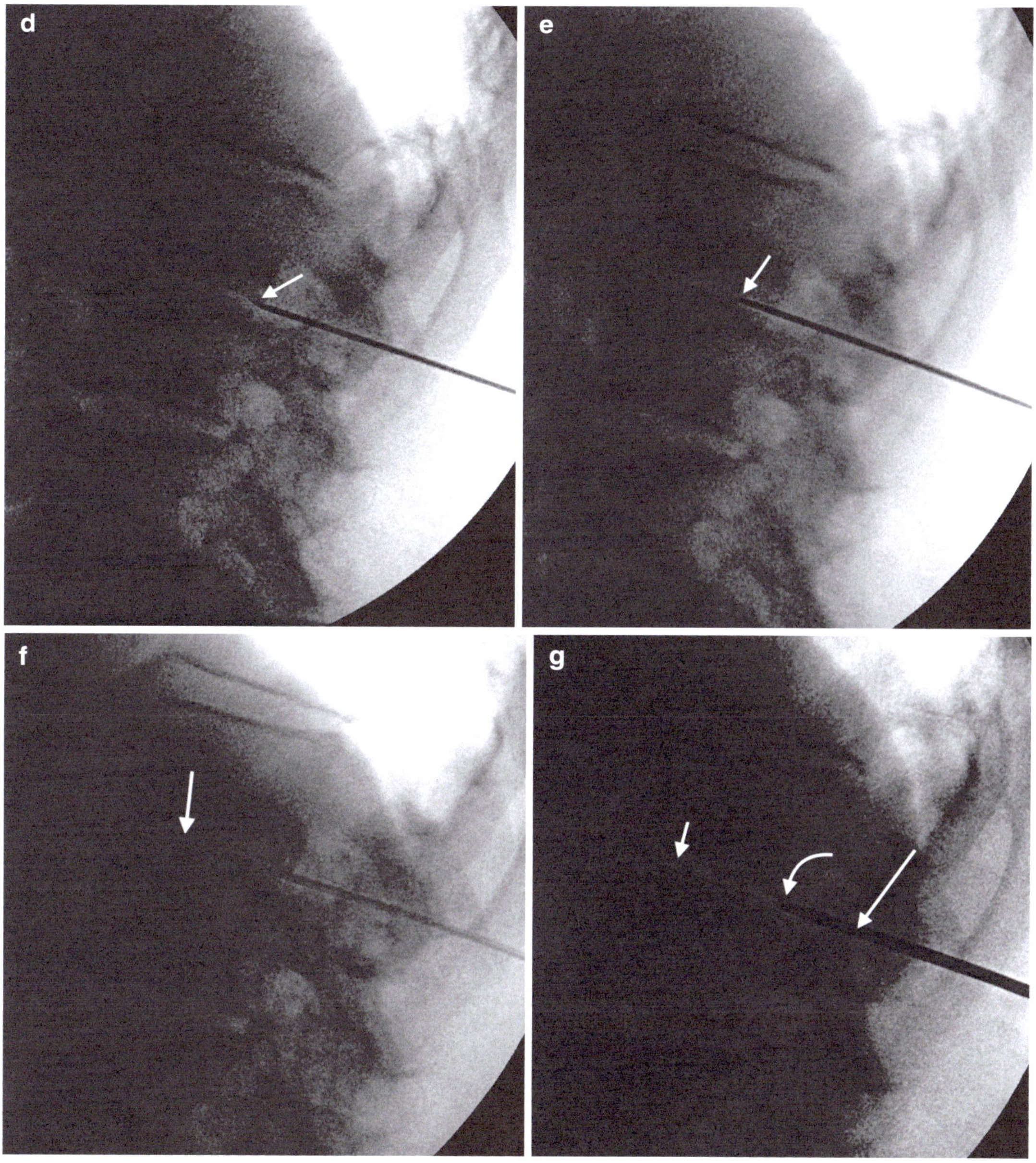

Fig. 9.16 (continued)

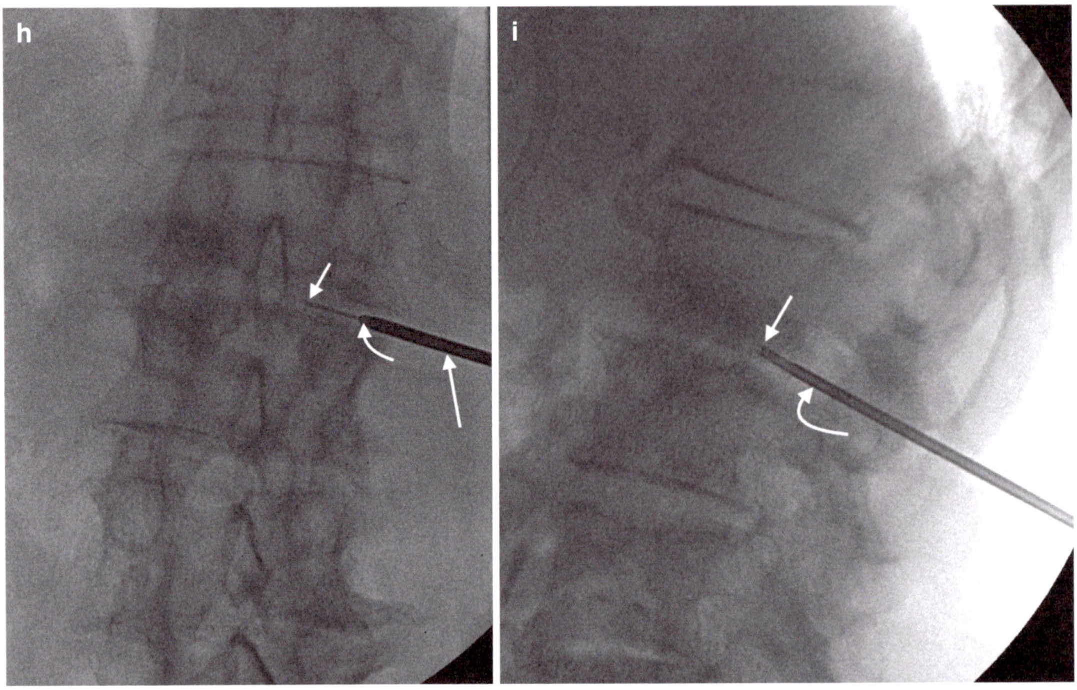

Fig. 9.16 (continued)

References

Akiyama T, Chikuda H, Yasunaga H, Horiguchi H, Fushimi K, Saita K. Incidence and risk factors for mortality of vertebral osteomyelitis: a retrospective analysis using the Japanese diagnosis procedure combination database. BMJ Open. 2013;3:e002412.

Berbari EF, Kanj SS, Kowalski TJ, Darouiche RO, Widmer AF, Schmitt SK, Hendershot EF, Holtom PD, Huddleston III PM, Petermann GW, Osmon DR. Executive summary: 2015 Infectious Diseases Society of America (IDSA) clinical practice guidelines for the diagnosis and treatment of native vertebral osteomyelitis in adults. Clin Infect Dis. 2015;6:859–63.

Bhavan KP, Marschall J, Olsen MA, Fraser VJ, Wright NM, Warren DK. The epidemiology of hematogenous vertebral osteomyelitis: a cohort study in a tertiary care hospital. BMC Infect Dis. 2010;10:158.

Boden SD, Davis DO, Dina TS, Sunner JL, Wiesel SW. Postoperative diskitis: distinguishing early MR imaging findings from normal postoperative disk space changes. Radiology. 1992;184:765–71.

Brigden ML. Clinical utility of the erythrocyte sedimentation rate. Am Fam Physician. 1999;60:1443–50.

De Lucas EM, Gonzalez Mandly A, Gutierrez A, Pellon R, Martin-Cuesta L, Izquierdo J, Sanchez E, Ruiz E, Quintana F. CT-guided fine-needle aspiration in vertebral osteomyelitis: true usefulness of a common practice. Clin Rheumatol. 2009;28:315–20.

Dhale RP, Dharmadhikari CA, Kulkarni RD, Powar RM. Role of anti-teichoic acid antibodies in the diagnosis of *Staphylococcus aureus* infections using counter-immunoelectrophoresis. Indian J Med Microbiol. 2003;21:213.

Diehn FE. Imaging of Spine infection. Radiol Clin North Am. 2012;50:777–98.

Duarte RM, Vaccaro AR. Spinal Infection: state of the art and management algorithm. Eur Spine J. 2013;22:2787–99.

Enoch DA, Cargill JS, Laing R, Herbert S, Corrah TW, Brown NM. Value of CT-guided biopsy in the diagnosis of septic discitis. J Clin Pathol. 2008;61:750–3.

Garces J, Hidalgo G. Lateral access for CT-guided percutaneous biopsy of the lumbar Spine. AJR Am J Roentgenol. 2000;174:425–6.

Garg V, Kosmas C, Young PC, Togaru UK, Robbin MR. Computed tomography-guided percutaneous biopsy for vertebral osteomyelitis: a department's experience. Neurosurg Focus. 2014;37:E10.

Go JL, Rothman S, Prosper A, Sibergleit R, Lerner A. Spine infections. Neuroimaging Clin N Am. 2012;22:755–72.

Govender S. Spinal infections. Bone Joint. 2005;11:1454–8.

Gupta RK, Cheung YK, Al Ansari AG, Naran S, Lallu S, Fauck R. Diagnostic value of image-guided needle aspiration cytology in the assessment of vertebral and intervertebral lesions. Diagn Cytopathol. 2002;27:191–6.

Heyer CM, Al-Hadari A, Mueller KM, Stachon A, Nicolas V. Effectiveness of CT-guided percutaneous biopsies of the spine: an analysis of 202 examinations. Acad Radiol. 2008;15:901–11.

Heyer CM, Brus LJ, Peters SA, Lemburg SP. Efficacy of CT-guided biopsy of the spine in patients with spondylitis-an analysis of 164 procedures. Eur J Radiol. 2012;81:244–9.

Jain NK, Dao K, Ortiz AO. Postoperative spine paraspinal fluid collections. Neuroimaging Clin N Am. 2014;24:375–8.

Jimenez-Mejias ME, Dios Colmenero J, Sanchez-Lora FJ, Palomino-Nicas J, Reguera JM, Garcia de la Heras J, Garcia-Ordonez MA, Pachon J. Postoperative spondylodiskitis: etiology, clinical findings, prognosis, and comparison with nonoperative pyogenic spondylodiskitis. Clin Infect Dis. 1999;29:339–45.

Kim BJ, Lee JW, Kim SJ, Lee GY, Kang HS. Diagnostic yield of fluoroscopy-guided biopsy for Infectious Spondylitis. ANJR Am J Neuroradiol. 2013;34:233–8.

Kim CJ, Kang SJ, Yoon D, Lee MJ, Kim M, Song KH, Jang HC, Jung SI, Kim ES, Kim HB, Oh MD, Park KH, Kim NJ. Factors influencing culture positivity in pyogenic vertebral osteomyelitis patients with prior antibiotic exposure. Antimicrob Agents Chemother. 2015;59:2470–3.

Kim CJ, Song KH, Park WB, Kim ES, Park SW, Kim HB, Oh MD. Microbiologically and clinically diagnosed vertebral osteomyelitis: impact of prior antibiotic exposure. Antimicrob Agents Chemother. 2012;56:2122–4.

Ledbetter LN, Salzman KL, Shah LM. Imaging psoas sign in lumbar spinal infections: evaluation of diagnostic accuracy and comparison with established imaging characteristics. AJNR Am J Neuroradiol. 2016;37:336–41.

Marschall J, Bhavan KP, Olsen MA, Fraser VJ, Wright NM, Warren DK. The impact of prebiopsy antibiotics on pathogen recovery in hematogenous vertebral osteomyelitis. Clin Infect Dis. 2011;52:867–72.

Mazzie JM, Brooks MK, Gnerre J. Imaging and management of postoperative Spine infection. Neuroimaging Clin N Am. 2014;24:365–74.

Michel SCA, Pfirrmann CWA, Boos N, Hodler J. CT-guided core biopsy of subchondral bone and intervertebral space in suspected spondylodiskitis. AJR Am J Roentgenol. 2006;186:977–80.

Patel KB, Poplawski MM, Pawha PS, Naidich TP, Tanenbaum LN. Diffusion –weighted MRI "Claw Sign" improves differentiation of infectious from degenerative Modic Type 1 signal changes of the spine. AJNR Am J Neuroradiol. 2014;35:647–52.

Pigrau C, Rodriguez-Pardo D, Fernandez-Hidalgo N, Moreto L, Pellise F, Larrosa MN, Puig M, Almirante B. Health care associated hematogenous pyogenic vertebral osteomyelitis: a severe and potentially preventable infectious disease. Medicine. 2015;94:e365.

Rankine JJ, Barron DA, Robinson P, Millner PA, Dickson RA. Therapeutic impact of percutaneous spinal biopsy in spinal infection. Postgrad Med J. 2004;80:607–9.

Rimondi E, Staals EL, Errani C, Bianchi G, Casadei R, Alberghini M, Malaguti MC, Rossi G, Durante S, Mercuri M. Percutaneous CT-guide biopsy of the spine: results of 430 biopsies. Eur Spine J. 2008; 17:975–81.

Ross JS, Zepp R, Modic MT. The postoperative lumbar spine: enhanced MR evaluation of the intervertebral disk. AJNR Am J Neuroradiol. 1996;17:323–31.

Singh G. C-reactive protein and erythrocyte sedimentation rate: continuing role for erythrocyte sedimentation rate. Adv Biol Chem. 2014;4:5–9.

Sucu HK, Bezircioglu H, Ciek C, Ersahin Y. Computerized tomography-guided percutaneous transforamino-discal biopsy sampling of vertebral body lesions. J Neurosurg. 2003;99:51–5.

Tehranzadeh J, Tao C, Browning CA. Percutaneous needle bBiopsy of the Spine. Acta Radiol. 2007;48:860–8.

Terreaux W, Geoffroy M, Ohl X, Job L, Carl P, Eschard JP, Salmon JH. Diagnostic contribution of a second percutaneous needle biopsy in patients with spontaneous diskitis and negative blood cultures and first biopsy. Joint Bone Spine 2016. pii: S1297-319X(16)00050-6. doi:10.1016/j.jbspin.2016.02.006. [Epub ahead of print].

Wattamwar AS, Ortiz AO. Use of a percutaneous diskectomy device to facilitate the diagnosis of infectious spondylitis. ANJR Am J Neuroradiol. 2010;31:1157–8.

Wu JS, Gorbachova T, Morrison WB, Haims AH. Imaging-guided bone biopsy for osteomyelitis: are there factors associated with positive or negative cultures? AJR Am J Roentgenol. 2007;188:1529–34.

Wu R, Tseng YA, Drexler S, Ortiz O. Image-guided percutaneous cervical spine biopsies: A review of techniques, results, and complication avoidance. Neurographics 4;2014:78–85.

Spine Infection Mimics

10

Joseph P. Mazzie and A. Orlando Ortiz

Learning Objectives

1. To introduce and describe several pathologic entities with imaging manifestations in the spine that simulate spine infection
2. To learn to identify and discriminate these mimics from spine infection
3. To understand the utility of image-guided percutaneous spine biopsy when indicated to assess for possible spine infection

10.1 Introduction

The diagnosis of spine infection can be challenging on either a clinical basis or even with highly sensitive imaging studies such as magnetic resonance imaging (MRI). With back pain as a very ubiquitous patient complaint, it is not uncommon to encounter clinical situations in which the imaging study shows findings that resemble, but are not, spine infection. The diagnosis of spine infection cannot always be solely based upon imaging findings. It is in the context of this clinical management dilemma that this chapter intends to describe and analyze diagnostic entities that may mimic the imaging presentation of spine infection. In general, the radiologic differential diagnosis for spine infection includes degenerative disk disease, diskectomy, spondyloarthropathy, and, less commonly, trauma and neoplasm. The findings of some of these so-called spine infection mimics simulate the appearance of infection so closely that, in many instances, a spine biopsy is required to exclude the possibility of spine infection. It is important to understand that the clinical management of these entities is different than what would be seen with spine infection. Hence, a spine biopsy may be required in order to facilitate arriving at the correct clinical diagnosis.

Table 10.1 Spine infection: radiologic differential diagnosis

Common	Less common

Degenerative disk disease
  Type 1 reactive vertebral endplate changes
  Schmorl's nodes
	Trauma
	  Spine trauma
	  Osteoporotic vertebral compression fracture
	Chronic low-grade trauma
	  Neuropathic osteoarthropathy

Disk intervention
  Diskectomy
  Disk injection procedures
Other spine surgery
	Neoplasm
	  Primary neoplasm (chordoma)
	  Metastatic disease
	  Lymphoma, myeloma

Spondyloarthropathy
  Gout
  Chronic hemodialysis
  Seronegative spondyloarthritis
	Other
	Sarcoid

A.O. Ortiz, *Image-Guided Percutaneous Spine Biopsy*, DOI 10.1007/978-3-319-43326-4_10

> The radiologic differential diagnosis for spine infection includes degenerative disk disease, diskectomy, spondyloarthropathy, and, less commonly, trauma and neoplasm.

10.2 Degenerative Disk Disease

This condition is encountered in the majority of spine imaging examinations that are performed in the adult population. The frequency and severity of imaging findings tend to increase with the age of the patient. Given the increased weight-bearing stress that is placed upon the lumbar spine, degenerative disk disease is often seen within the lower lumbar intervertebral disk spaces, including L4–L5 and L5–S1.One or more of the intervertebral disk space levels may be affected. Disk space narrowing at the affected level is usually present. Anterior spur formation may be seen particularly in elderly patients. A disk bulge, protrusion, or extrusion may also be present. Fibrovascular changes in the adjacent vertebral endplates result in varying amounts of T1 hypointensity and T2 hyperintensity within the affected endplates, the so-called type 1 change (Modic et al. 1988). These MR signal changes may occur in a horizontal band-like or triangular pattern. Because there is altered vascularity within the endplates, contrast enhancement is observed and is more pronounced on fat-suppressed T1-weighted MR images. Intradiskal post-contrast enhancement is distinctly absent. Another pattern (type 2) is due to fat deposition within the affected vertebral endplates resulting in T1 hyperintensity and T2 iso- or hypointensity with no associated contrast enhancement. The degenerative cascade ultimately progresses to osseous growth within the vertebral endplates that is manifested as sclerosis on radiographic or CT examinations and on MRI is hypointense on both T1 and T2 sequences (type 3 change). Thus, it is the type 1 reactive endplate change in degenerative disk disease that can at times be confused for spine infection, especially when the reactive change is exuberant (Fig. 10.1). The disk-endplate margin remains relatively intact in early reactive endplate changes which may help to distinguish this entity from spondylodiskitis. A focal diffusion pattern, or "claw" sign, on MR diffusion-weighted sequences is reported to be present in type 1 reactive endplate change (Fig. 10.1) (Patel et al. 2014). Some authors postulate that disk infection with *Propionibacterium acnes* bacteria, a low-virulence skin microbe, may play a role in the development of these reactive endplate changes and have reported improvement in low back pain and disability following treatment with antibiotics in a double-blind randomized clinical trial (Albert et al. 2013). In the presence of aggressive reactive endplate changes in patients with degenerative disk disease, if there is a reasonable clinical suspicion for spine infection, then the possibility of a spine biopsy may be considered.

> Type 1 reactive endplate change in degenerative disk disease, consisting of fibrovascular replacement, can at times be confused for spine infection, especially when the reactive change is exuberant.

10.3 Schmorl's Nodes (Intravertebral Disk Prolapse)

A Schmorl's node is a focal prolapse of disk material (annulus fibrosis and/or nucleus pulposus) through the superior or inferior vertebral endplate into the vertebral body. Schmorl's nodes have a bimodal age distribution and are seen in young adolescents and patients in their sixth decade of life and beyond (Stabler et al. 1997). Males are affected much more frequently (76% of cases) than females (Mattei and Rehman 2014). The etiology of this acquired condition is variable and includes trauma, degenerative disk disease, and metabolic and neoplastic disorders. Schmorl's nodes can be found anywhere along the spinal axis, but are most frequently

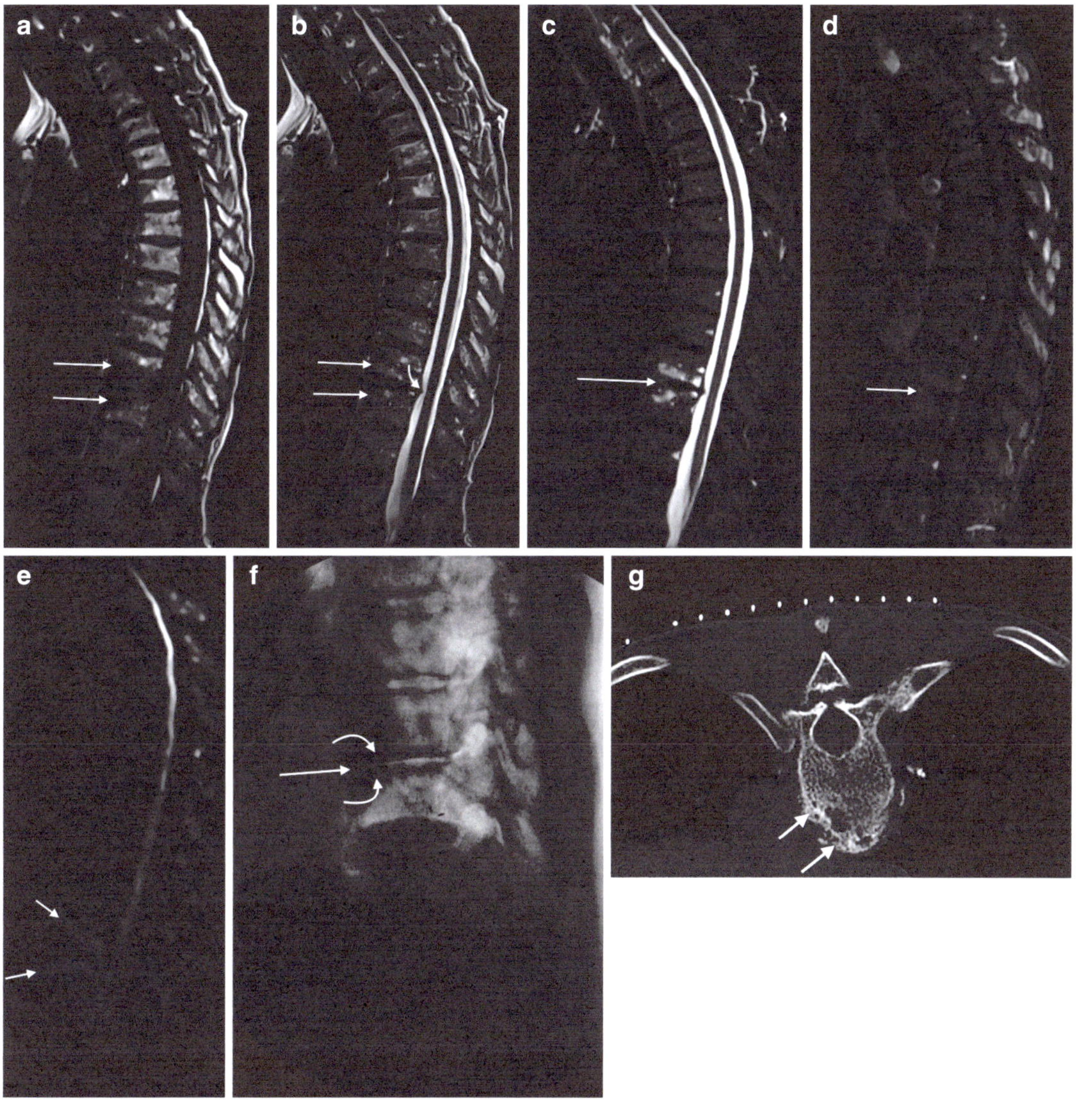

Fig. 10.1 A 75-year-old female with severe mid-back pain. T1-weighted sagittal image (**a**) shows triangular areas of low signal intensity (*arrows*) at the T10–T11 level. These show mixed hypo- and hyperintensity (*arrows*) on the T2-weighted sequence (**b**) as well as a small disk protrusion (*curved arrow*). The inversion recovery sagittal image (**c**) shows focal hyperintensity within the anterior aspect of the disk (*arrow*). The fat-suppressed contrast-enhanced T1-weighted sagittal image (**d**) shows enhancement within the anterior disk and in the endplates (*arrow*). The patient was referred for a spine biopsy for suspected spine infection. A serum infection profile (WBC with differential, ESR, and CRP) was drawn and was normal. Therefore, the MR study was repeated with a diffusion-weighted sequence (**e**) which shows the presence of a "claw" sign (*arrows*) – indicating the presence of reactive endplate change. A lateral fluoroscopic image of the thoracic spine (**f**) shows disk space narrowing (*arrow*) and endplate sclerosis (*curved arrows*). An axial CT image (**g**) in bone window algorithm obtained during a subsequent thoracic epidural steroid injection procedure shows scattered sclerotic foci (*arrows*)

encountered within the lower thoracic spine and the upper lumbar spine. They are most commonly located within the mid-portion of vertebral body (Mattei and Rehman 2014). When trauma is the precipitating event, an axial loading mechanism is responsible for Schmorl's node formation (Wagner et al. 2000a). The other etiologic entities are thought to weaken the vertebral endplate, subsequently leading to intraosseous extension of the disk material. Schmorl's nodes can be associated with focal axial back pain that localizes to the vertebral body level of the Schmorl's node. Alternatively, they may be incidental findings that are seen during spine imaging examinations performed for other clinical indications.

Regardless of the etiology and the patient's clinical presentation, Schmorl's node imaging presentation on MR examinations can be quite striking and may even simulate infection. The prolapsed disk material elicits an inflammatory response in the surrounding bone (Fig. 10.2). This manifests as a zone or band of T1 hypointensity and T2 hyperintensity. There may be alternating zones of inflammation with Schmorl's node at the center, which may create a target-like appearance. Since the vertebral endplates are vascularized structures, the inflammatory reaction surrounding Schmorl's node may create a vascular response at the margin of Schmorl's node. This zone of vascular proliferation will show enhancement on contrast-enhanced MRI studies (Stabler et al. 1997). To a certain extent, there is an overlap in this type of reactive endplate process and what is seen in the degenerative disk reactive endplate change cascade. MR may show Schmorl's nodes with surrounding fatty replacement or sclerotic reaction (which can also be seen on plain radiographs or CT examinations). Additionally, the two processes, degenerative disk disease and Schmorl's node formation, may be superimposed. But when there is prominent signal alteration and enhancement within and about the affected disk and Schmorl's node, the MR imaging findings may mimic spondylodiskitis.

Fortunately, in the case of Schmorl's nodes, there are a few imaging findings that may indicate the diagnosis. First, the preponderance of pathologic findings in Schmorl's node formation is within the affected vertebral endplate and the adjacent portion of the vertebral trabeculae and marrow. This is where the corresponding MR signal and enhancement findings will be encountered with Schmorl's node formation. In contrast, disk space infection shows signal and enhancement abnormalities within the disk. A target-like pattern of alternating zones of signal change with peripheral enhancement adjacent to the vertebral endplate as seen on multiplanar MR images may also indicate the presence of Schmorl's node. The focal location within the mid-portion of the vertebral endplate may also suggest the presence of Schmorl's node. Lastly, Schmorl's nodes can occur at multiple vertebral levels within the same patient and may also show some variation in MR signal and enhancement characteristics. This constellation of imaging findings with respect to MR signal and enhancement pattern, location, and lesion multiplicity may strongly suggest the diagnosis and obviate the requirement for spine biopsy.

> A target-like pattern of alternating zones of signal change with peripheral enhancement adjacent to the vertebral endplate as seen on multiplanar MR images may suggest the presence of Schmorl's node.

10.4 Disk Intervention

The MR imaging appearance in patients who have recently undergone a diskectomy or disk injection procedure can have features that overlap those that are seen with disk space infection (Fig. 10.3). Patients, who have undergone other spine surgical procedures whether open or percutaneous, may also demonstrate postsurgical imaging findings that can overlap with those of spine infection (Fig. 10.4). The diskectomy procedure is being performed on a disk that has already been injured; fissuring of the annulus fibrosis is associated with protrusion or extrusion of disk material. The herniated disk fragment is resected, a mechanical excision that further disturbs the normal architecture of the disk and vertebral endplate. Therefore, it is expected that the disk signal on T1- and T2-weighted images will be altered as compared to nearby normal disks. Additionally, contrast-enhanced MRI will show focal enhancement at the surgical site. Two thin bands of linear enhancement that extend within the disk annulus parallel

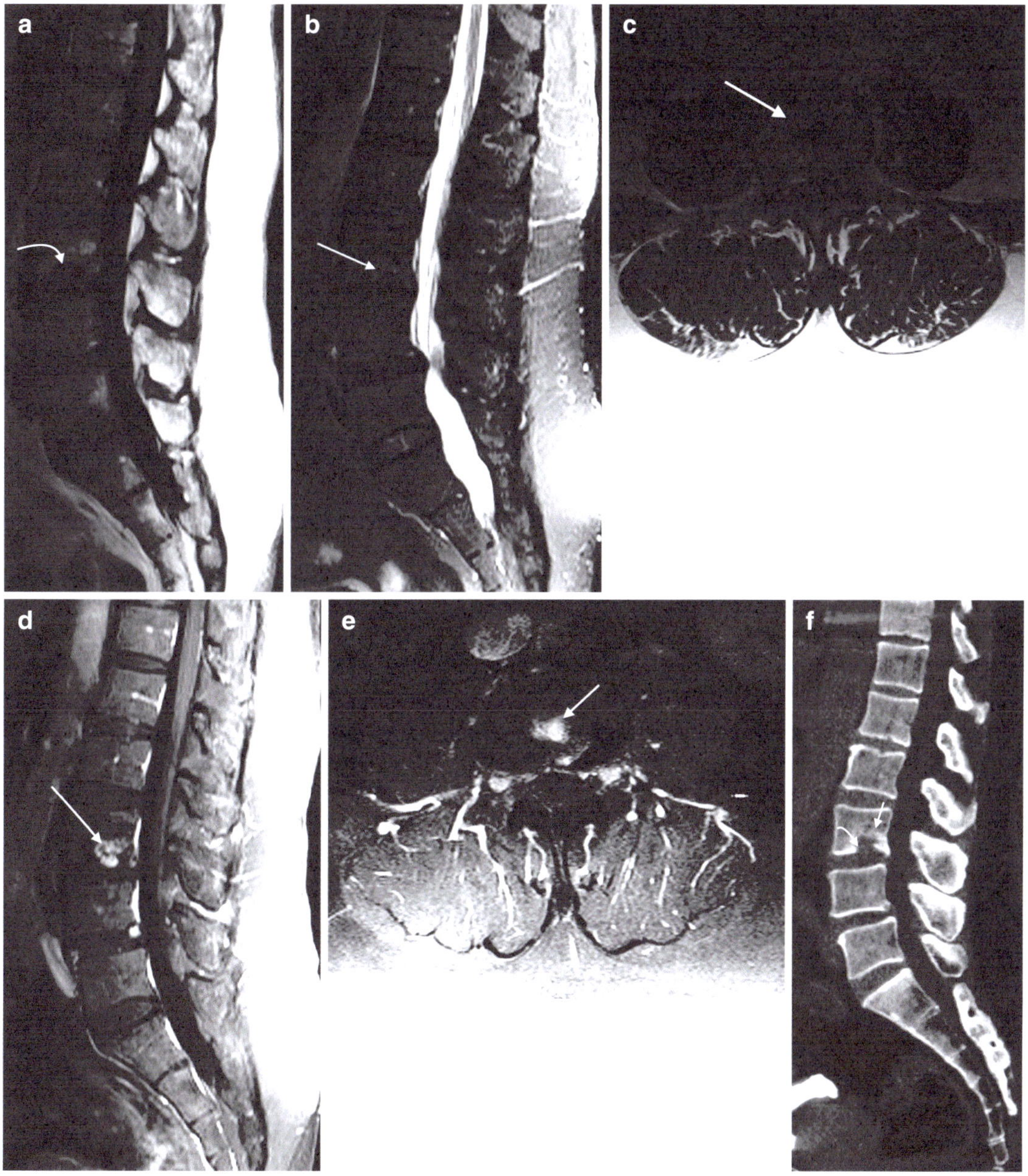

Fig. 10.2 A 78-year-old male with history of prostate cancer. T1-weighted sagittal image (**a**) shows a Schmorl's node (*curved arrow*) involving the inferior endplate of L3. A peripheral zone of T2 hyperintensity (arrow) surrounds the Schmorl's node (**b**). The T1 axial image (**c**) shows a round zone of hyperintensity (*arrow*) surrounding the Schmorl's node. The fat-suppressed contrast-enhanced T1-weighted sagittal (**d**) and axial (**e**) image shows focal enhancement within the Schmorl's node and adjacent marrow (*arrows*). A sagittal CT reformation in bone window algorithm (**f**) shows the focal endplate defect (*curved arrow*) and the patchy reactive bone formation (*arrow*) along the margin of this intravertebral disk protrusion

to the vertebral endplates, with or without enhancement in the endplates, have been reported in 20% of asymptomatic post-diskectomy patients (Ross et al. 1996). It is when this pattern of signal and enhancement change starts to extend beyond the surgical site that the possibility of infection should be considered (Bittane et al. 2014; Boden et al. 1992).

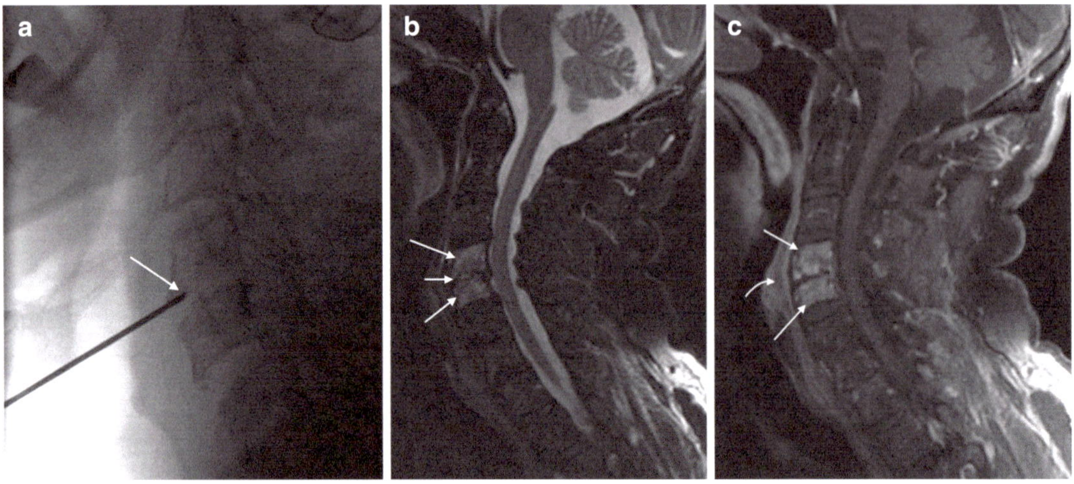

Fig. 10.3 A 73-year-old male with neck pain. Lateral fluoroscopic image (**a**) obtained during C4–C5 anesthetic injection (*arrow*). Patient's pain improved, and a follow-up MRI for evaluation of prostate cancer shows diffuse-increased signal within the vertebral bodies (*large arrows*) and C4–C5 disk (*small arrow*) on the T2 sagittal image (**b**). The fat-suppressed contrast-enhanced T1-weighted sagittal image (**c**) shows vertebral body enhancement (*arrows*) and prevertebral soft tissue enhancement (*curved arrow*). The patient remained asymptomatic and his serum infection profile was normal

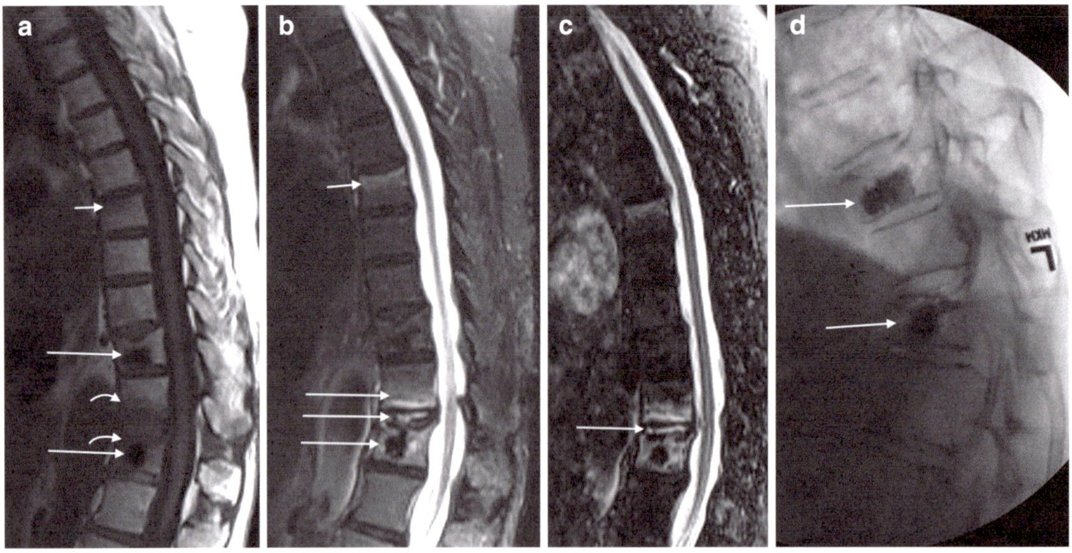

Fig. 10.4 A 70-year-old female with history of osteoporosis and recent lower thoracic vertebral augmentation presents with severe upper thoracic back pain. T1-weighted sagittal image (**a**) shows round hypointense foci of low signal intensity (*large arrows*) at T9 and T11 from the recent vertebral augmentation procedures. Additionally, T1 hypointensity (*curved arrows*) is seen at the T10–T11 endplates. A subtle hypointense band of marrow edema is associated with mild height loss at T6 (*small arrow*). The T2 sagittal image (**b**) shows areas of hyperintense signal within the T11 vertebral body, T10–T11 disk, and T10 endplate (*large arrows*). A hyperintense band of marrow edema (*small arrow*) is seen within the T6 vertebral body. The signal changes are further accentuated at T10–T11 (*arrow*) on the STIR sagittal image (**c**). A lateral fluoroscopic image (**d**) shows the treated T9 and T11 vertebral compression fractures (*arrows*); there was no tenderness to palpation on physical examination at these levels. The patient's back pain was due to the acute T6 vertebral compression fracture

Distinguishing between "normal" post-diskectomy changes and an infected diskectomy site is challenging, the latter being suggested by extensive intradiskal and vertebral endplate enhancement on contrast-enhanced MR images.

10.5 Spondyloarthropathies

10.5.1 Gout

Gout is the most common crystalline type of arthropathy in the United States, and its incidence and prevalence are steadily increasing (Lawrence et al. 2008). Gout typically affects the appendicular skeleton resulting in the deposition of monosodium urate crystals within intra- or extra-articular sites. The intra-articular deposition of these monosodium urate crystals results in an acute inflammatory response; this leads to osseous erosions and progressive destruction of bones and joints. When long-standing and severe, gout can progress to form chalky white tophi (chronic tophaceous gout). When examined under polarized light, urate crystals characteristically demonstrate a needle shape with strong negative birefringence.

Establishing a diagnosis of gout is most commonly performed on the basis of clinical and laboratory findings and is usually straightforward. However, with atypical manifestations, the clinical diagnosis can be delayed, thus affecting patient morbidity (Ning and Keenan. 2010). The most common clinical presentation of an acute gout attack is the rapid onset of a painful mono-arthropathy often in the first metatarsophalangeal joint (podagra). While urate crystal deposition is commonly encountered in the appendicular skeleton, involvement of the axial skeleton is rare but does occur. In one retrospective review, the authors found that approximately 48% of the axial gout patients had involvement of the lumbar vertebrae, 29% involved the cervical spine, 20% involved the thoracic spine, and 8.7% involved the sacroiliac joints (Konatalapalli et al. 2009). Involvement of the spine has been reported to occur in the posterior elements, sacroiliac joints, paravertebral soft tissues, and the intervertebral disk (Popovich et al. 2006). Involvement of the axial skeleton may occur at multiple levels with both osseous and extra-osseous imaging findings. These findings include osseous erosions or destruction as well as paravertebral soft tissue masses. Axial skeleton gouty arthropathy may have a confusing clinical presentation and can be readily mistaken for an infectious or malignant etiology (Fig. 10.5). Therefore, differential diagnostic considerations prior to biopsy would include infection, lymphoma, myeloma, or metastatic disease (Popovich et al. 2006).

CT is sometimes used to evaluate back pain. Gouty tophus on CT has been measured to be approximately 160 Hounsfield units secondary to the monosodium urate crystals (Gerster et al. 2002). Facet joint erosions in the lumbar spine in a patient with gout should raise suspicion for axial gouty arthropathy (Saketkoo et al. 2009). With the advent and increasing use of dual-energy CT, and with the inherent capabilities of dual-energy CT, it is now possible to distinguish clusters of urate crystals from other calcifications, i.e., hydroxyapatite crystals. Urate crystals can be uniquely color coded, allowing for improved depiction. As such, dual-energy CT may be used in patients with an unclear diagnosis or in excluding gout (Desai et al. 2011). Since dual-energy CT may directly depict urate crystal deposition, it can be specifically used to evaluate for gout regardless of patients' serum urate levels; as such, dual-energy CT findings can confirm a diagnosis of gout in patients with normal serum urate levels or even exclude it in patients with hyperuricemia (Desai et al. 2011). While MRI maybe helpful in establishing a diagnosis, the overall imaging findings are nonspecific. One study found that 13 patients with axial gout demonstrated lesions to be hypo- to iso-intense on T1- weighted images and variable on T2-weighted images. The degree of T2 signal intensity was thought to be related to the degree of calcium within the tophi (Yu et al. 1997). This study also found that nearly all gouty tophi

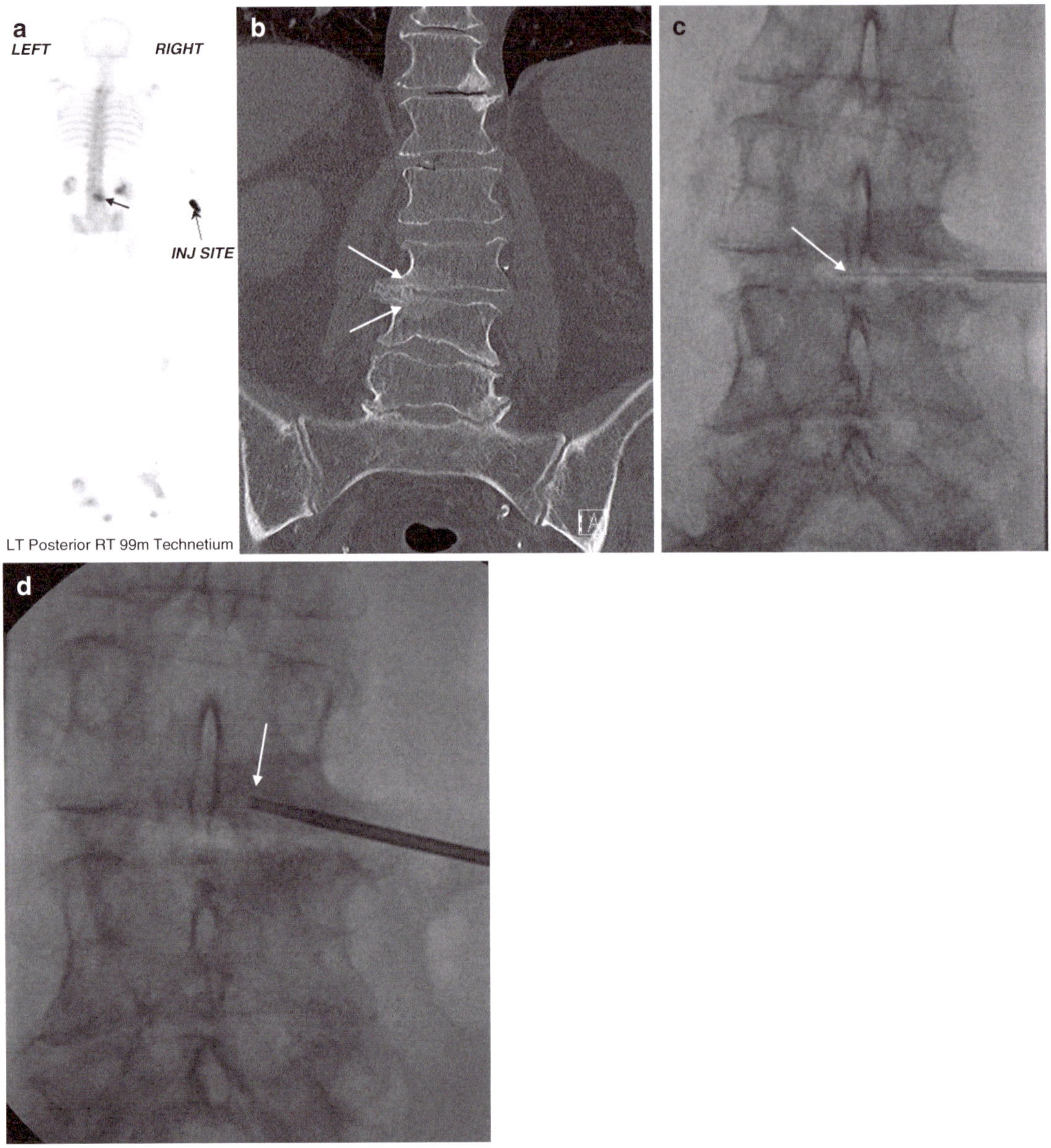

Fig. 10.5 A 67-year-old female with history of breast cancer and low back pain. Focal radionuclide uptake (*arrow*) is seen within the lumbar spine on the static image from the bone scan (**a**). Coronal CT reformation in bone window algorithm (**b**) shows focal asymmetric sclerotic change adjacent to a prominent lateral osteophyte at L3–L4 (*arrows*); this finding is present at other spinal levels. Fluoroscopic frontal projection (**c**) shows an insert needle (*arrow*) within the L3–L4 disk. Fluoroscopic frontal projection (**d**) shows a biopsy needle within an area of sclerosis at L3–L4 (*arrow*). The disk and endplate biopsies were submitted for both microbiologic and pathologic analysis; the latter showed the presence of urate crystals. A subsequent radiograph of the foot showed the presence of gout

demonstrated near-homogeneous enhancement on contrast-enhanced MR examinations. It can be difficult to differentiate axial gouty arthropathy from infectious spondylodiskitis as epidural collections have also been reported with gouty arthropathy (Fig. 10.6) (Yen et al. 2005). FDG-PET has recently been reported to be positive in axial gouty arthropathy demonstrating hyper-

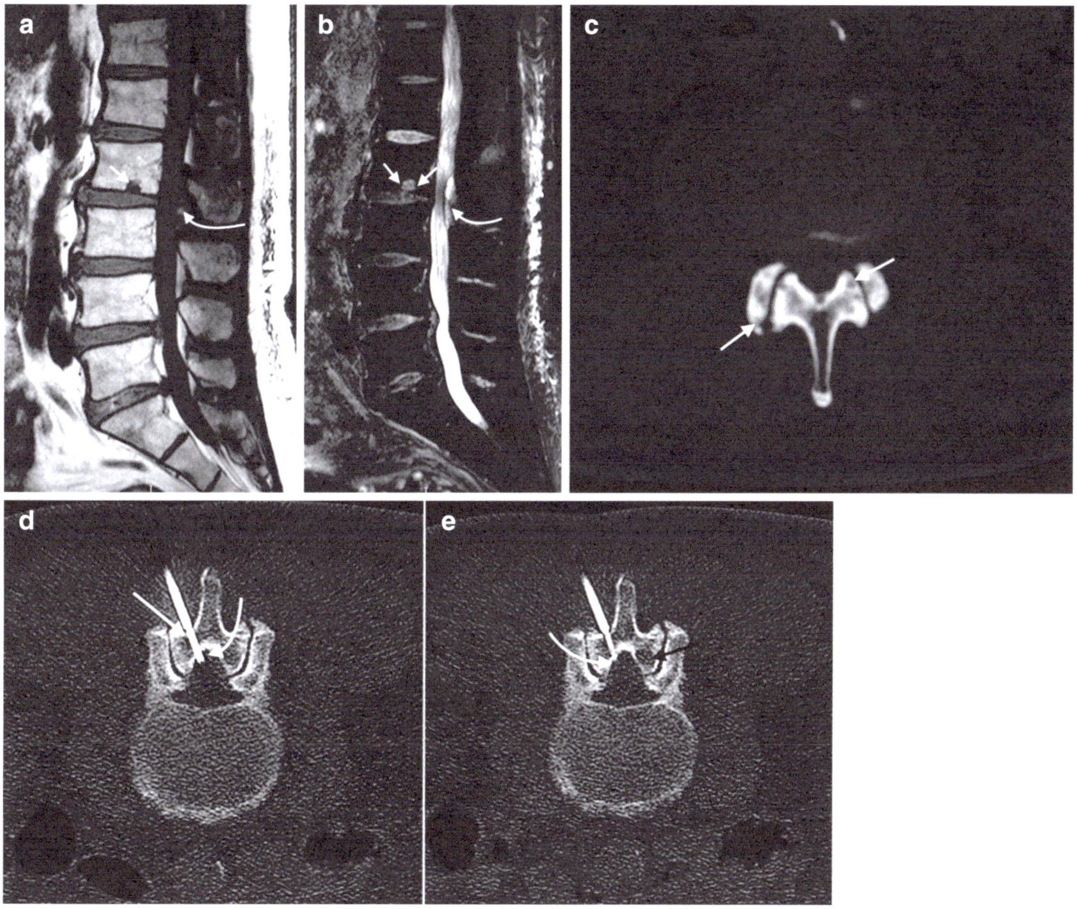

Fig. 10.6 A 72-year-old male with prior history of diabetes, chronic renal failure, and gout presents with severe, crippling back pain. An elevated ESR (83), CRP (32.8), and WBC (12.1) were noted at the time of clinical presentation. A T1-weighted sagittal image (**a**) shows a subtle hypointense dorsal epidural collection at L2–L3 (*curved arrow*). What appears to be Schmorl's node (*arrow*) involves the inferior endplate of L2. The epidural fluid collection (*curved arrow*) is hyperintense on the T2 sagittal image (**b**). The small round hyperintense focus within the inferior endplate of L2 (*small arrows*) appears separate from the adjacent disk and may not be Schmorl's node. Axial CT image (**c**) in bone window algorithm at L2–L3 shows multiple small periarticular erosions (*arrows*) within the facet joints. Because of the patient's multiple comorbidities and poor medical condition, a percutaneous aspiration of the epidural collection was requested. Axial CT image (**d**) shows a bone needle traversing the lamina (*arrow*) and entering the dorsal epidural space (*curved arrow*) at L2–L3. A percutaneous aspiration device was then carefully inserted into the dorsal epidural space (*curved arrow*) as shown on the axial CT image (**e**) in order to aspirate thick viscous material; note the focal erosion (*arrow*) within the facet joint. Subsequent pathologic analysis showed the presence of urate crystals and confirmed a diagnosis of gout

metabolism within the lytic bone lesions and paraspinal masses. The authors postulate that macrophages and other growth factors play a role in the resolution of urate crystals in an acute gouty attack. High uptake of FDG has been correlated with macrophage/growth factor activity accounting for increased FDG uptake (Popovich et al. 2006).

10.5.2 Spondyloarthropathy of Chronic Hemodialysis: Dialysis-Related Amyloidosis

Patients receiving long-term hemodialysis therapy may develop an erosive and destructive spondyloarthropathy (Kiss et al. 2005). This spondyloarthropathy can involve one or more components of the spinal column and can affect on or more levels of the spinal axis. The lower cervical spine is involved more frequently than the thoracic or lumbar spine. The etiology of this condition is due to β2-microglobulin amyloid deposits which accumulate at the sites of spinal involvement (Otsubo et al. 2009). Non-spinal sites of involvement include the hips, wrists, shoulders, and knees (Lim and Ong 2013). This spondyloarthropathy has a somewhat indolent presentation with pain and neurologic symptoms referable to the affected spine level(s). The MR imaging findings, however, can be quite striking and may closely simulate those of spine infection (Fig. 10.7). The vertebral endplates will show low T1 signal intensity and high T2 signal intensity. Additionally focal or diffuse T2

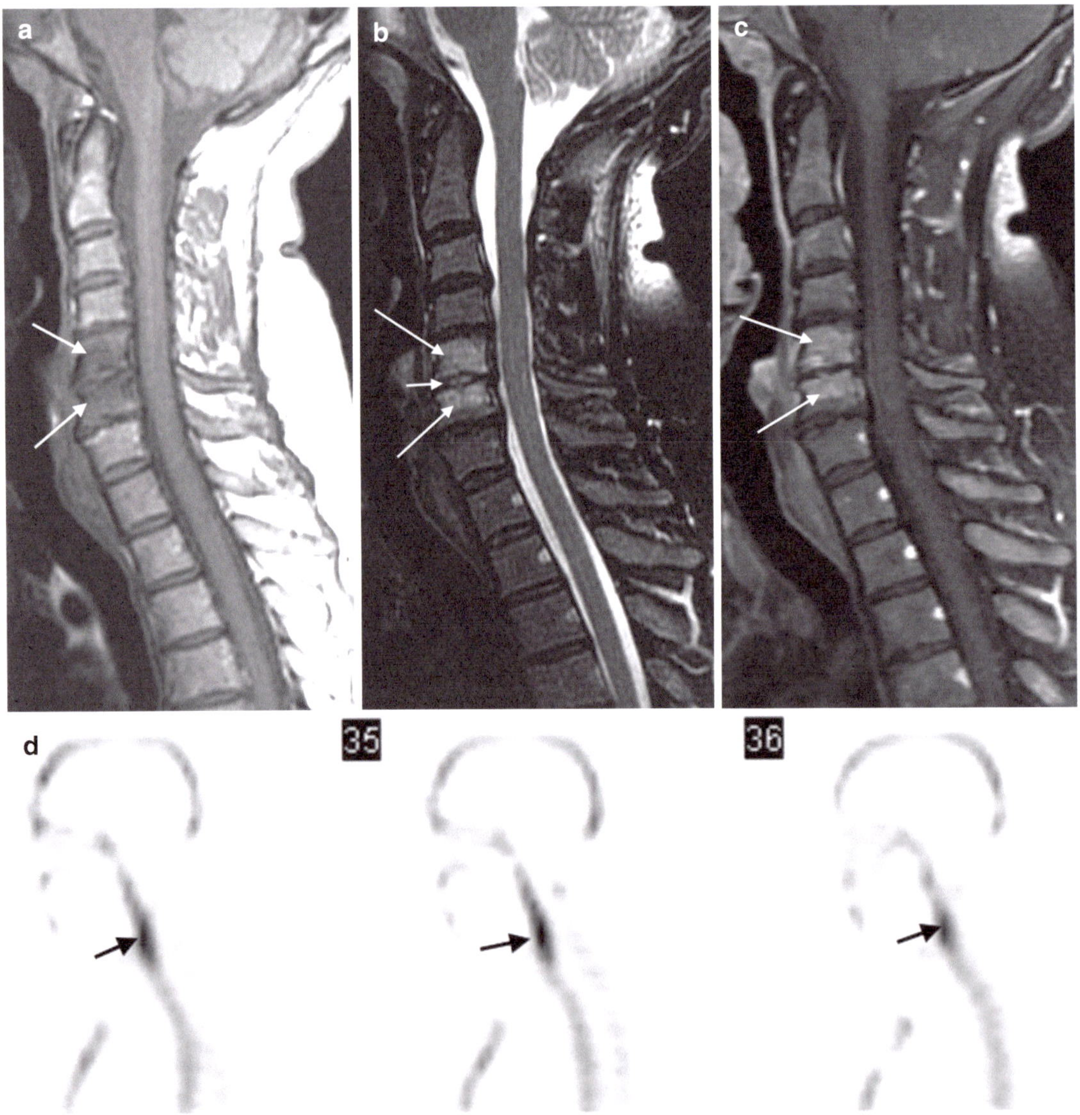

Fig. 10.7 A 44-year-old female with neck pain. T1-weighted sagittal image (**a**) shows hypointense signal within the C5 and C6 vertebral bodies (*arrows*). The T2 sagittal image (**b**) shows hyperintense signal (*arrows*) within these vertebral bodies and within the intervening disk (*small arrow*). The fat-suppressed contrast-enhanced T1-weighted sagittal image (**c**) shows vertebral body enhancement (*arrows*). Lateral static images from a SPECT bone scan (**d**) shows increased radionuclide uptake (*arrows*) within the lower cervical spine. Axial CT image (**e**) obtained during biopsy shows focal endplate erosions (*small arrow*). A C5–C6 biopsy (**f**) was performed using an anterior approach (*arrow*); this revealed amyloid deposition

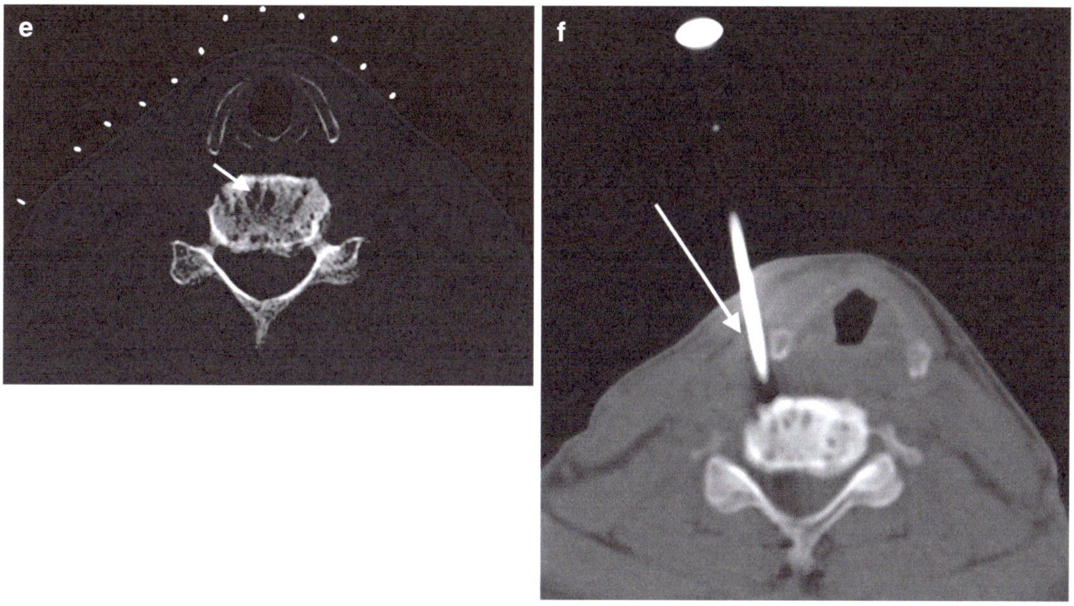

Fig. 10.7 (continued)

hypointensity or hyperintensity can be seen within the disk. Low T2 signal within the disk, when present, is helpful in distinguishing this entity from diskitis. When dialysis patients were routinely being administered intravenous gadolinium-based contrast agents to evaluate for possible infection, prominent enhancement could be seen within the affected disk and adjacent vertebral endplates. Amyloid deposits may also involve the facet joints and the ligamentum flavum (Kiss et al. 2005). Plain radiographs may show disk space narrowing associated with vertebral endplate irregularity (Theodorou et al. 2002). CT will show focal erosions within the vertebral endplate or articular facet with or without a surrounding sclerotic rim. The paraspinal soft tissues are relatively spared by the amyloid deposits, but synovial involvement at joint interfaces can be quite prominent. With progression of the disease, vertebral body collapse may occur, which can result in spinal instability and possible spinal canal compromise with spinal cord compression.

An increased serum β2-microglobulin is not diagnostic. Therefore, a spine biopsy is often required for definitive diagnosis. Nevertheless, the combination of a history of chronic hemodialysis and unenhanced MRI findings suggesting a focal erosive spondyloarthropathy with other musculoskeletal sites of involvement may avoid the need for a spine biopsy.

> When a spondyloarthropathy is suspected, the histopathologic analysis should include the appropriate analytic techniques; i.e., assess for birefringent urate crystals or amyloid deposition.

10.5.3 Seronegative Spondyloarthritis

Seronegative spondyloarthritis consists of a group of inflammatory disorders of the musculoskeletal system in which the serum rheumatoid factor is absent. Many of these disorders, however, are associated with another positive antigen, HLA-B27. These disorders include ankylosing spondylitis, psoriatic arthritis, arthritis associated with inflammatory bowel disease, reactive arthritis (Reiter syndrome), and undifferentiated arthritis (Canella et al. 2013; Hermann et al. 2005). These disorders affect both the axial and appendicular skeleton, with enthesopathy or inflammation at the junction between the bone and adjacent connective tissue (tendon, ligament, or fascia). Individually, these entities are also associated with specific extraarticular manifestations, such as uveitis, that may suggest their diagnosis. Sacroiliac joint involvement is not uncommon;

facet joint involvement may also be observed (Hermann et al. 2005). The C-reactive protein may also be elevated and can be used as a marker of disease activity. In approximately one-third of patients, inflammatory lesions may occur within the vertebral endplates associated with variable intervertebral disk involvement. The signal changes on MRI, T1 hypointensity, T2 hyperintensity, and contrast enhancement can resemble those seen in early infectious spondylodiskitis. The location near the vertebral corner and the relative sparing of the vertebral endplate cortical margin, and/or the presence of multi-spinal level involvement, may distinguish a seronegative spondylodiskitis from infection (Fig. 10.8). Alternatively, the presence of paraspinal and/or epidural soft tissue involvement or the destruction of the disk-endplate cortical margin is more in keeping with a diagnosis of spine infection. The additional clinical information, including patient history, clinical findings, and laboratory tests, can be used to differentiate these inflammatory spondyloarthropathies from spine infection. Additionally, review of extremity (hands, wrists, feet) and/or sacroiliac joint radiographs can be very helpful.

10.6 Trauma

Traumatic injury to the spine can affect the vertebral body and intervertebral disk. This is often seen with flexion or axial load mechanisms, but can be observed in any type of traumatic insult to the spinal axis. Disruption of the disk – vertebral endplate complex will be associated with morphologic and signal and enhancement changes on MRI that can simulate infectious spondylitis. It is therefore important to look at the plain radiographs and CT examinations of the spinal axis that are commonly performed in these patients in order to identify fracture deformities and fracture lines. Equally as important is the requirement for obtaining an accurate history of recent significant trauma. The combination of clinical history and radiographic information (plain film and CT) can usually be used to distinguish a traumatic etiology from an infectious cause.

Osteoporotic vertebral compression fractures can occur insidiously or as a result of a fall or sudden bending or lifting movement (Fig. 10.9). These patients are often elderly and female. Acute and subacute osteoporotic vertebral compression fractures are associated with a high incidence of vertebral endplate fracture and disk injury as demonstrated on MRI studies (Ortiz and Bordia. 2011). MR will show a disruption of the vertebral endplate with angulation or overt fracture line and a variable amount of marrow edema or vertebral body cleft formation. The superior endplate, inferior endplate, or both endplates may be affected depending on the type of fracture morphology. The affected intervertebral disk will show alteration of morphology and may show either focal or diffuse T2 hyperintensity. Contrast-enhanced MRI studies are infrequently performed during the evaluation of these patients, but when they are, band-like contrast enhancement or more diffuse enhancement will be seen within the affected portions of the vertebral body. Evaluating the scout sagittal image in these patients can be helpful in identifying other chronic vertebral compression deformities, which in combination with the appropriate clinical history (i.e., a history of osteoporosis) may suggest the correct diagnosis. Additionally, reviewing prior imaging studies will also help to

Fig. 10.8 A 45-year-old female with low back pain. T1-weighted sagittal image (**a**) shows multiple large areas of hypointense endplate signal (*arrows*) at several levels. Focal areas of endplate deformity are seen throughout the lumbar spine. These areas are hyperintense on the T2 sagittal image (**b**) and located near the corners of the vertebral bodies (*arrows*). The fat-suppressed contrast-enhanced T1 sagittal image (**c**) shows prominent enhancement (*arrows*) in these areas of presumed inflammation. The reformatted sagittal CT image (**d**) in bone window algorithm shows subtle foci of endplate erosion (*curved arrows*) and sclerosis (*small arrows*). A CT-guided biopsy (**e**) was performed using a posterolateral approach (*arrow*) with an unremarkable microbiologic and pathologic analysis. A follow-up rheumatologic evaluation confirmed a diagnosis of ankylosing spondylitis

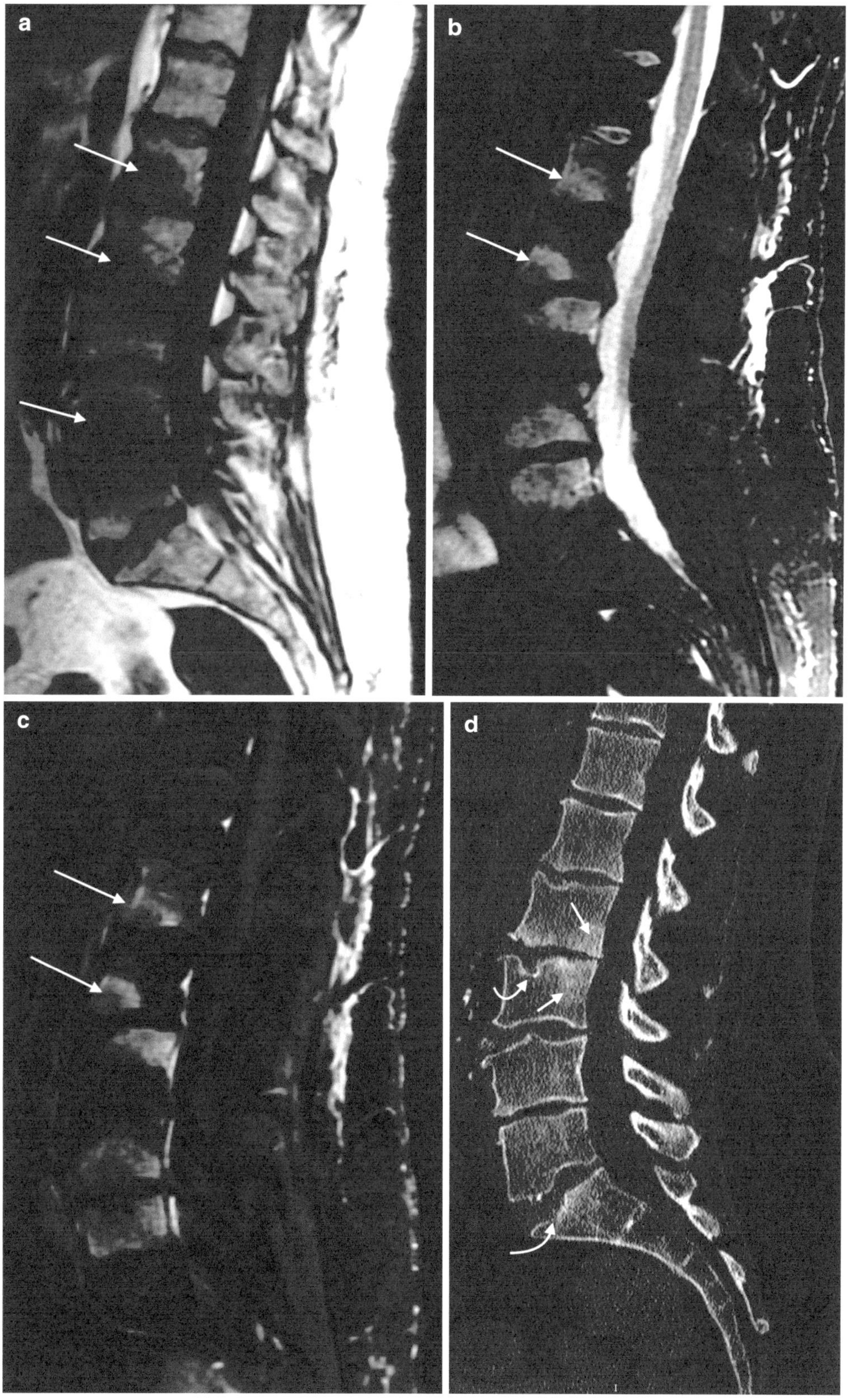
a
b
c
d

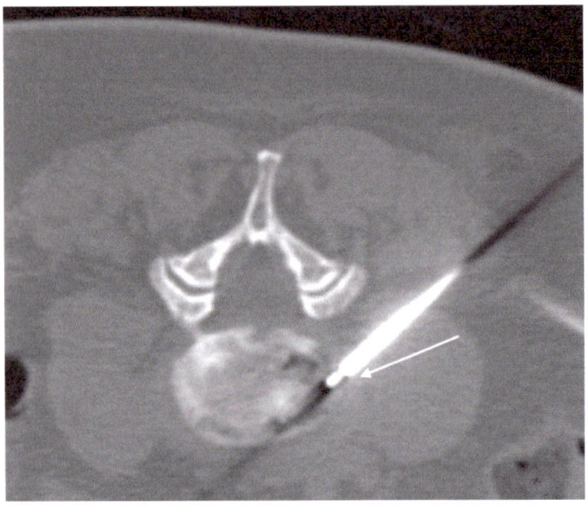

Fig. 10.8 (continued)

suggest the diagnosis, as osteoporotic vertebral compression deformities, while initially occult on plain radiographs, will gradually progress over a relatively short period of time (weeks to months).

Vertebral endplate and disk injury are associated with spine fractures and can therefore be confused for spine infection on MRI examinations. Radiographic and/or CT correlation, in addition to a history of recent trauma or osteoporosis, can help to suggest the appropriate diagnosis.

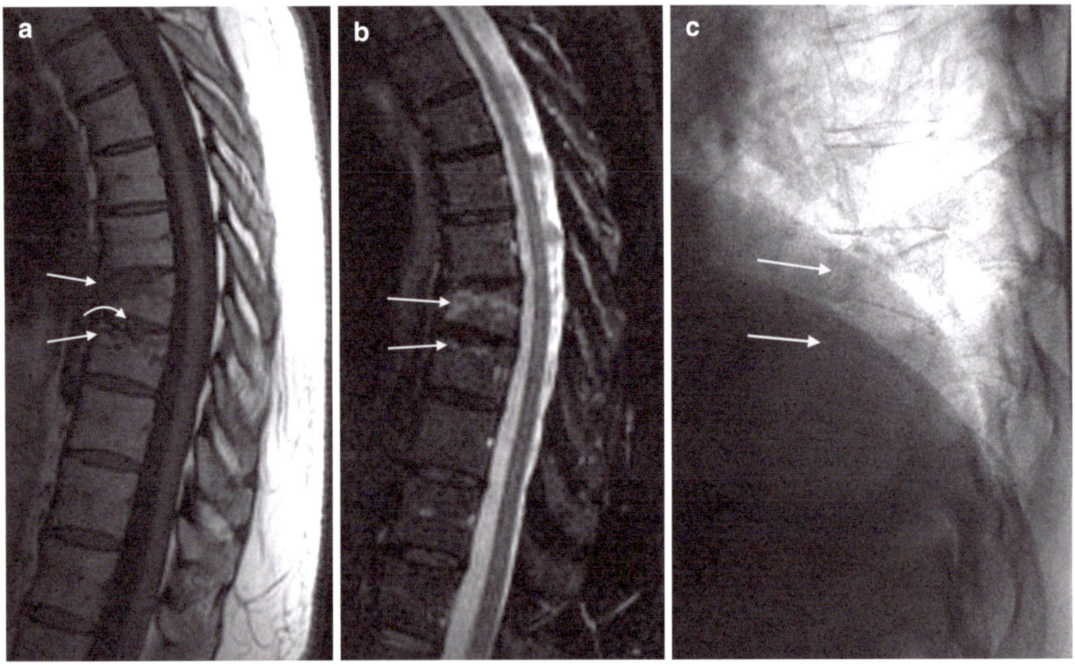

Fig. 10.9 A 55-year-old female with 10/10 mid-back pain after a fall at work. T1-weighted sagittal image (**a**) shows two vertebral body compression fractures (*arrows*) with signal abnormality within the intervertebral disk (*curved arrow*). STIR sagittal image (**b**) shows endplate signal abnormality (*arrows*). Lateral radiograph (**c**) of thoracic spine shows the vertebral compression deformities (*arrows*)

10.7 Neuropathic Osteoarthropathy

Neuropathic osteoarthropathy consists of a spectrum of bone and joint destruction that is associated with a significant neurosensory deficit including loss of proprioception (Jones et al. 2000). This impairment of normal sensory feedback is thought to lead to repetitive mechanical trauma to the axial and appendicular skeleton. Another possible mechanism for this osteoarthropathy is that compromised sympathetic innervation results in loss of vascular tone; the resulting vasodilation and hyperemia lead to bone resorption at joint or disk interfaces. Thus, pathologic alteration of the normal sensory mechanism either affecting the peripheral nervous system or the central nervous system, or both, results in neuropathic bone disease that affects one or more components of the axial and/or appendicular skeleton. Some conditions that may predispose to the development of neuropathic osteoarthropathy include spinal cord injury, syringomyelia, meningomyelocele, congenital insensitivity to pain, and diabetes mellitus (Jones et al. 2000). Diabetes mellitus is the most common cause of neuropathic osteoarthropathy, affecting the foot. Hypertrophic and atrophic forms of neuropathic osteoarthropathy may be seen; the former is characterized by osseous fragmentation, sclerosis, and osteophytosis, whereas the latter consists of osseous resorption. When the osteoarthropathy affects the spinal axis, the imaging findings on radiography, CT, or MRI will reflect injury to the intervertebral disk, the adjacent vertebral bodies, and the facet joints (Wagner et al. 2000b). Disk space height loss tends to be associated with vacuum phenomena; rim enhancement of the residual disk tissue may be seen on contrast-enhanced MR images. The vertebral body and endplates will show sclerosis, osseous fragmentation, osseous debris, and disorganization. Spondylolisthesis is due to both disk space and facet joint involvement. A key radiologic finding in neuropathic osteoarthropathy is the absence of soft tissue swelling or edema in the setting of such extensive disk and osseous involvement. Without the appropriate clinical history, the imaging findings in neuropathic osteoarthropathy can be strikingly similar to and be interpreted as possible spine infection (Jones et al. 2000).

> The presence of disk space height loss, vertebral endplate destruction with debris and fragmentation, increased density due to sclerosis, and osteophytosis, in the appropriate clinical setting, may indicate the presence of neuropathic osteoarthropathy.

10.8 Neoplasm

For the most part, neoplastic processes that involve the spinal axis can usually be differentiated from spine infection. When two adjacent vertebral bodies, however, are involved by a neoplastic process, the imaging findings can be indistinguishable from spine infection (Gabe et al. 2010). These overlapping imaging appearances become even more similar when the involved spinal segment is affected by the presence of a pathologic fracture. By far the two most common neoplastic processes that can involve the spine and result in this diagnostic dilemma are metastatic disease and multiple myeloma (Fig. 10.10). In the case of metastatic disease, the clinical history of a known primary with a predilection for osseous metastatic spread, and the involvement of other skeletal or organ sites of metastatic spread, can be used to suggest the diagnosis

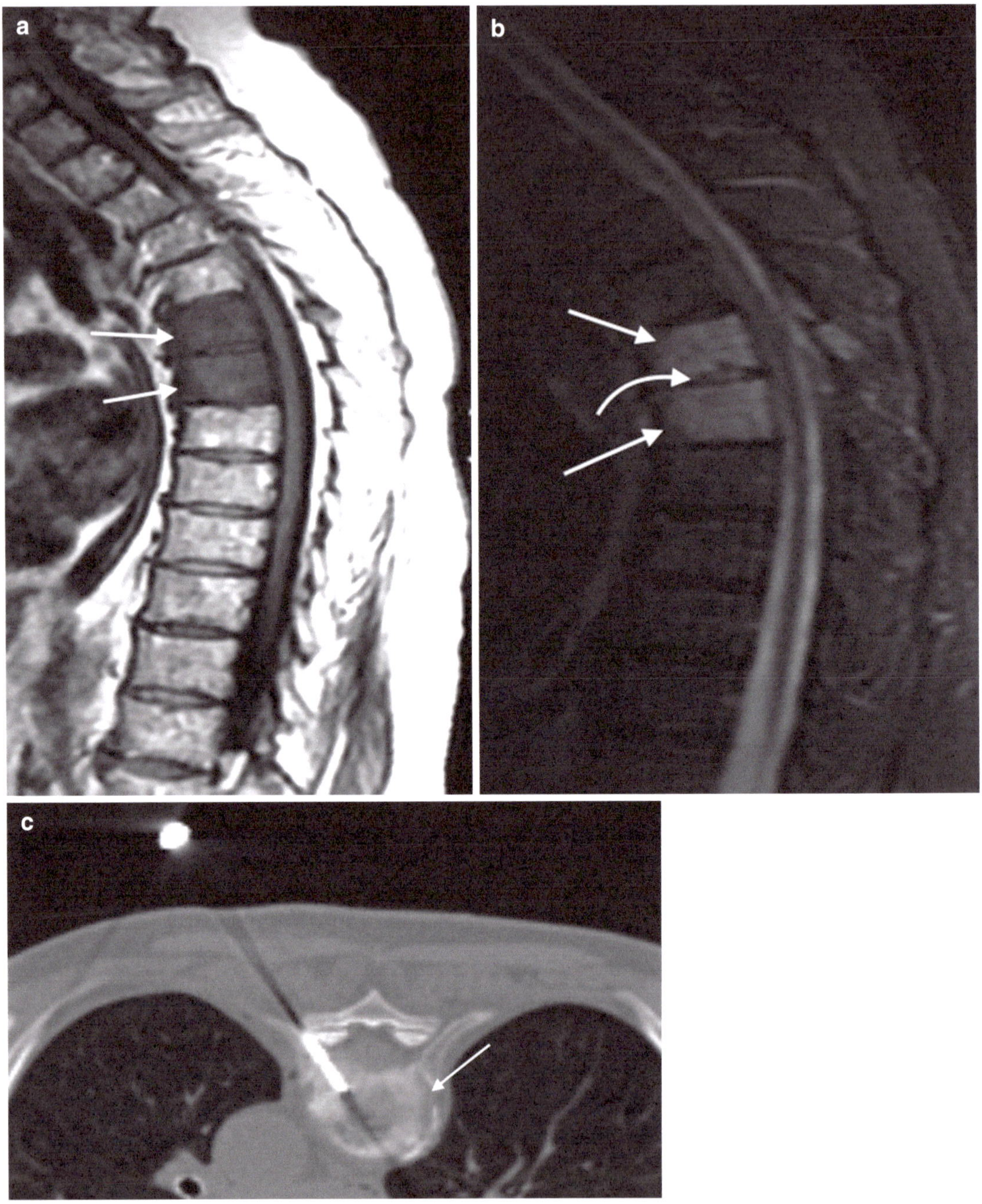

Fig. 10.10 A 91-year-old female with remote history of pancreatic cancer presents with burning back pain. T1-weighted sagittal image (**a**) shows diffuse hypointense signal (*arrows*) within two adjacent vertebral bodies. The STIR sagittal image (**b**) shows hyperintense signal within the vertebral bodies (*arrows*) and the intervening disk (*curved arrow*). Axial CT image (**c**) from the spine biopsy procedure performed using a transcostovertebral approach shows diffuse vertebral endplate irregularity with mild soft tissue swelling (*arrow*). The initial clinical concern was spine infection, but the biopsy demonstrated metastatic pancreatic cancer

(Fig. 10.11). Yet it is in those situations in which a neoplasm is first presenting with metastatic involvement of the axial skeleton that it can be difficult to distinguish between metastases and infection. This clinical scenario can also be seen in multiple myeloma which may not yet be diagnosed until the occurrence of a pathologic vertebral compression fracture (Fig. 10.12).

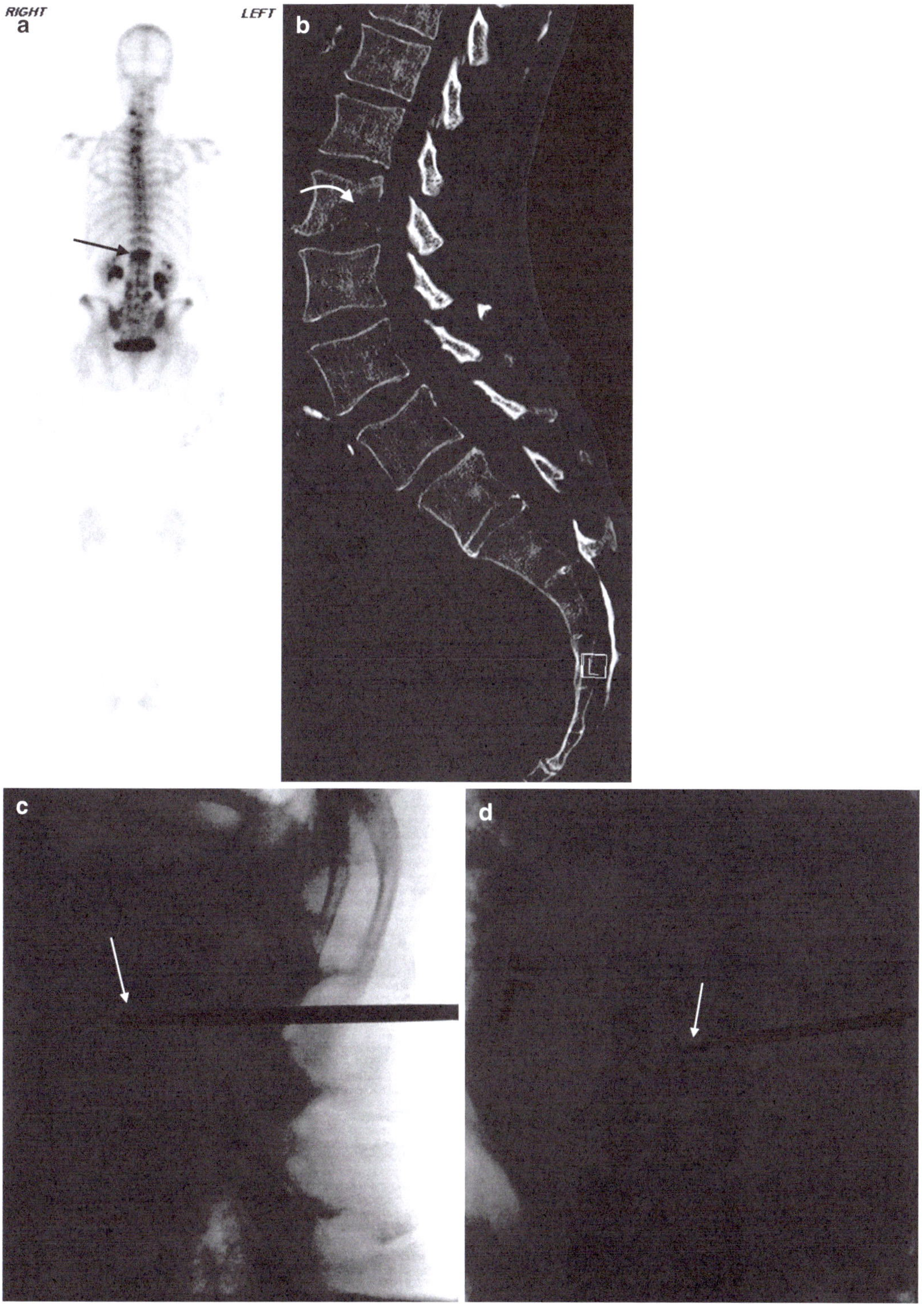

Fig. 10.11 A 69-year-old female with a history of breast cancer presents with 10/10 low back pain. Skeletal scintigraphy (**a**) shows focal radionuclide uptake within the upper lumbar spine (*arrow*). Reformatted sagittal CT image in bone window algorithm (**b**) shows a lytic lesion (*curved arrow*) within the posterior aspect of the inferior endplate of L1. Lumbar spine biopsy performed through a transpedicular approach using coaxial technique shows the biopsy needle within the posterior vertebral body (*arrow*) on this lateral projection (**c**). Frontal projection (**d**) shows inferior angulation of the coaxial biopsy needle system (*arrow*). The biopsy confirmed the presence of metastatic breast cancer

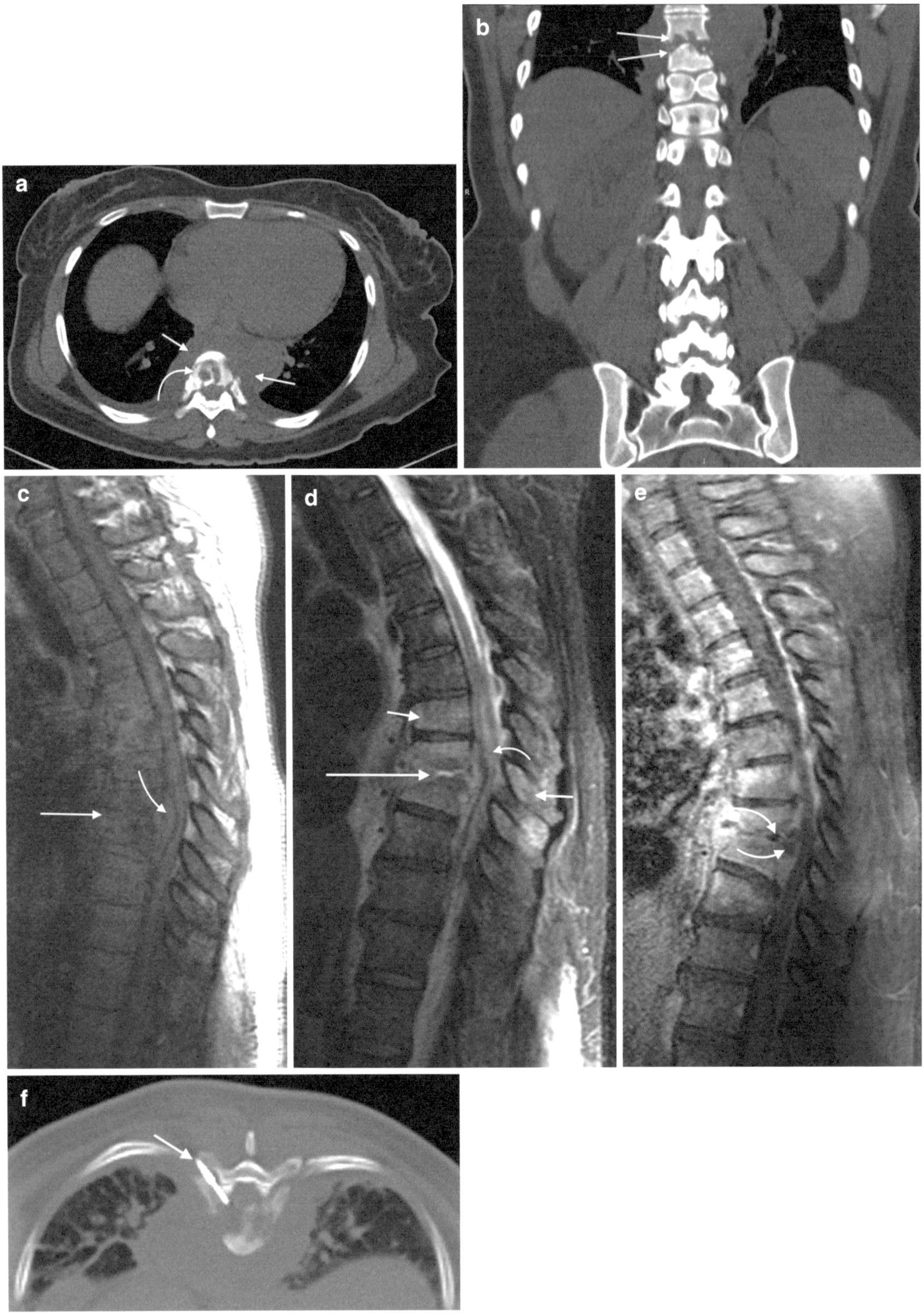
a
b
c
d
e
f

Fig. 10.12 A 41-year-old female with history of intravenous drug abuse and severe thoracic and abdominal pain. Axial CT image (**a**) from an abdomen CT study shows concentric areas of osteolysis within a thoracic vertebral body (*curved arrows*) surrounded by extensive paraspinal soft tissue (*arrows*). A reformatted coronal image (**b**) shows that the lytic change involves adjacent vertebral endplates (*arrows*). A T1-weighted sagittal image (**c**) shows loss of the disk-endplate margins (*arrow*) and a ventral epidural soft tissue component (*curved arrows*). The diffuse hypointense marrow signal reflects the patient's chronic anemia. The T2 sagittal image (**d**) shows destruction of the disk space (*large arrow*) and abnormal vertebral marrow signal involving three vertebral bodies and the posterior elements (*small arrows*). Spinal cord compression with edema is also noted (*curved arrow*). A fat-suppressed contrast-enhanced T1-weighted sagittal image (**e**) shows prominent enhancement surrounding a necrotic area in the disk and ventral epidural space (*curved arrows*). An image-guided biopsy was requested to assess for a presumed spine infection. The axial CT image (**f**) from the biopsy procedure shows the use of the costotransverse approach (*arrow*) to access this extensive area of pathology. The operator was able to obtain multiple specimens, which were submitted for not only microbiologic analysis but also for pathologic analysis. The biopsy results showed plasmacytoma and no evidence of infection. This altered the patient's clinical management, and she underwent surgical decompression and spinal stabilization along with clinical management of myeloma

Indeed, additional clinical evaluation may be required in these cases especially when the patient does not manifest the clinical signs of infection. Lymphoma and leukemia, especially the extranodal form of lymphoma, can also involve the vertebral body, paraspinal soft tissues, and/or the epidural space and, rarely, can simulate the appearance of infectious spondylitis (Fig. 10.13). Primary bone tumors such as chordoma or sarcoma, for example, can occasionally mimic the appearance of an infected spinal segment.

The medical literature is replete with case reports in which any number of neoplasms that can involve the spinal axis present initially with an imaging appearance that masquerades as infection. Alternatively, there is also a long list of case reports in which an infectious process simulates a neoplastic process. For example, scattered foci of vertebral osteomyelitis can look just like metastatic disease on MRI (Hsu et al. 2008). How then should we best approach this type of diagnostic challenge from both an imaging and an interventional perspective? In clinical situations where pathologic diagnostic categories may overlap, then it is critical to recognize the value of differential diagnosis and to at least consider the diagnostic possibility of an infectious or neoplastic entity and to observe a meticulous process for either including or excluding a given diagnostic entity. First, it is important to obtain the patient's prior medical history, in particular, querying for a history of cancer. Second, all prior imaging studies on that patient should be reviewed as this may help to distinguish progression of a neoplastic process from spine infection. Third, all pertinent clinical laboratory analyses to assess for both neoplastic and infectious states should be performed. When an intervention, such as a biopsy of the spine, is warranted, then it is important to obtain an adequate volume of specimen. This will be necessary as specimens should be submitted for both pathologic and microbiologic analysis. Such a strategy will enable the operator to utilize spine biopsy to its fullest potential as a problem-solving procedure.

10.9 Other

Sarcoid can occasionally involve the spinal axis. One or more of the spinal compartments may be affected, and rarely the imaging appearance can be similar to that seen with spine infection (Valencia et al. 2009).

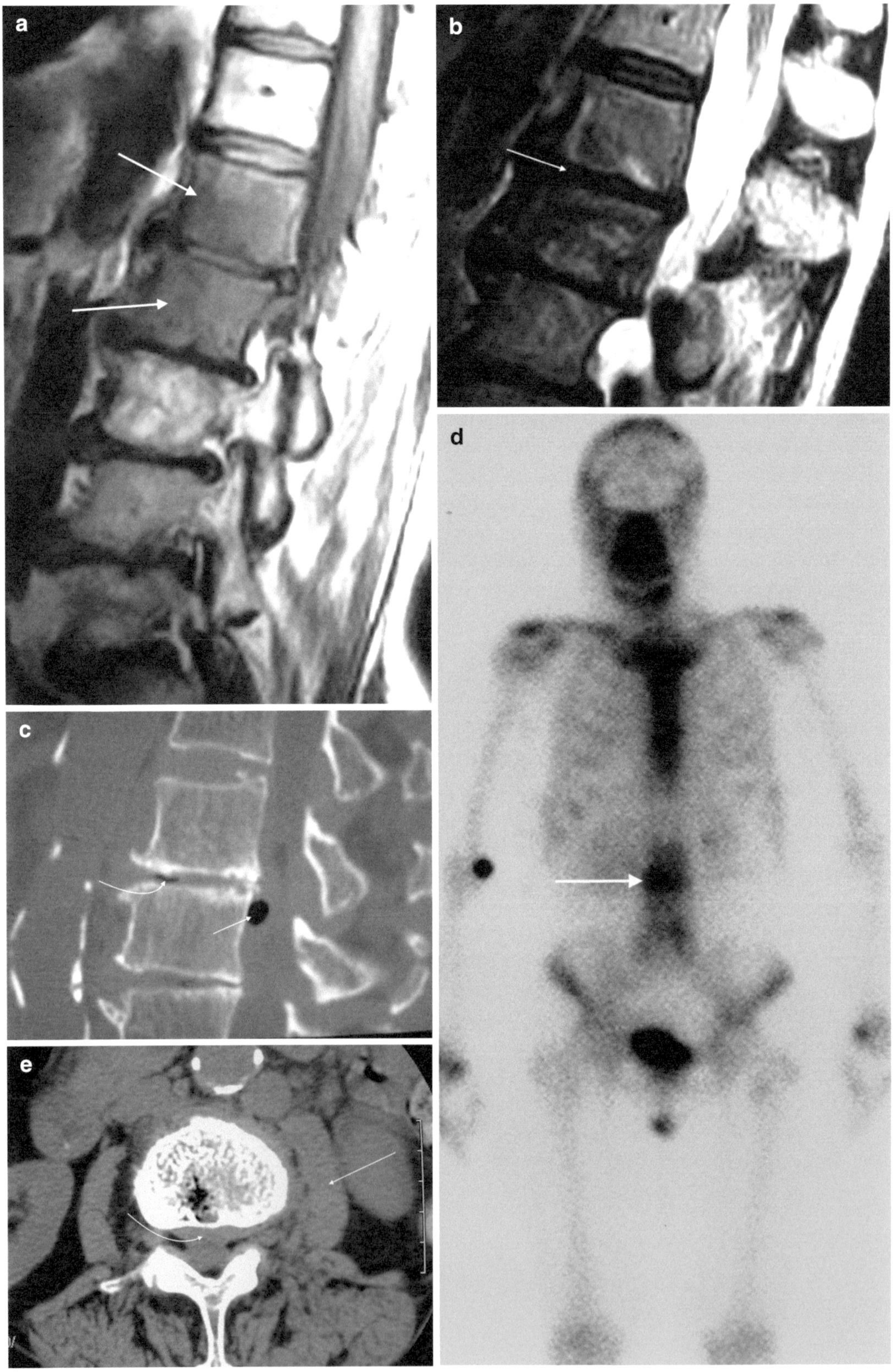
a
b
c
d
e

Fig. 10.13 An 81-year-old female with low back pain. T1-weighted sagittal image (**a**) shows diffuse hypointense signal within two vertebral bodies (*large arrows*) and the intervening disk space (*small arrow*). Close-up view of upper lumbar spine on T2-weighted sagittal image (**b**) shows no signal abnormality within the disk (*arrow*) and a small disk protrusion (*curved arrow*). Close-up view of reformatted sagittal CT image (**c**) in bone window algorithm shows intradiskal gas (*curved arrow*), focal epidural gas (*small arrow*), as well as intact vertebral endplates. Static image from bone scan (**d**) shows focal uptake of radionuclide within the upper lumbar spine (*arrow*). Axial CT image (**e**) in soft tissue algorithm shows a disk protrusion (*curved arrow*) and left paraspinal soft tissue fullness (*arrow*). A biopsy was performed and demonstrated leukemia

Key Review Points

1. Degenerative disk disease, recent diskectomy, and spondyloarthropathy are common conditions that share a similar imaging appearance with spine infection.
2. Trauma, neuropathic osteoarthropathy, and neoplasm can also mimic the imaging appearance of infectious spondylitis.
3. Type 1 degenerative disk disease is often seen within the lower lumbar spine (L4–L5 or L5–S1); T2 signal loss is part of the degenerating disk cascade, whereas T2 signal increase is seen within the infected disk.
4. The focal target-like imaging appearance of Schmorl's nodes can be used to distinguish this entity from infection.
5. In acute diskectomy patients, the signal alterations and enhancement findings are confined to the diskectomy site with parallel linear bands of enhancement seen within the disk annulus.
6. In patients with suspected gout or seronegative spondyloarthropathy, it is important to look at other imaging studies such as radiographs of the hands, feet, and sacroiliac joints.
7. Spondyloarthropathy of chronic hemodialysis has an imaging appearance that strikingly resembles infection. An important observation is to note that the patient is not undergoing the contrast portion of the MRI study because they have kidney failure and are on long-term hemodialysis.
8. Clinical history and prior studies (plain radiographs and/or CT) are useful in identifying trauma patients or patients with osteoporotic vertebral compression fractures that have concomitant vertebral endplate and disk injuries.
9. A useful imaging finding that might suggest neuropathic osteoarthropathy of the spine as the diagnosis, instead of spine infection, is the paucity of soft tissue swelling or involvement in the presence of extensive vertebral body destruction and debris.
10. When trying to differentiate between spine infection and a neoplastic process, always obtain as much specimen as possible so that samples can be sent for microbiologic and histopathologic analysis.

References

Albert HB, Sorensen JS, Christensen BS, Manniche C. Antibiotic treatment in patients with chronic low back pain and vertebral bone edema (Modic type 1 changes): a double-blind randomized clinical controlled trial of efficacy. Eur Spine J. 2013;22:697–707.

Bittane RM, de Moura AB, Lien RJ. The postoperative spine: what the spine surgeon needs to know. Neuroimaging Clin N Am. 2014;24:295–303.

Boden SD, Davis DO, Dina TS, Sunner JL, Wiesel SW. Postoperative diskitis: distinguishing early MR imaging findings from normal postoperative disk space changes. Radiology. 1992;184:765–71.

Canella C, Schau B, Ribeiro E, Sbaffi B, Marchiori E. MRI in seronegative spondyloarthritis: imaging features and differential diagnosis in the spine and sacroiliac joints. AJR Am J Roentgenol. 2013;200:149–57.

Desai MA, Peterson JJ, Garner HW, Kransdorf MJ. Clinical utility of dual-energy CT for evaluation of tophaceous gout. Radiographics. 2011;5:1356–75.

Gabe MJ, Allmendinger AM, Krauthamer A, Spektor V, Destian S, Zablow B. Imaging manifestations of malignant neoplasia mimicking pyogenic osteodiscitis. Clin Imaging. 2010;34:309–15.

Gerster JC, Landry M, Dufresne L, Meuwly JY. Imaging of tophaceous gout: computed tomography provides specific images compared with magnetic resonance imaging and ultrasonography. Ann Rheum Dis. 2002;61:52–4.

Hermann KGA, Althoff CE, Schneider U, Zuhlsdorf S, Lembcke A, Hamm B, Bollow M. Spinal changes in patients with spondyloarthritis: comparison of MR imaging and radiographic appearances. Radiographics. 2005;25:559–70.

Hsu CY, Yu CW, Wu MZ, Chen BB, Huang KM, Shih TT. Unusual manifestations of vertebral osteomyelitis: intraosseous lesions mimicking metastases. AJNR Am J Neuroradiol. 2008;29:1104–10.

Jones EA, Manaster BJ, May DA, Disler DG. Neuropathic osteoarthropathy: diagnostic dilemmas and differential diagnosis. Radiographics. 2000;20:S279–93.

Kiss E, Keusch G, Zanetti M, Jung T, Schwarz A, Schocke M, Jaschke W, Czermak BV. Dialysis-related amyloidosis revisited. AJR Am J Roentgenol. 2005;185:1460–7.

Konatalapalli RM, Demarco PJ, Jelinek JS, Murphey M, Gibson M, Jennings B, Weinstein A. Gout in the axial skeleton. J Rheumatol. 2009 Mar;36:609–13.

Lawrence RC, Felson DT, Helmick CG, Arnold LM, Choi H, Deyo RA, Gabriel S, Hirsch R, Hochberg MC, Hunder GG, Jordan JM, Katz JN, Kremers HM, Wolfe F. Estimates of the prevalence of arthritis and other rheumatic conditions in the United States. Part II. Arthritis Rheum. 2008;58:26–35.

Lim CY, Ong KO. Various musculoskeletal manifestations of chronic renal insufficiency. Clin Radiol. 2013;68:e397–411.

Mattei TA, Rehman AA. Schmorl's nodes: current pathophysiological, diagnostic and therapeutic paradigms. Neurosurg Rev. 2014;37:39–46.

Modic MT, Steinberg PM, Ross JS, Masaryk TJ, Carter JR. Degenerative disk disease: assessment of changes in vertebral body marrow with MR imaging. Radiology. 1988;166:193–9.

Ning TC, Keenan RT. Unusual clinical presentations of gout. Curr Opin Rheumatol. 2010;22:181–7.

Ortiz AO, Bordia R. Injury to the vertebral endplate-disc complex associated with osteoporotic vertebral compression fractures. AJNR Am J Neuroradiol. 2011;32:115–20.

Otsubo S, Kimata N, Okutsu I, Oshikawa K, Ueda S, Sugimoto H, Mitobe M, Uchida K, Otsubo K, Nitta K, Akiba T. Characteristics of dialysis-related amyloidosis in patients on haemodialysis therapy for more than 30 years. Nephrol Dial Transplant. 2009;24:1593–8.

Patel KB, Poplawski MM, Pawha PS, Naidich TP, Tanenbaum LN. Diffusion – weighted MRI "claw sign" improves differentiation of infectious from degenerative modic type 1 signal changes of the spine. AJNR Am J Neuroradiol. 2014;35:647–52.

Popovich T, Carpenter JS, Rai AT, Carson LV, Williams HJ, Marano GD. Spinal cord compression by tophaceous Gout with Fluorodeoxyglucose-Positron-Emission Tomographic/MR Fusion Imaging. Am J Neuroradiol. 2006;27:1201–3.

Ross JS, Zepp R, Modic MT. The postoperative lumbar spine: enhanced MR evaluation of the intervertebral disk. AJNR Am J Neuroradiol. 1996;17:323–31.

Saketkoo LA, Robertson HJ, Dyer HR, Virk Z, Ferreyro HR, Espinoza LR. Axial gouty arthropathy. Am J Med Sci. 2009;338:140–6.

Stabler A, Bellan M, Weiss M, Gartner C, Brossmann J, Reiser MF. MR imaging of enhancing intraosseous disk herniation (Schmorl's Nodes). AJR Am J Roentgenol. 1997;168:933–8.

Theodorou DJ, Theodorou SJ, Resnick D. Imaging in dialysis spondyloarthropathy. Semin Dial. 2002;15:290–6.

Valencia MP, Deaver PM, Mammarappallil MC. Sarcoidosis of the thoracic and lumbar vertebrae, mimicking metastasis or multifocal osteomyelitis by MRI: case report. Clin Imaging. 2009;33:478–81.

Wagner AL, Murtagh FR, Arrington JA, Stallworth D. Relationship of Schmorl's nodes to vertebral body endplate fractures and acute endplate disk extrusions. AJNR Am J Neuroradiol. 2000a;21:276–81.

Wagner SC, Schweitzer ME, Morrison WB, Przbylski GJ, Parker L. Can imaging findings help differentiate spinal neuropathic arthropathy from disk space infection? Initial experience. Radiology. 2000b;214:693–9.

Yen PS, Lin JF, Chen SY, Lin SZ. Tophaceous gout of the lumbar spine mimicking infectious spondylodiscitis and epidural abscess: MR imaging findings. J Clin Neurosci. 2005;12:44–6.

Yu JS, Chung C, Recht M, Dailiana T, Jurdi R. MR imaging of tophaceous gout. AJR Am J Roentgenol. 1997;168:523–7.

Image-Guided Percutaneous Spine and Rib Biopsy: Pathology

11

Steven A. Drexler and A. Orlando Ortiz

11.1 Introduction

A biopsy procedure does not necessarily start and end with the performance of the procedure. The objective of a biopsy is to obtain pathologic tissue in a sufficient amount so as to enable a pathologist and/or a microbiologist to make the diagnosis. The assumption that all that is necessary is to provide them with a specimen and that they will make the diagnosis can be equated with the request for an imaging study and the typical poor/vague history that presents itself at the radiologist's reading station. Neither of these scenarios results in excellent medical care.

11.2 What Does the Operator Expect from the Pathologist?

Prior to an image-guided percutaneous spine or rib biopsy procedure, the operator may be considering a specific pathologic diagnosis based upon the patient's imaging examinations and clinical presentation. At this time, the operator may want to discuss the case with the pathologist to determine how to proceed with the biopsy procedure. For example, if the operator is concerned about spine infection, then the majority of the specimen may be sent to microbiology. If the operator is suspecting lymphoma, then the specimen may be prepared for flow cytometry. A special stain may be required based upon the suspected pathologic diagnosis. The operator can also review the imaging findings with the pathologist, and this will in turn assist the pathologist in their subsequent analysis of the biopsy specimens. During the procedure, the pathologist's assistance can be quite valuable. The presence of a pathologist is particularly helpful when assessing FNA samples for specimen adequacy and for cytologic diagnosis. After the procedure, the pathologist owns the major responsibility of trying to make the correct diagnosis. It may be helpful in certain instances for the operator to review the slides and images with the pathologist.

11.3 What Does the Pathologist Expect from the Operator?

A spine or rib biopsy procedure is requested. This presents the operator with significant opportunities to discuss the case not only with the clinician but also with the pathologist and microbiologist. There may be special circumstances when the operator should discuss the case with the pathologist or microbiologist prior to the procedure. It is important for the operator to not only communicate with these clinical associates after the biopsy procedure, not just to get the results, but prior to the procedure in order to optimize the results. The pathologist may want to discuss the case with the operator in order to obtain more clinical information. The operator should inform the pathologist if the patient has undergone any prior biopsies or surgeries and at

A.O. Ortiz, *Image-Guided Percutaneous Spine Biopsy*, DOI 10.1007/978-3-319-43326-4_11

which institution or facility these were performed. This will improve the pathologist's chances of establishing the correct diagnosis. Similarly, the microbiologist should be informed whether or not the patient is being treated with antibiotics and, if so, which ones and for how long. Providing adequate clinical and radiologic information is also helpful to the pathologist. It is sometimes beneficial for the pathologist to review the prior imaging studies with the operator in order to assist in optimal biopsy planning. For instance, it is helpful for the pathologist to know if the lesion is lytic, cystic, solid, or enhancing. A radiologic differential diagnosis is quite useful and should be provided to the pathologist. If the operator suspects a specific diagnosis based upon a pathognomonic radiologic presentation, then the pathologist should be informed (Fig. 11.1).

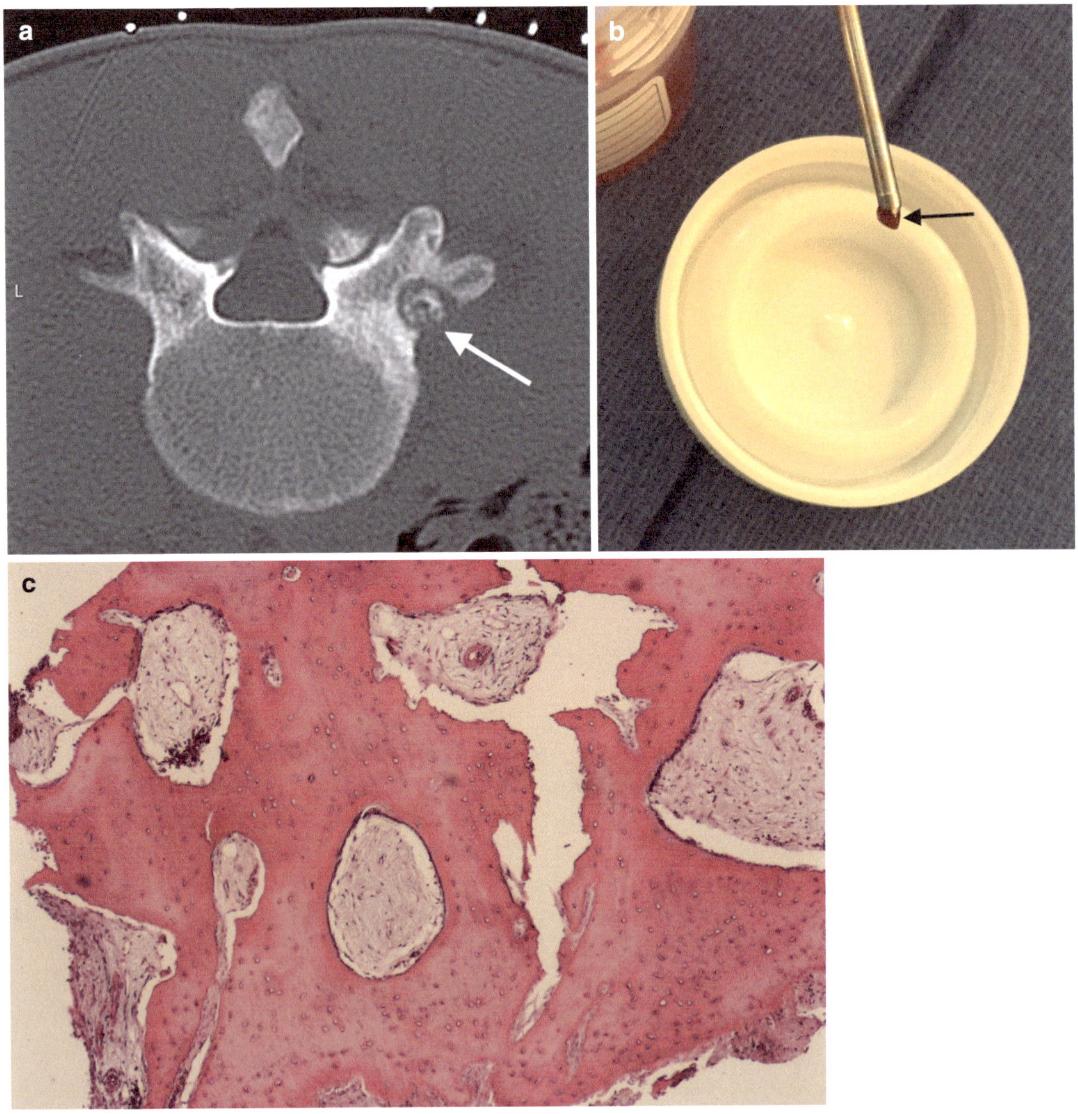

Fig. 11.1 An 18-year-old male with nocturnal low back pain (same patient as in Fig. 12 in Chap. 6). Axial CT image in bone window algorithm (**a**) shows a small, well-circumscribed hypodense lesion within a sclerotic right lumbar pedicle (*arrow*); the lesion contains a small central mixed density nidus. Close-up photograph of biopsy specimen (**b**) shows red-brown bone core (*arrow*). Photomicrograph with H/E stain (**c**) shows circumscribed area of disorganized, sclerosed bone with marrow fibrosis. The histologic findings were consistent with an osteoid osteoma

Diagnostic tissue is best obtained from the nonnecrotic component of a given lesion (Omura et al. 2011). After all, the goal of an image-guided percutaneous spine or rib biopsy procedure is to obtain specimen. The optimum biopsy procedure should yield as much tissue from the pathologic structure or region as possible. FNA is suitable for rapid answers in lesions that are easily biopsied using needle aspiration (Fig. 11.2) (Gupta et al. 2002). Cohesive or fibrous lesions may not be easily aspirated (e.g., schwannoma or fibrosarcoma). The small amount of tissue from FNA may not be sufficient for special studies including immunohistochemistry, flow cytometry, or molecular studies. The size of the needle that is used or additional FNA passes in order to obtain more tissue can alleviate this concern (Kreula 1990). Fine-needle aspirates are submitted in 50% alcohol. FNAs can be

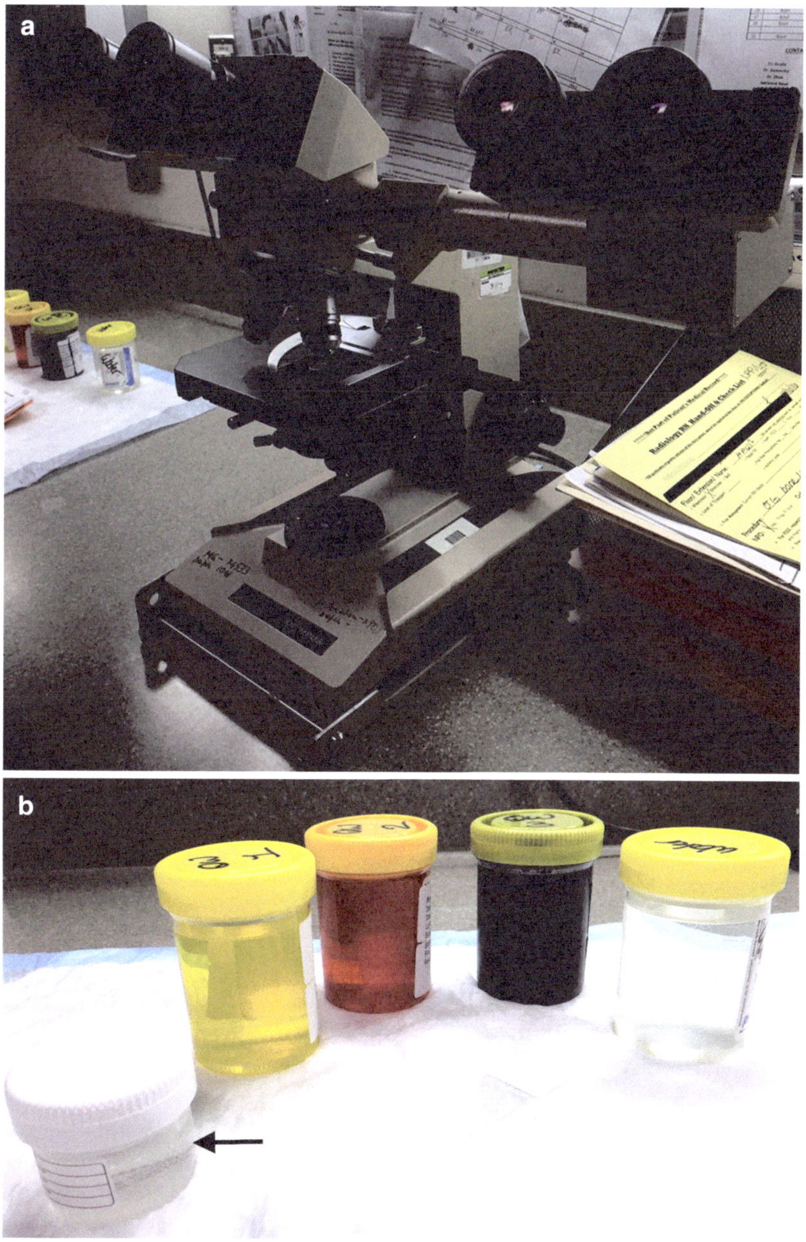

Fig. 11.2 Photograph (**a**) of a dual-viewer microscope that is located within the procedure area. This enables the cytotechnologist and pathologist to immediately confirm the absence or presence of a diagnostic FNA specimen. Photograph (**b**) of rapid staining agents that allow the cytotechnologist or pathologist to quickly process an FNA specimen and air-dry the slides. The slides can be prepared and reviewed within a few minutes. This technology contributes to the efficiency and safety of the biopsy procedure. A specimen cup (*arrow*) is kept on standby for any core biopsy material. Furthermore, the operator can directly convey additional information to the pathology department at the time of the biopsy

also performed during some bone biopsy procedures (Schweitzer et al. 1996). For FNA procedures, small cell clusters from the tissue that is sampled are desirable. The objective is to avoid contamination of the FNA sample with the patient's blood. It is difficult to detect an abnormal cell in a virtual "sea" of blood. For this reason, it is important to perform the FNA procedure prior to the core biopsy procedure, as the latter can of cause an intralesional hemorrhage of sufficient quantity so as to contaminate a subsequent FNA pass. Soft tissue cores generate a much larger sample of the lesion than FNA which enables the performance of special studies with fewer needle passes (Yang and Damron 2004). A soft tissue cutting needle can be useful for lytic lesions. Small lesions require a short needle "throw" or excursion, while larger lesions can accommodate a longer needle "throw." The pathologist is looking for as much tissue as possible from the soft tissue components of a given lesion. That being said, at least 2 mm in each dimension is preferred. Large bone cores by increasing the volume and area of sampling are desirable (Ortiz et al. 2010). However, the larger needle size and diagnostic benefit of larger specimens must be balanced against the increased risk of procedure-related hemorrhage. Tissue cores are submitted in 10% formalin. When performing bone biopsies, the operator must try to not only obtain as many bone cores as possible but also to handle the specimens as carefully as possible. This applies to transferring the specimen from the bone biopsy cannula into the transport media. Crush artifact may be created when obtaining core specimens, and this can cause diagnostic dilemmas. The likelihood of crush artifact can be reduced by trying not to impact the bone biopsy needle with one single specimen. Some lytic osseous lesions are very soft, and an FNA or soft tissue core biopsy may need to be performed in order to obtain a specimen. In certain situations, the only specimen that can be obtained is an aspirate of bloody material. This specimen should not be discarded and should be analyzed for the presence of neoplastic cells.

> Always try to perform the FNA procedure prior to the core biopsy procedure.

11.4 Special Situations

Specimens for flow cytometry to diagnose lymphoma are submitted fresh on ice as quickly as possible to the lab, preferably early in the day to allow for specimen handling. FNA specimens that cannot be immediately assessed by the pathologist can be placed in an alcohol-based transport medium. If there is a concern for an inflammatory process such as gout, the specimen can be placed on a small piece of non-adherent dressing that is soaked in normal saline (Fig. 11.3). Infection is best verified by Gram stain and culture (Howard et al. 1994). Bacterial, fungal, and mycobacterial cultures should be submitted directly to the microbiology department separately from the specimen submitted for tissue processing. An operator ought to consider sending specimens to both microbiology and pathology for analysis for lesions that involve multiple spinal levels and/or when the clinical and laboratory parameters (white blood cell count, erythrocyte sedimentation rate, and C-reactive protein) are abnormal. Another clinical scenario in which both types of analyses should be performed is in patients who are immunocompromised.

11.5 Optimizing Specimen Volume and Transport Media

One of the most deflating reports to receive, after a spine or rib biopsy procedure, often reads as one of the following:

> "Non-diagnostic specimen. Blood only in smears. Cell block shows minute fragments of benign cartilage and benign cortical bone. No marrow elements are present in the smears or cell block."
> Or
> "QNS: quantity not sufficient for diagnosis."

It must be understood that this biopsy result can occur with any biopsy procedure (Hwang et al. 2011). Hence, pre-procedure disclosure to the patient about the possibility of a nondiagnostic biopsy should always be discussed. This will prevent the patient from becoming frustrated or disappointed if the result of the procedure is less

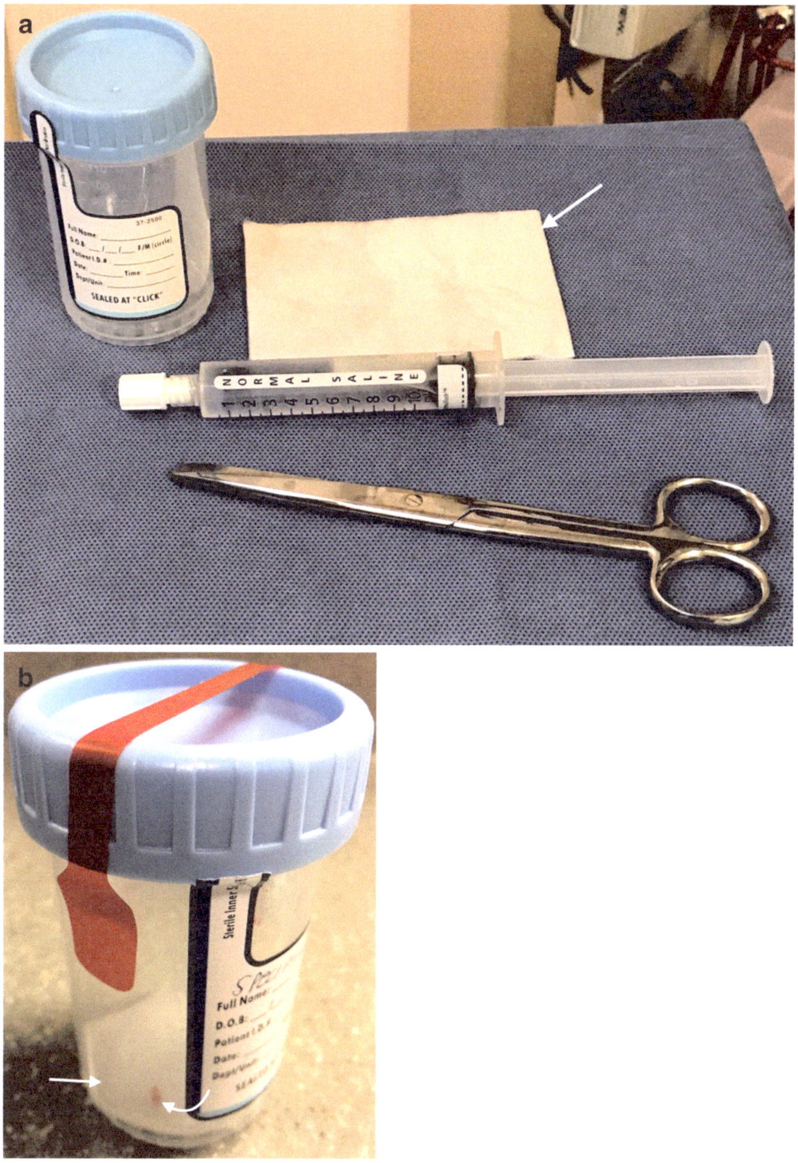

Fig. 11.3 Photograph (**a**) of non-adherent dressing (*arrow*) and 10 mL normal saline. The scissors are used to cut a small piece from the pad and place the small piece of the pad within the sealable container. The normal saline is used to soak the non-adherent dressing. Photograph (**b**) of saline-soaked non-adherent dressing (*arrow*) within a sealed container. A specimen core (*curved arrow*) has been placed on top of the non-adherent dressing; this was submitted to assess for urate crystals

than what was expected. The patient will also be aware that they may require another biopsy procedure. The biopsy procedure represents sampling of a small portion of a spine or rib lesion. If there is scant tissue within the sampled volume, then the likelihood of achieving a pathologic diagnosis is reduced. If the lesion is not completely sampled or not sampled at all, then the possibility of a confirmatory diagnosis is reduced (Figs. 11.4 and 11.5). Even more frustrating is the improper handling of specimens from the time of their acquisition (e.g., placing the specimen in the wrong transport medium) to the time of transport and delivery (the specimen is lost).

The goals then are to maximize the amount of pathologic tissue that can be reasonably acquired during the biopsy procedure, to place the harvested material in the appropriate labeled specimen containers, and to expeditiously transport these containers to the appropriate destinations for processing and analysis. Limited specimen volume due to small gauge sampling devices may be an issue. At times the operator may not have a choice in this matter due to factors such as small lesion size or a suspected hypervascular lesion. Small lesions may limit the number and size of specimen samples. Whenever possible, the use of larger-gauge needles enables the operator to harvest more specimens (Fig. 11.6). This translates into better statistical sampling of the lesion with a higher likelihood of obtaining diagnostic tissue.

The most useful pathology information is obtained from biopsy samples that include at least one core of bone or soft tissue. In order to optimize pathologic evaluation and diagnosis, it is best to submit as many cores as possible (Wu et al. 2008). At least three bone cores, if possible, should be obtained and placed in 10% formalin for submission to pathology. Of note, bone biopsy specimens must undergo a 48-h period of

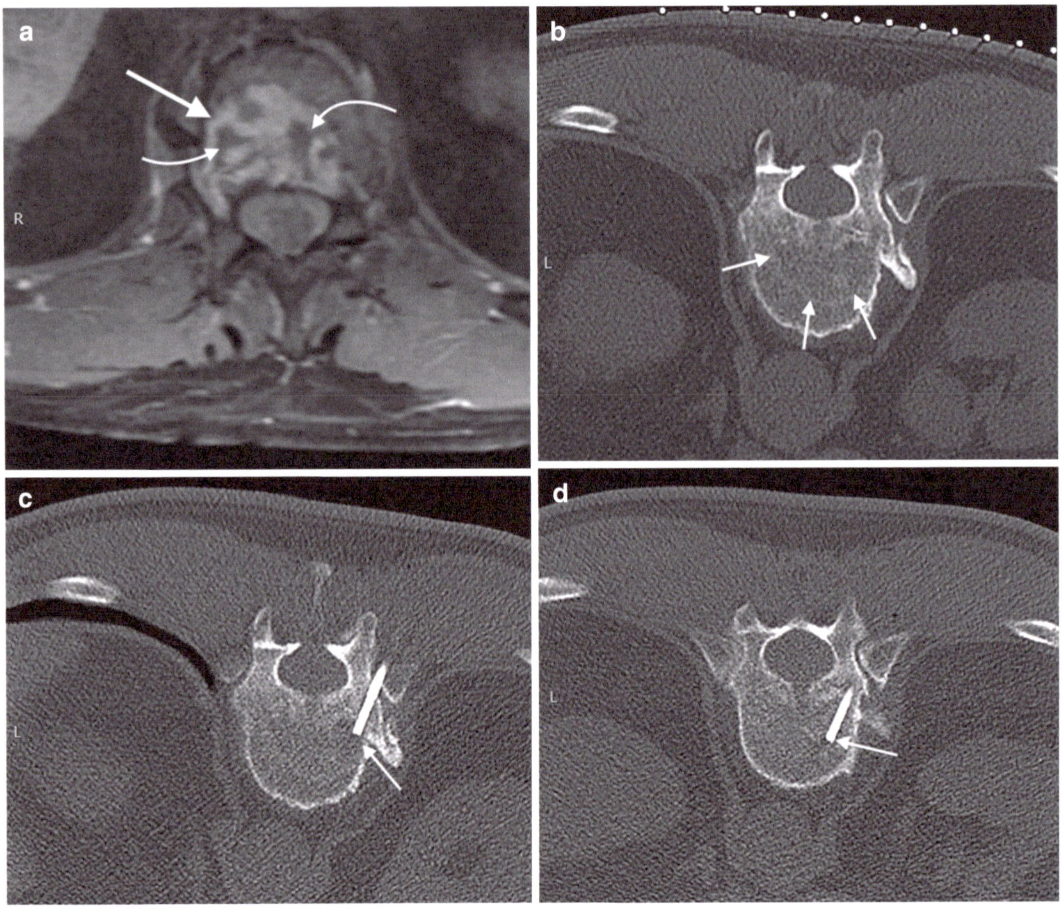

Fig. 11.4 A 58-year-old male with T12 bone lesion. Fat-suppressed contrast-enhanced T1-weighted axial image (**a**) shows large enhancing lesion (*arrow*) that contains several large necrotic or cystic foci (*curved arrows*). Axial CT image (**b**) with skin grid in place shows a subtle lesion (*arrows*). CT-guided coaxial biopsy (**c**, **d**) using costovertebral approach shows biopsy needle at the margin of lesion (*arrows*). An FNA (**e**) was then performed (*arrow*). The procedure yielded three bone cores and one FNA specimen. The FNA specimen (**f**) was nondiagnostic with only blood present on the smears. That the latter showed only blood is no surprise as the FNA was performed after the bone biopsy. Moreover, if the needle tip is within the vertebral marrow, blood will be aspirated (think of the vertebral body as a large trabeculated venous structure with marrow elements). The cell block (**g**), which was obtained from the bone cores, showed only minute fragments of calcified tissue (*arrow*), most likely representing the bone. In this case, the peripheral location of the biopsy needle relative to the center or "meat" of the lesion may account for this nondiagnostic biopsy. A steeper approach to the lesion would have yielded access to the epicenter of the lesion with the possibility of a diagnostic biopsy

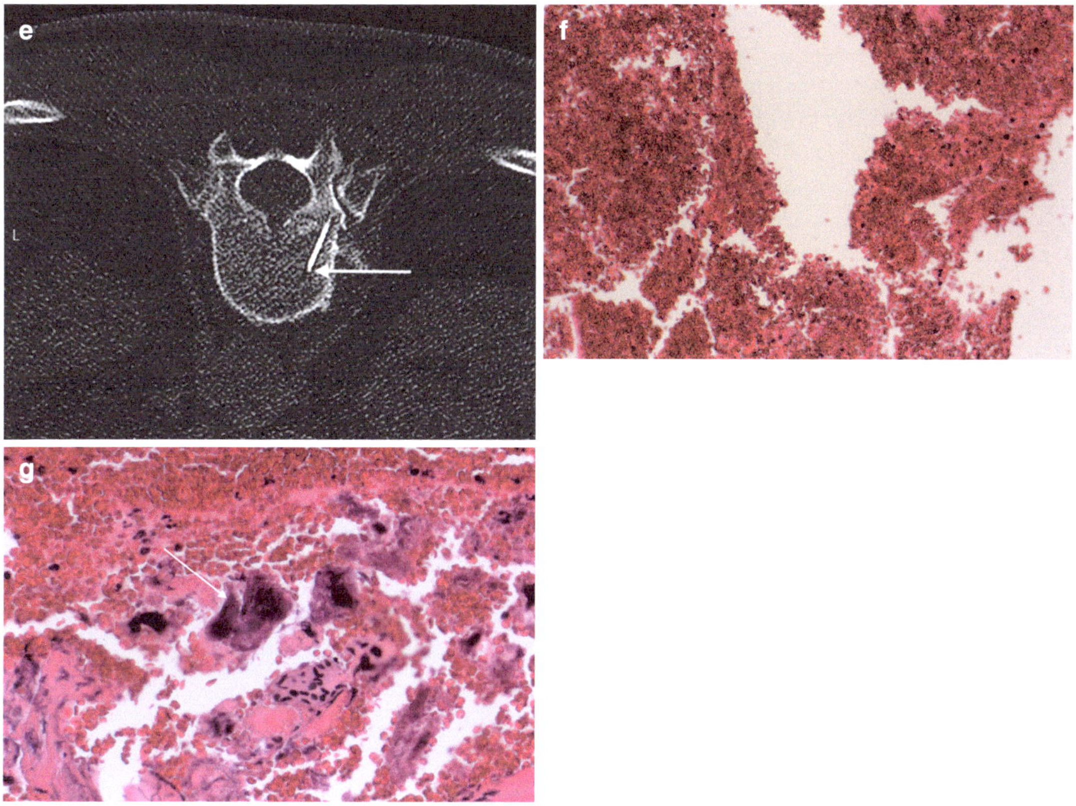

Fig. 11.4 (continued)

decalcification in 7% formic acid prior to sectioning and staining. Thus, it is important to obtain enough tissue such that an adequate amount remains after decalcification for histological analysis. Never discard marrow aspirates as these may harbor representative tissue from the lesion in question (Hewes et al. 1983). For soft tissue or lytic lesion soft tissue biopsies, at least four soft tissue cores, if possible, should be obtained; these also can be submitted in 10% formalin. The type of imaging guidance (i.e., CT vs. fluoroscopy) does not appear to be a factor in obtaining core samples and arriving at a pathologic diagnosis.

Pre-procedure disclosure to the patient about the possibility of a nondiagnostic biopsy should always be discussed.

11.6 Basic Histopathology

The pathologist will utilize certain basic staining techniques for analyzing spine or rib osseous lesions or paraspinal or extraosseous rib lesions. The initial stain that is used is the H/E or hematoxylin-eosin stain (Fig. 11.1). The results of this stain will help determine which additional staining techniques, if any, might be of benefit.

Common stains used for bone biopsy procedures:

1. H/E is the primary screen used to evaluate the pathology and decide if additional staining or testing is warranted.
2. Immunohistochemistry for tumor types or infection—antibody binding

to antigens present in the tissue linked to a chromagen. For example, schwannomas are S100 positive; lymphomas are positive for LCA (CD20).
3. For bacteria, Gram stain will stain Gram negatives purple and Gram positives black.
4. For mycobacterium, Ziehl-Neelsen stain will stain the organisms red.
5. For fungus, PAS (pink) or GMS (black).

11.7 Histopathology of Commonly Encountered Spine and Rib Lesions

While a variety of pathologic conditions may be encountered within the spine, ribs, or their adjacent soft tissues, there are certain neoplasms that have a propensity to occur within these sites (Table 11.1) (Mills et al. 2015).

Certain special stains are helpful in the identification of specific tumor types (Table 11.2). The

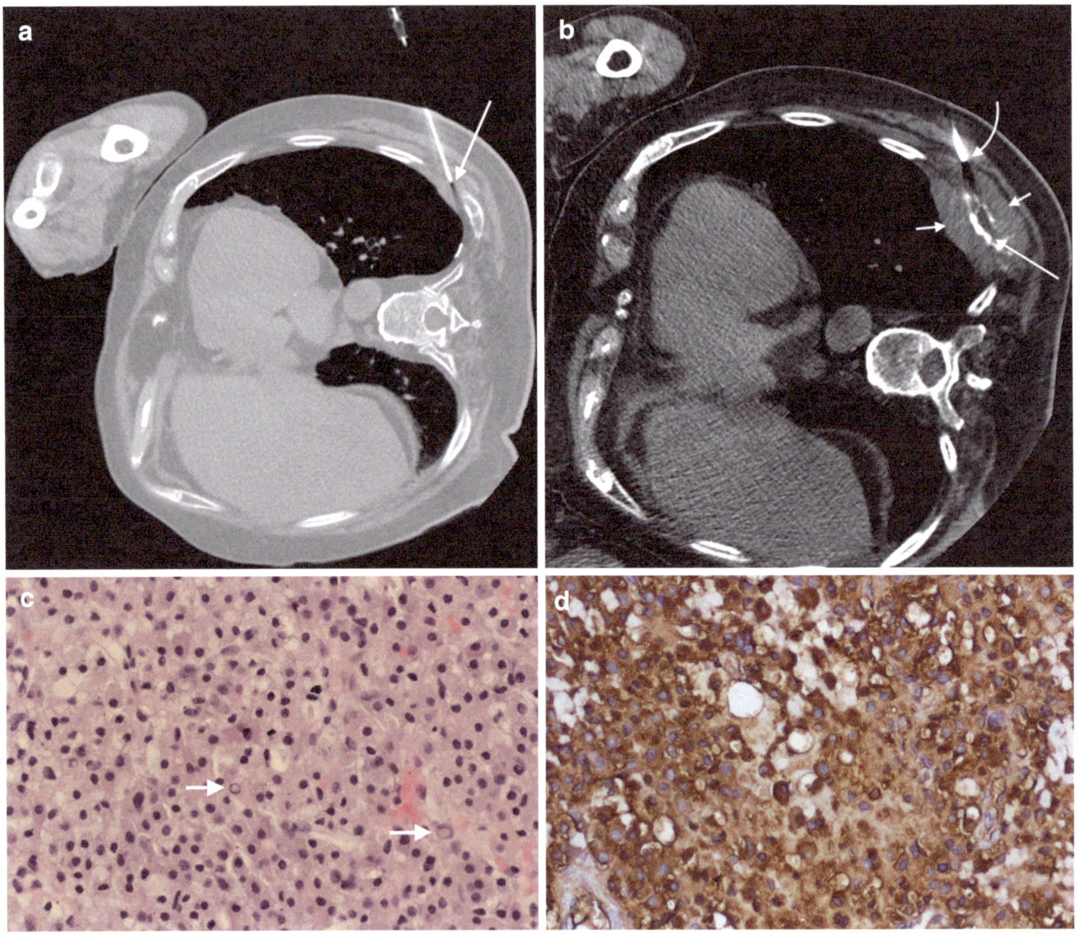

Fig. 11.5 An 86-year-old male with prior history of asbestos exposure presents with focal left pleural thickening and a rib lesion. Axial CT image (**a**) shows FNA (*arrow*) of extraosseous soft tissue component. The results of this biopsy were negative for malignant cells and consisted of a relatively hypocellular specimen. The patient returned 7 months later for a repeat biopsy. Axial CT image (**b**) shows a marked increase in the size of the rib lesion (*arrow*) and its extraosseous extension (*small arrows*). A guide needle (*curved arrow*) is in place for FNA. The repeat biopsy consisted of two FNA touch preps which showed the presence of sheets of atypical plasma cells (**c**) with numerous Dutcher bodies (*arrows*). Immunoperoxidase stains that were performed on the cell block, from the soft tissue biopsy cores, included a positive kappa stain (**d**). The immunoprofile excluded malignant mesothelioma and was consistent with a plasmacytoma with kappa restriction

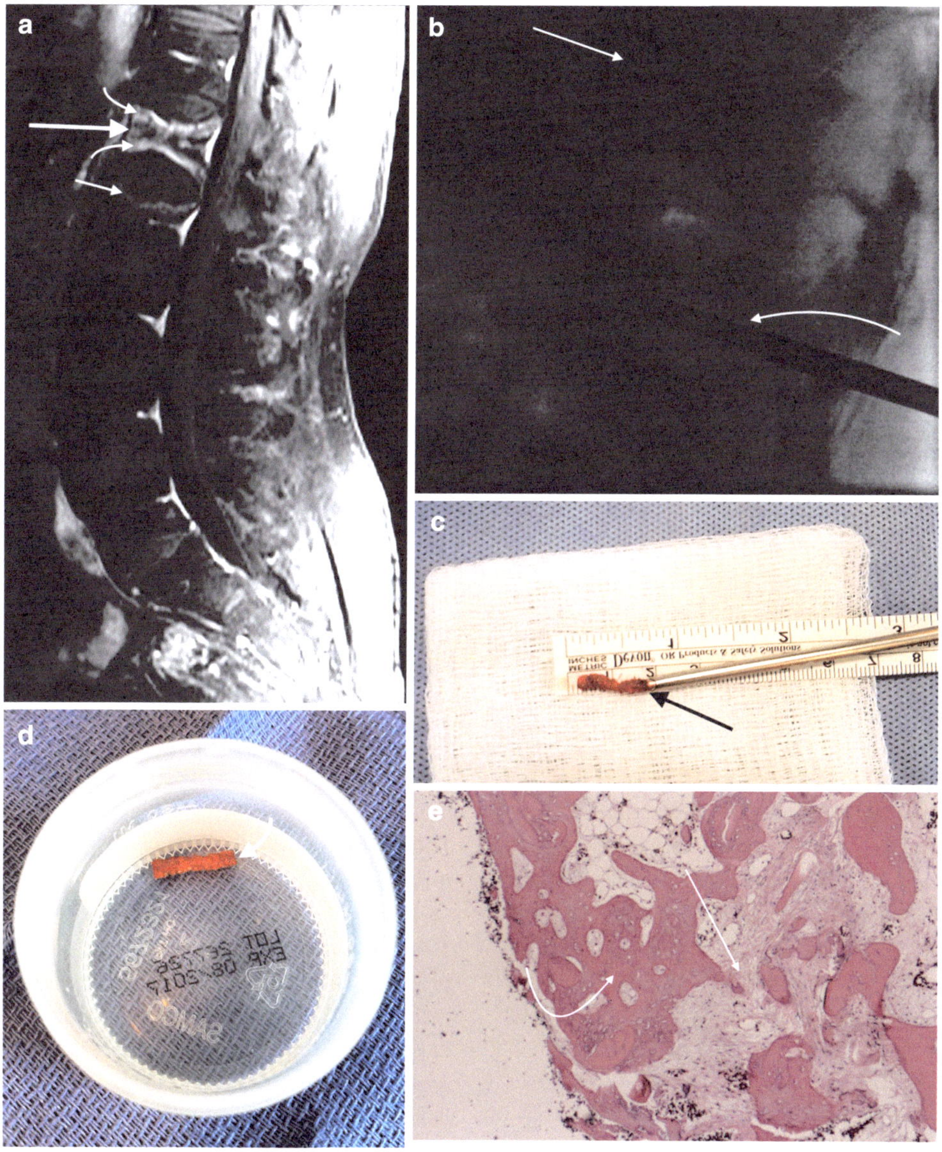

Fig. 11.6 A 68-year-old male with history of metastatic prostate cancer and painful lumbar vertebral compression fractures. Contrast-enhanced fat-suppressed T1-weighted sagittal image (**a**) shows a partial impaction-type vertebral compression deformity of L1 (*arrow*) with band-like enhancement along the vertebra endplates (*curved arrows*). Superior endplate enhancement is also seen involving the L2 vertebral body (*small arrow*). Lateral fluoroscopic image (**b**) shows use of an 8-gauge bone biopsy system (*curved arrow*) with transpedicular technique at L2; L1 (*arrow*) was also biopsied, but did not yield any diagnostic tissue. Photograph (**c**) of a large 1.5 cm length bone core being expressed from the biopsy cannula (*arrow*). Photograph (**d**) of the tan-red bone core (*arrow*) within the 10% formalin specimen container. Photomicrograph (**e**) with H/E stain shows changes consistent with a healing fracture, fracture callous including fibrosis (*arrow*) and reorganizing bony spicules (*curved arrow*)

Table 11.1 Lesions Commonly Encountered at Biopsy

Spine
1. Metastasis: lung, breast, prostate, gastrointestinal
2. Myeloma
3. Lymphoma
4. Primary: giant cell tumor, chordoma

Rib
1. Metastasis
2. Primary: chondrosarcoma

staining pattern, positive or negative, on specific immunohistochemistry studies contributes to the immunoprofile of the tissue and may narrow if not determine the histopathologic diagnosis (Kabiraj et al. 2015).

11.7.1 Metastasis

The vertebral column is the most common site for osseous metastases, with about 70% of lesions found within the thoracic spine (Ross 2005). The most common primary sites to metastasize to the spine include carcinomas of the prostate, lung, and breast (Murphy et al. 1981). It is therefore important to notify the pathologist if the patient has either a prior history of cancer or suspicious concurrent imaging findings in another location. Additionally, lesion multiplicity will increase the probability that a given spine or rib lesion might represent a metastatic process (Jakanani and Saifuddin 2013). It is in this latter situation where skeletal scintigraphy may be of value in screening the skeleton. Metastases are initially characterized into one of the groups of carcinoma, lymphoma, or sarcoma and then further subcategorized using histological and immunohistochemical means (Figs. 11.7, 11.8, 11.9, and 11.10). Some tumors require molecular studies utilizing fluorescent in situ hybridization (FISH) or sequencing.

11.7.2 Myeloma

Multiple myeloma is a clonal B-cell tumor consisting of differentiated plasma cells (Angtuaco et al. 2004). Since it accounts for approximately

Table 11.2 Special Stains (Dabbs 2014)

Metastasis	Carcinoma—CK7 and CK20 to narrow source site
Lung	TTF1 adenocarcinoma, P63 squamous cell carcinoma, CAM 5.2. small cell carcinoma
Breast	ER/PR/GCDFP/E-cadherin for lobular vs. ductal, GATA-3
Prostate	PAP, PSA
Thyroid	TTF1, thyroglobulin
Myeloma	CD138, Kappa/Lambda—via IHC or SISH
Lymphoma	LCA CD20, CD3, and other lymphoid markers
Leukemia	IHC myeloperoxidase, C34, lysozyme, TdT, CD117, and FISH (various for deletions and translocations)
Primary bone tumor	
Chordoma	S100
Giant cell tumor	CD68, S100
Sarcoma	Vimentin, CD99+, various other markers to narrow type
	Chondrosarcoma—S100 positive, IDH1, and IDH2

10% of hematologic cancers, it is common for this condition to involve the skeletal system, including the spine and ribs (Stoker and Kissin 1985). Myeloma is identified initially by the presence of dense aggregates of atypical plasma cells and then subcategorized using stains for kappa and lambda studies (Fig. 11.5). This may include immunohistochemistry and/or in situ hybridization studies.

11.7.3 Lymphoma

Lymphoma is identified by the presence of aggregates of atypical lymphocytes (Fig. 11.11). Immunohistochemical staining with B-cell, T-cell, and other markers is needed to confirm the diagnosis of lymphoma. Lymphoma may either present with secondary involvement of the spine or ribs or, less commonly, with primary involvement of these osseous structures. Primary lymphoma of the bone is rare and accounts for less than 5% of all primary osseous neoplasms (Krishnan et al. 2003).

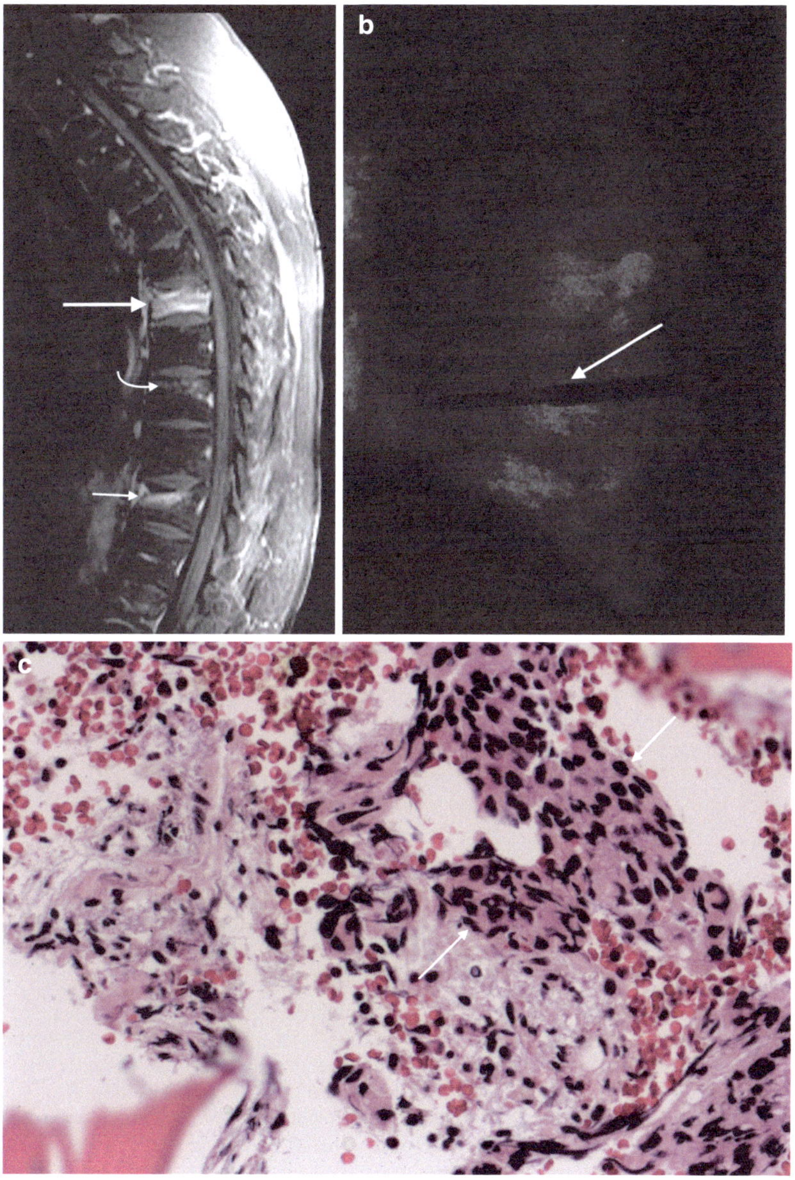

Fig. 11.7 A 68-year-old male with metastatic prostate cancer and painful thoracic vertebral compression fractures (same patient as in Fig. 6). Contrast-enhanced fat-suppressed T1-weighted sagittal image (**a**) of the thoracic spine shows a partial compression deformity of T7 (*large arrow*) with diffuse vertebral body enhancement, subtle superior endplate enhancement within the T9 vertebral body (*curved arrow*), and focal enhancement within a partially compressed T11 vertebral body (*small arrow*). Lateral fluoroscopic image (**b**) shows coaxial bone biopsy of the T9 vertebra with a 10-gauge bone biopsy system (*arrow*); the height loss at T9 has progressed as compared to the MRI study (**a**). Photomicrograph of biopsy specimen (**c**) with H/E stain shows fragments of bone with foci of metastatic carcinoma (*arrows*), consistent with prostate carcinoma

11.7.4 Giant Cell Tumor

Giant cell tumor is identified by the presence of osteoclast like giant cells evenly distributed in a background of polyhedral or oval mononuclear cells (Fig. 11.12). These tumors occur most frequently within the appendicular skeleton, arising in the epiphyses of long bones, especially about the knee. Giant cell tumors, however, can be found within the spine or sacrum (Chakarun et al. 2013). This neoplasm tends to be large and multilobular and contains foci of hemorrhage, cyst formation, and pale necrosis. Though histologically benign, giant cell tumors are locally aggressive and have a fairly high recurrence rate (15–25%).

11.7.5 Chordoma

These tumors are derived from notochordal rests that are present along the craniospinal axis from the skull base to the sacrum. Indeed, the central

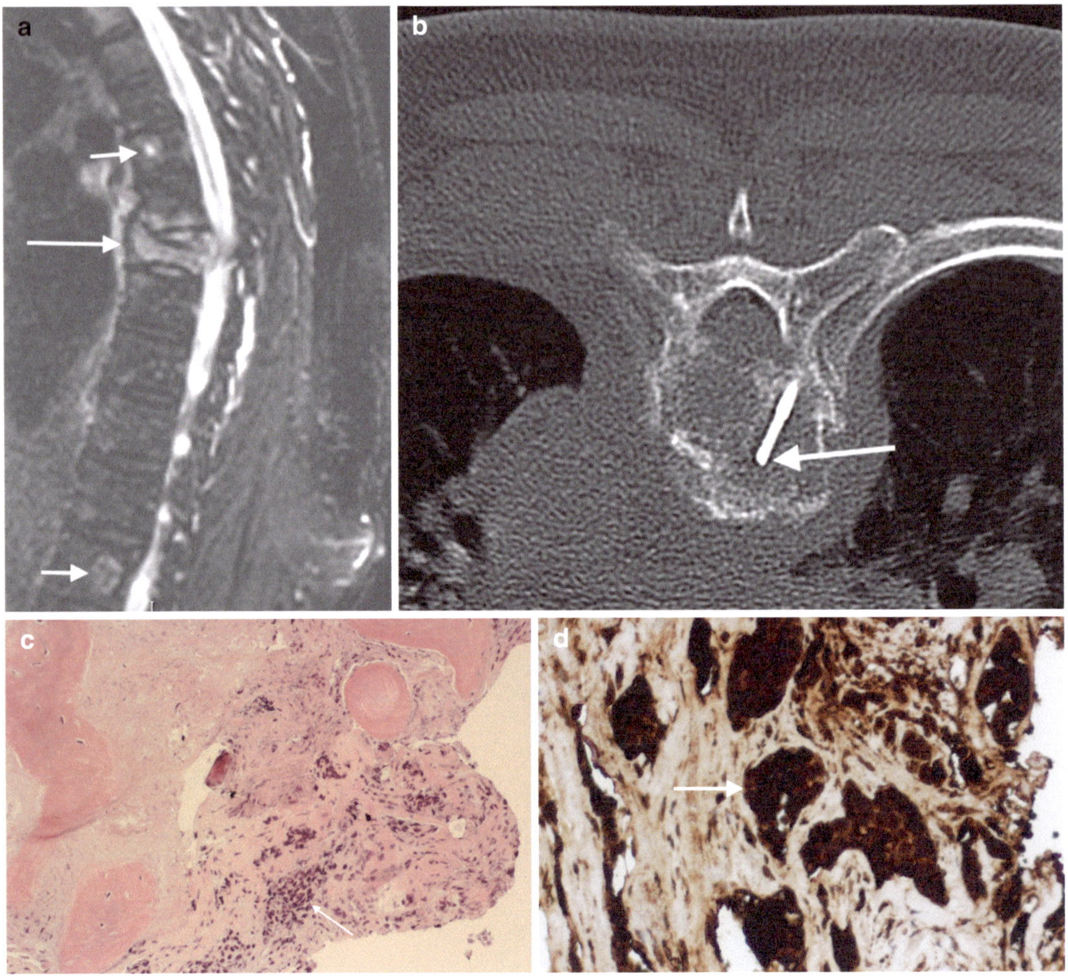

Fig. 11.8 A 65-year-old female with history of breast cancer presents with back pain and a T7 vertebral compression fracture (same patient as in Fig. 3 in Chap. 5). T2-weighted sagittal image (**a**) shows a pathologic T7 vertebral compression deformity (*arrow*) as well as small lesions (*small arrows*) within other vertebra. Axial CT image (**b**) obtained during a T7 biopsy with coaxial technique shows a bone needle within the lesion (*arrow*). Photomicrograph (**c**) with H/E stain is positive for malignant cells (*arrow*). Photomicrograph (**d**) of positive immunohistochemical stain for cytokeratin 7 (CK7) (*arrow*) confirmed a diagnosis of metastatic breast carcinoma

skull base and sacrum are two common locations for these neoplasms. Upon gross inspection, these tumors show a glistening off-white chondroid, fleshy appearance. Their histopathology shows large PAS-positive vacuoles within the cellular cytoplasm which accounts for the "physaliphorous cell" terminology (Fig. 11.13). The dense connective tissue trabeculae within the lesion contribute to its lobulated appearance. These slow-growing neoplasms show locally invasive characteristics that result in bone destruction. This limits tumor resection and contributes to their unfavorable prognosis. CSPGY is a tumor biomarker that may be associated with an increased risk of metastatic disease (Schoenfeld et al. 2016).

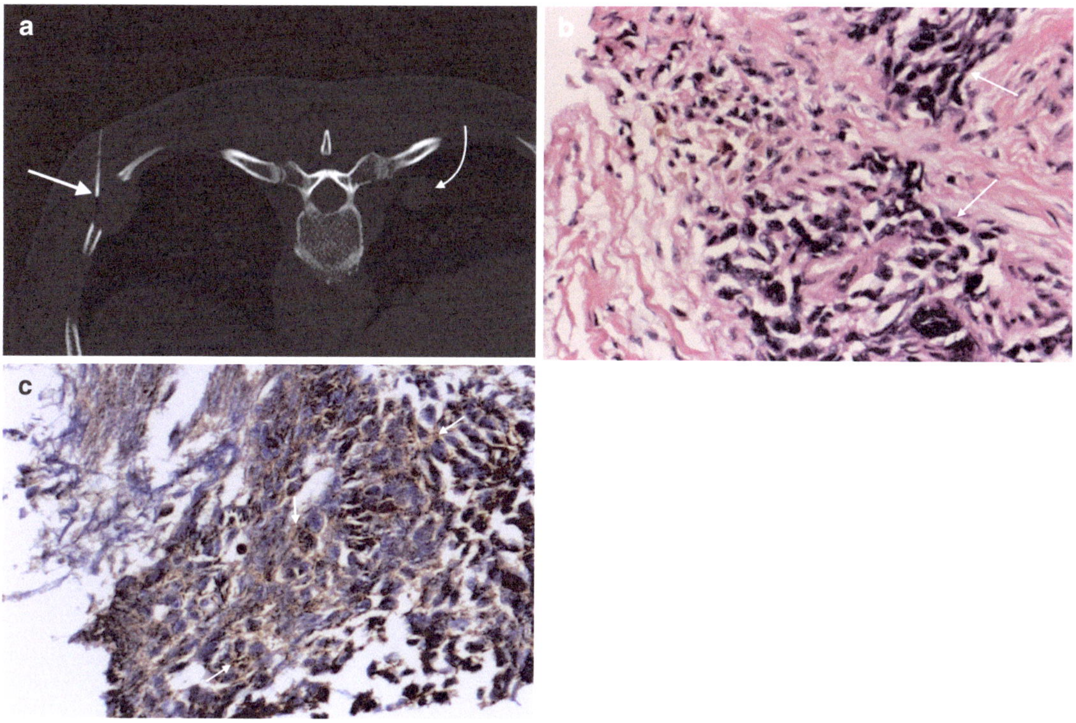

Fig. 11.9 A 53-year-old male with multiple pulmonary nodules and a rib lesion seen on a chest CT (same patient as in Fig. 14, Chap. 8). Axial CT image (**a**) from rib biopsy procedure shows a 19-gauge guide needle within a soft tissue mass (*arrow*) that has destroyed a portion of the posterior ninth rib; a posterior lung mass is present (*curved arrow*). Photomicrograph (**b**) with H/E stain is positive for malignant cells (*arrows*). Photomicrograph (**c**) shows positive immunocytochemical stain for synaptophysin (*arrows*). The cytomorphological and immunophenotypic features (also positive for TTF-1 and CK7) of this tumor were consistent with a primary lung small cell carcinoma

11.7.6 Chondrosarcoma

This is the third most common malignant bone tumor and a small percentage can be located within the spine (7%) and ribs (8%) (Murphey et al. 2003). They may occur as primary tumors or be secondarily superimposed on preexisting lesions such as enchondromas or osteochondromas. Chondrosarcoma is heterogeneous in appearance depending on the type of chondrosarcoma and grade. However, generally it is composed of atypical chondrocyte-like cells in a background of malignant myxoid-type matrix. The tumor usually presents as a lytic bone lesion with or without calcifications (Fig. 11.14). Diagnosis and classification are highly dependent on location and radiological appearance (including lesion size, extent (within the bone as well as the extraosseous soft tissue component), margins, matrix, and the presence or absence of metastases). So communicating that history to the pathologist is important. A pathologist that has expertise in orthopedic pathology may be needed to review the case.

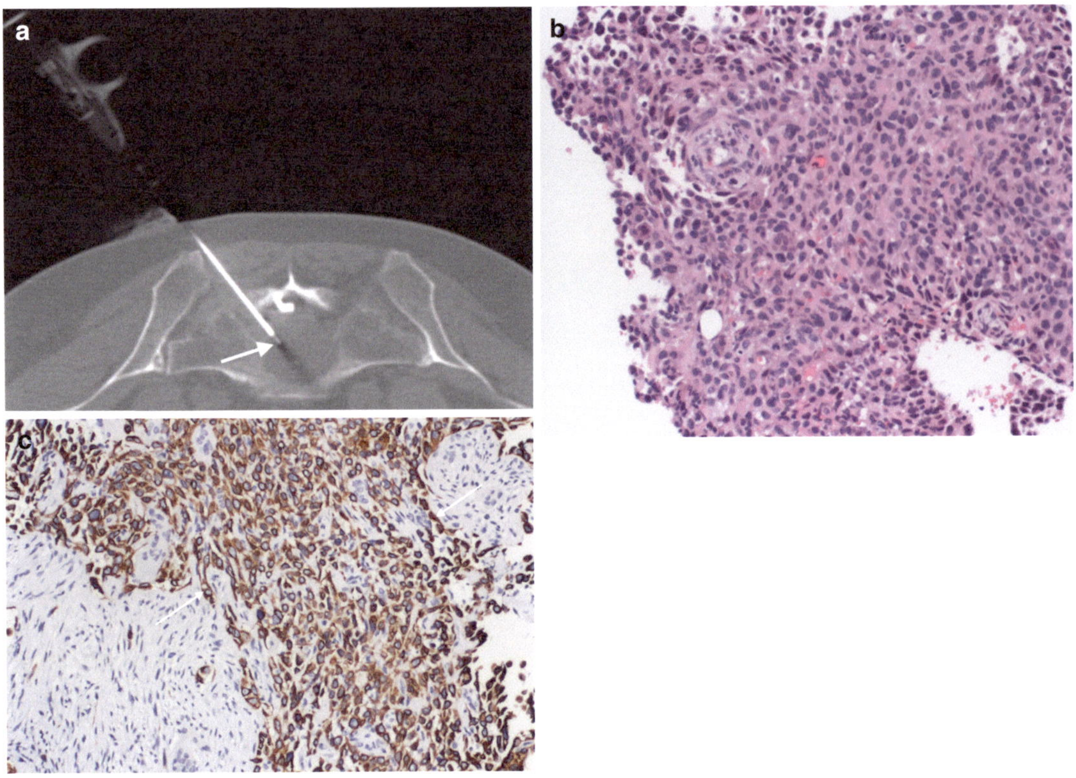

Fig. 11.10 An 81-year-old female with severe low back pain and a lung mass (same patient as in Fig. 12, Chap. 7). Axial CT image (**a**) from coaxial biopsy procedure shows the tip of a cutting needle (*arrow*) within a large lytic soft tissue mass at S1. Photomicrograph (**b**) with H/E stain is positive for malignant cells (carcinoma). Photomicrograph (**c**) shows positive immunocytochemical stain (*arrows*) for CK7. The tumor was focally positive for CA 125 (not shown). The pathologic differential diagnosis for the primary site included the ovary, uterus, or lung; clinical and radiographic correlation were recommended

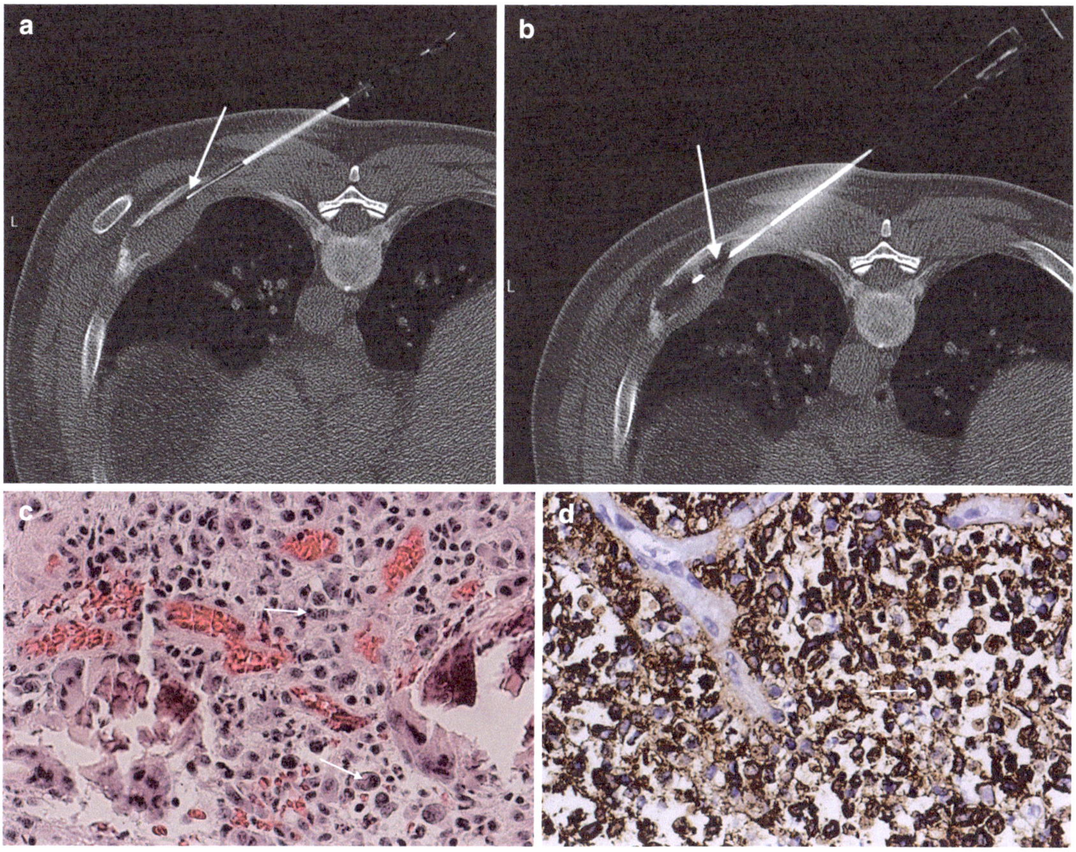

Fig. 11.11 A 56-year-old male with painful lytic rib lesion and no known primary tumor. Axial CT image (**a**) during biopsy procedure with coaxial technique shows fine-needle aspiration (*arrow*) of soft tissue component of the rib lesion. Axial CT image (**b**) shows a soft tissue core biopsy needle within the lesion (*arrow*). Photomicrograph (**c**) with high-power view is positive for malignant cells (*arrows*). Immunoperoxidase stains were performed on the cell block from the soft tissue core biopsy. Photomicrograph (**d**) shows positive stain (*arrow*) for CD20 (a B-cell marker). The immunoprofile of the tumor (CD10, CD20, bc16, and MUM1 positive) and a high proliferative index were consistent with a large cell lymphoma

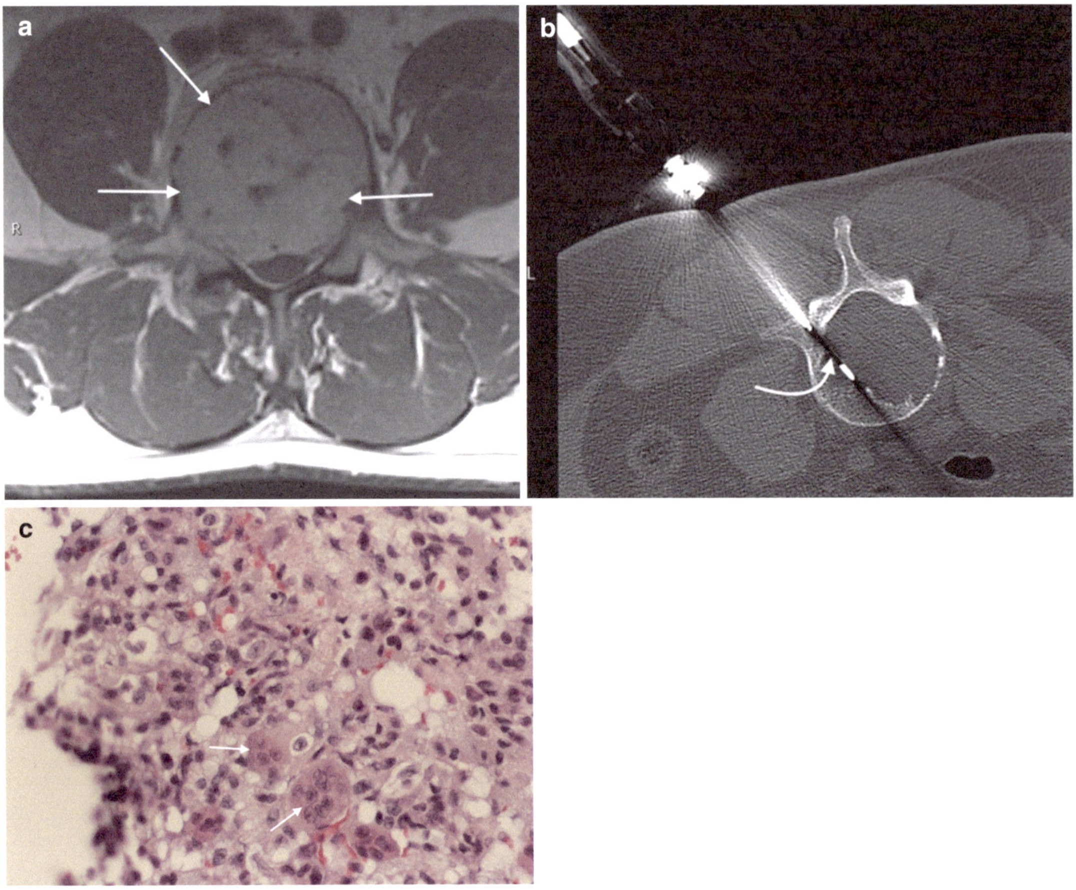

Fig. 11.12 A 47-year-old male with low back pain (same patient as in Fig. 5, Chap. 6). Contrast-enhanced T1-weighed axial image (**a**) shows large enhancing mass (*arrows*) within the L4 vertebral body. Axial CT image (**b**) shows transpedicular coaxial placement of a soft tissue core biopsy needle (*arrow*) into this lytic lesion. Photomicrograph of biopsy specimen (**c**) shows the presence of multinucleated giant cells (*arrows*) within the tumor matrix consistent with giant cell tumor

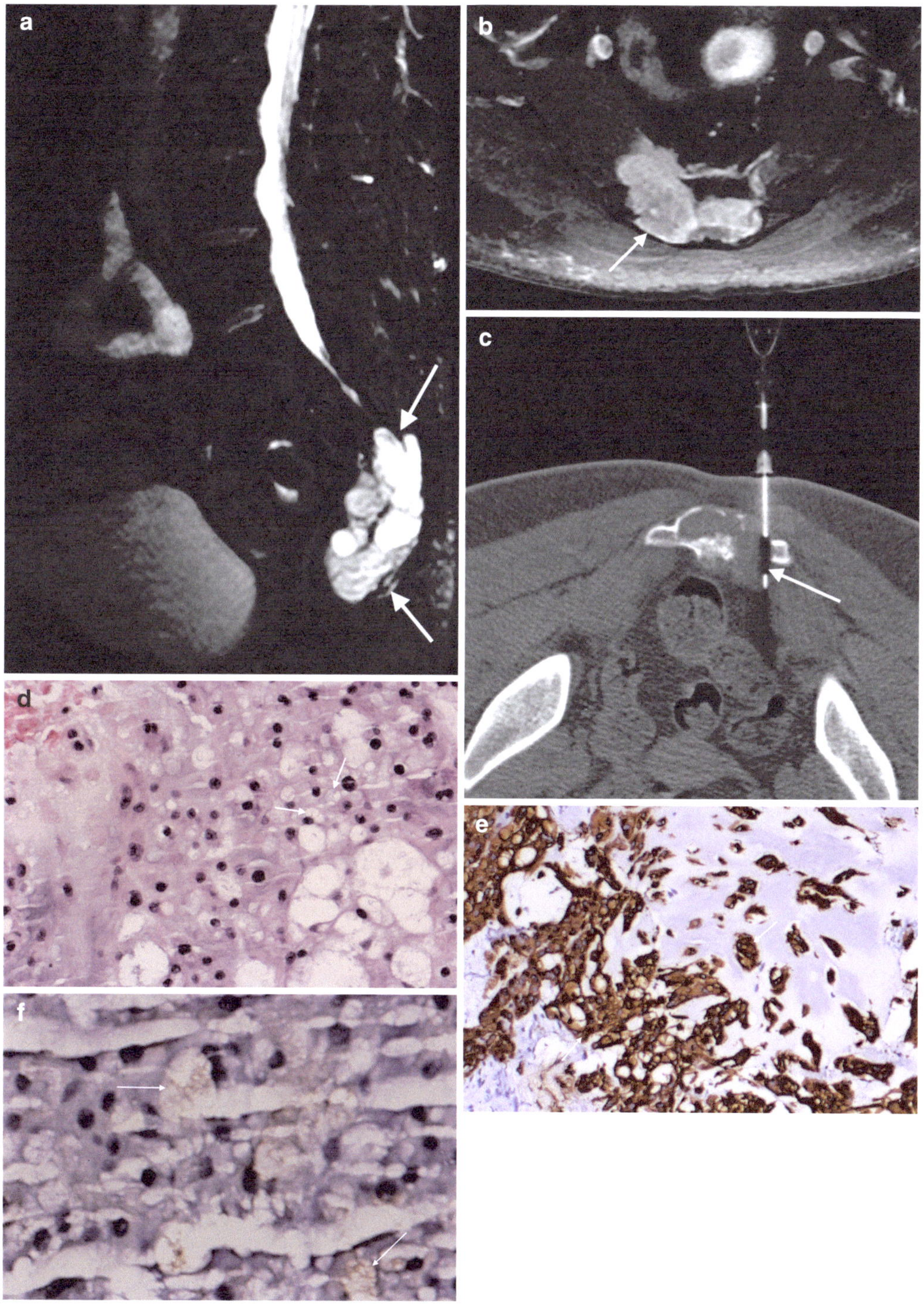

Fig. 11.13 A 57-year-old female with 3 year history of pain radiating to the lower extremities. Fat-suppressed T2-weighted sagittal image (**a**) shows large lobulated hyperintense sacral mass (*arrows*). Fat-suppressed contrast-enhanced T1-weighted axial image (**b**) shows an enhancing sacral mass (*arrow*) at the S5 level. Axial CT image (**c**) during biopsy procedure with coaxial technique shows soft tissue core biopsy needle (*arrow*) within the destructive sacral lesion. Photomicrograph (**d**) with H/E stain shows prominent cytoplasmic vacuoles (*arrows*). Photomicrographs show positive staining for CAM5.2 (**e**) (*arrows*) and s100 (**f**); the latter shows a focal weak cytoplasmic stain (*arrows*). The immunoprofile (positive CAM 5.2, AE1/AE3, EMA, S100) was consistent with chordoma

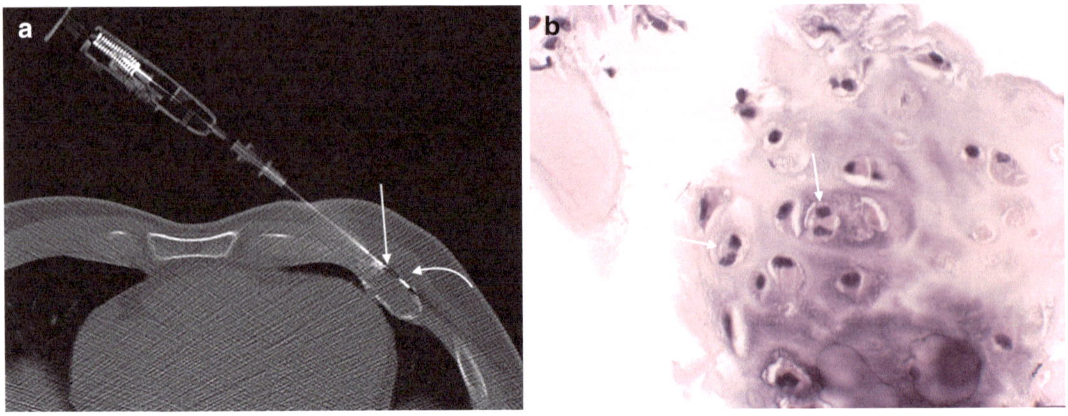

Fig. 11.14 A 70-year-old male with a palpable chest wall mass. Axial CT image (**a**) from a rib biopsy procedure shows a soft tissue core biopsy needle (*arrow*), inserted via coaxial technique, within the substance of an expansile lytic rib lesion with an extraosseous soft tissue component (*curved arrow*). Photomicrograph (**b**) with H/E stain showed a chondroid neoplasm with enlarged nuclei and binucleate chondroid cells (*arrows*) consistent with a chondrosarcoma

Key Review Points

1. The objective of a biopsy procedure is to obtain pathologic tissue in a sufficient amount so as to enable a pathologist and/or a microbiologist to make the diagnosis.
2. Whether considering a specific diagnosis or if uncertain how to process or transport a specimen, the most optimal opportunity for the operator to discuss the case with the pathologist is prior to performing the biopsy procedure.
3. Always discuss the possibility of a non-diagnostic biopsy with the patient prior to obtaining informed consent.
4. Important objectives for the operator and his/her team are to maximize the amount of pathologic tissue that can be reasonably acquired during the biopsy procedure, to place the specimens in correctly labeled containers, and to expeditiously transport these labeled containers to the appropriate destinations for processing and analysis.
5. The hematoxylin-eosin (H/E) stain is the primary screening stain for evaluating biopsy specimens.
6. Immunohistochemistry is used to further assess tissue samples in order to determine the etiology of the neoplastic tissue that is identified on the H/E stain.
7. The pathologist does not interpret the gross and microscopic features of the biopsy specimen in a void; rather, the pathologist relies on the critical history that is provided by the operator as well as on the imaging findings that are reported by the radiologist.

References

Angtuaco AJ, Fassas ABT, Walker R, Sethi R, Barlogie B. Multiple myeloma: clinical review and diagnostic imaging. Radiology. 2004;231:11–23.

Chakarun CJ, Forrester DM, Gottsegen CJ, Patel DB, White EA, Matcuk GR. Giant cell tumor of bone: review, mimics and new developments in treatment. Radiographics. 2013;33:197–211.

Dabbs DJ. Diagnostic immunohistochemistry. 4th ed. Theranostic and genomic applications, expert consult: online and print. Philadelphia: Elsevier; 2014.

Gupta RK, Cheung YK, Al Ansari AG, Naran S, Lallu S, Fauck R. Diagnostic value of image-guided needle aspiration cytology in the assessment of vertebral and intervertebral lesions. Diagn Cytopathol. 2002;27:191–6.

Hewes RC, Vigorita VJ, Freiberger RH. Percutaneous bone biopsy: the importance of aspirated osseous blood. Radiology. 1983;148:69–72.

Howard CB, Einhorn M, Dagan R, et al. Fine-needle bone biopsy to diagnose osteomyelitis. J Bone Joint Surg Br. 1994;76-B:311–4.

Hwang S, Lefkowitz RA, Landa J, Zheng J, Moskowitz CS, Maybody M, Hameed M, Panicek DM. Percutaneous CT-guided bone biopsy: diagnosis of malignancy in lesions with initially indeterminate biopsy results and CT features associated with diagnostic or indeterminate results. AJR Am J Roentgenol. 2011;197:1417–25.

Jakanani GC, Saifuddin A. Percutaneous image-guided needle biopsy of rib lesions: a retrospective study of diagnostic outcome in 51 cases. Skeletal Radiol. 2013;42:85–90.

Kabiraj A, Gupta J, Khaitan T, Bhattacharya PT. Principle and techniques of Immunohistochemistry-a review. Int J Biol Med Res. 2015;6:5204–10.

Kreula J. Effect of sampling technique on specimen size in fine needle aspiration biopsy. Invest Radiol. 1990;25:1294–9.

Krishnan A, Shirkhoda A, Tehranzadeh J, Armin AR, Irwin R, Les K. Primary bone lymphoma: radiographic-MR imaging correlation. Radiographics. 2003;23:1371–83.

Mills SE, Greenson JK, Hornick JL, Longacre TA, Reuter VE. Sternberg s diagnostic surgical pathology. 6th ed. Philadelphia: Wolters Kluwer; 2015.

Murphey MD, Walker EA, Wilson AJ, Kransdorf MJ, Temple T, Gannon FH. Imaging of primary chondrosarcoma: radiologic-pathologic correlation. Radiographics. 2003;23:1245–78.

Murphy WA, Destouet JM, Gilula LA. Percutaneous skeletal biopsy 1981: a procedure for radiologists – results, review, and recommendations. Radiology. 1981;139: 545–9.

Omura MC, Motamedi K, Uybico S, Nelson SD, Seeger LL. Revisiting CT-guided percutaneous core needle biopsy of musculoskeletal lesions: contributors of biopsy success. AJR Am J Roentgenol. 2011;197: 457–61.

Ortiz AO, Zoarski G, Brook A. Image-guided percutaneous spine biopsy. In: Mathis JM, Golovac S, editors. Image-guided spine interventions. 2nd ed. New York: Springer; 2010. p. 75–106.

Ross JS. Neoplasms, pathways of spread. Blastic osseous metastases. Lytic osseous metastases. In: Ross JS, Brant-Zawadzki M, Moore KR, Crim J, Chen MZ, Katzman GL, editors. Diagnostic imaging spine, vol. IV-1. 1st ed. Salt Lake City: Amirsys; 2005. p. 1–13.

Schoenfeld AJ, Wang X, Wang Y, Hornicek FJ, Nielsen GP, Duan Z, Ferrone S, Schwab JH. CSPG4 as a prognostic biomarker in chordoma. Spine J; 2016;16:722–7.

Schweitzer ME, Gannon FH, Deely DM, O'Hara BJ, Juneja V. Percutaneous skeletal aspiration and core biopsy: complementary techniques. AJR Am J Roentgenol 1996; 166:415–8.

Stoker DJ, Kissin CM. Percutaneous vertebral biopsy: a review of 135 cases. Clin Radiol. 1985;36(6): 569–77.

Wu JS, Goldsmith JD, Horwich PJ, Shetty SK, Hochman MG. Bone and soft-tissue lesions: what factors affect diagnostic yield of image-guided core needle biopsy? Radiology. 2008;248:962–70.

Yang YJ, Damron TA. Comparison of needle core biopsy and fine needle aspiration for diagnostic accuracy in musculoskeletal lesions. Arch Pathol Lab Med. 2004;128(7):759–64.

Erratum to: Chapter 1 in Pre- and Periprocedural Planning and Patient Management for Spine or Rib Biopsies

Richard Silbergleit and A. Orlando Ortiz

Erratum to:
Chapter 1 in A. Orlando Ortiz, *Image-Guided Percutaneous Spine Biopsy*.
DOI: 10.1007/978-3-319-43326-4_1.

The first author information on the chapter opening page of chapter 1 was incorrect.

First author for this chapter is:
Richard Silbergleit

The updated version of the original chapter can be found under
DOI 10.1007/978-3-319-43326-4_1

A.O. Ortiz, *Image-Guided Percutaneous Spine Biopsy*, DOI 10.1007/978-3-319-43326-4_12

Index

A.O. Ortiz, *Image-Guided Percutaneous Spine Biopsy*, DOI 10.1007/978-3-319-43326-4

MIX
Papier aus verantwortungsvollen Quellen
Paper from responsible sources
FSC® C105338

If you have any concerns about our products,
you can contact us on
ProductSafety@springernature.com

In case Publisher is established outside the EU,
the EU authorized representative is:
Springer Nature Customer Service Center GmbH
Europaplatz 3, 69115 Heidelberg, Germany

Printed by Libri Plureos GmbH
in Hamburg, Germany